Contemporary Cardiology

Series Editor:

Peter P. Toth
Ciccarone Center for the Prevention of Cardiovascular Disease
Johns Hopkins University School of Medicine
Baltimore, MD
USA

For more than a decade, cardiologists have relied on the Contemporary Cardiology series to provide them with forefront medical references on all aspects of cardiology. Each title is carefully crafted by world-renown cardiologists who comprehensively cover the most important topics in this rapidly advancing field. With more than 75 titles in print covering everything from diabetes and cardiovascular disease to the management of acute coronary syndromes, the Contemporary Cardiology series has become the leading reference source for the practice of cardiac care.

More information about this series at http://www.springer.com/series/7677

Arrigo F.G. Cicero • Manfredi Rizzo

Editors

Nutraceuticals and Cardiovascular Disease

An Evidence-based Approach
for Clinical Practice

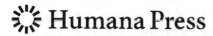 Humana Press

Editors
Arrigo F.G. Cicero
S. Orsola-Malpighi University Hospital
University of Bologna
BOLOGNA, Bologna
Italy

Manfredi Rizzo
School of Medicine
University of Palermo
Palermo, Palermo
Italy

ISSN 2196-8969   ISSN 2196-8977   (electronic)
Contemporary Cardiology
ISBN 978-3-030-62634-1   ISBN 978-3-030-62632-7   (eBook)
https://doi.org/10.1007/978-3-030-62632-7

This Humana imprint is published by the registered company Springer Nature Switzerland AG
The registered company address is: Gewerbestrasse 11, 6330 Cham, Switzerland

Contents

Contributors

Mustafa Cesur, MD Department of Endocrinology and Metabolism, Ankara Guven Hospital, Ankara, Turkey

Roberta Chianetta, BSc PROMISE Department, School of Medicine, University of Palermo, Palermo, Italy

Arrigo F.G. Cicero, MD, PhD Medicine and Surgery Sciences Department, Alma Mater Studiorum University of Bologna, Bologna, Italy

Italian Nutraceutical Society (SINut), Bologna, Italy

Alessandro Colletti, PharmD Italian Nutraceutical Society (SINut), Bologna, Italy

Department of Drug Science and Technology, University of Turin, Turin, Italy

Andreea Corina Lipid and Atherosclerosis Unit, IMIBIC/Reina Sofia University Hospital/University of Cordoba, Cordoba, Spain

CIBER Fisiopatologia Obesidad y Nutricion (CIBEROBN), Instituto de Salud Carlos III, Madrid, Spain

Adriana Florinela Cătoi Pathophysiology Department, "Iuliu Hațieganu" University of Medicine and Pharmacy, Cluj-Napoca, Romania

Teoman Dogru, MD Department of Gastroenterology, Balıkesir University, Faculty of Medicine, Balıkesir, Turkey

Cemal Nuri Ercin, MD Department of Gastroenterology, University of Health Sciences, Gulhane Faculty of Medicine, Ankara, Turkey

Federica Fogacci, MD Medical and Surgical Sciences Department, University of Bologna, Bologna, Italy

Silvia Fogacci, MW Medical and Surgical Sciences Department, University of Bologna, Bologna, Italy

Francesco M. Galassi, MD Archaeology, College of Humanities, Arts and Social Sciences, Flinders University, Adelaide, SA, Australia

FAPAB Research Center, Avola, Siracusa, Sicily, Italy

Ornella Guardamagna, MD Department of Public Health and Pediatric Sciences, Università di Torino, Torino, Italy

Luca Marco Luzzu PROMISE Department, School of Medicine, University of Palermo, Palermo, Italy

Giulia Massini Department of Public Health and Pediatric Sciences, Università di Torino, Torino, Italy

Laura García Molina, RD Department of Preventive Medicine and Public Health, University of Granada, Granada, Spain

Dragana Nikolic, BSc, PhD PROMISE Department, School of Medicine, University of Palermo, Palermo, Italy

Nikolaos Papanas, MD Diabetes Centre, Second Department of Internal Medicine, Democritus University of Thrace, University Hospital of Alexandroupolis, Alexandroupolis, Greece

Theano Penlioglou, MD Diabetes Centre, Second Department of Internal Medicine, Democritus University of Thrace, University Hospital of Alexandroupolis, Alexandroupolis, Greece

Pablo Perez-Martinez, MD Lipid and Atherosclerosis Unit, IMIBIC/Reina Sofia University Hospital/University of Cordoba, Cordoba, Spain

CIBER Fisiopatologia Obesidad y Nutricion (CIBEROBN), Instituto de Salud Carlos III, Madrid, Spain

Orlando Petrini POLE Pharma Consulting, Breganzona, Switzerland

Laboratory of Applied Microbiology, Department of Environment, Constructions and Design, University of Applied Sciences of Southern Switzerland – SUPSI, Bellinzona, Switzerland

Nicolas F. Renna, MD, PhD Department of Cardiology, Spanish Hospital of Mendoza, Mendoza, Argentina

Laboratory of Cardiovascular Physiopathology, Department of Pathology, School of Medicine, National University of Cuyo, IMBECU-CONICET, Mendoza, Argentina

Manfredi Rizzo, MD, PhD PROMISE Department, School of Medicine, University of Palermo, Palermo, Italy

Italian Nutraceutical Society (SINut), Bologna, Italy

José René Romano Clínica Vrsalovic, Formosa, Argentina

Hospital Centraol de Formosa, Formosa, Argentina

Alexandros Sachinidis, MD, PhD PROMISE Department, School of Medicine, University of Palermo, Palermo, Italy

2nd Propaedeutics Department of Internal Medicine, Hippocration Hospital, Medical School of Aristotle University Thessaloniki, Thessaloniki, Greece

Alper Sonmez, MD Department of Endocrinology and Metabolism, University of Health Sciences, Gulhane Faculty of Medicine, Ankara, Turkey

Anca Pantea Stoian, MD Department of Diabetes, Nutrition and Metabolic Diseases, Carol Davila University of Medicine and Pharmacy, Bucharest, Romania

Larysa Strilchuk, MD Department of Therapy, Medical Diagnostics and Hematology and Transfusiology, Lviv National Medical University named after Danylo Halytsky, Lviv, Ukraine

Peter P. Toth, MD, PhD CGH Medical Center, Sterling, IL, USA

Cicarrone Center for the Prevention of Cardiovascular Disease, Johns Hopkins University School of Medicine, Baltimore, MD, USA

Rock Falls Medical Center, Rock Falls, IL, USA

Department of Preventive Cardiology, CGH Medical Center, Sterling, IL, USA

Elena Varotto Archaeology, College of Humanities, Arts and Social Sciences, Flinders University, Adelaide, SA, Australia

FAPAB Research Center, Avola, Siracusa, Sicily, Italy

Department of Humanities (DISUM), University of Catania, Catania, Sicily, Italy

Chapter 1
Cardiovascular Disease Epidemiology and Risk Factors: General Concepts

Peter P. Toth

Introduction

Cardiovascular disease (CVD) is epidemic throughout the world and includes atherosclerotic disease in its various forms (coronary artery disease [CAD], peripheral arterial disease, carotid artery disease), hypertension, stroke, and heart failure, among others. CVD is the leading etiology for global mortality and the most important source of morbidity. The most significant clinical sequelae of CVD include myocardial infarction (MI), both hemorrhagic and ischemic stroke, claudication and lower limb loss, chronic kidney disease and end-stage renal disease, heart failure, arterial aneurysm formation in the aorta and its tributaries, and, especially for patients with diabetes mellitus (DM) and/or hypertension (HTN), retinopathy and nephropathy. The diagnosis and management of CVD incurs enormous economic costs upon society worldwide and is responsible for considerable disability throughout all regions of the world [1, 2]. The World Heart Federation estimates that over 17.3 million people die of CVD annually, and by 2030 that number is expected to increase to 23 million people [3]. This represents 31% of all deaths annually. The World Health Organization estimates that 85% of deaths due to CV occur from MI and stroke [4].

Prepared for publication in
NUTRACEUTICALS AND CARDIOVASCULAR DISEASE: AN EVIDENCE BASED APPROACH FOR CLINICAL PRACTICE (Arrigo F.G. Cicero, Manfredi Rizzo, eds) Springer

P. P. Toth (✉)
CGH Medical Center, Sterling, IL, USA

Cicarrone Center for the Prevention of Cardiovascular Disease, Johns Hopkins University School of Medicine, Baltimore, MD, USA

Rock Falls Medical Center, Rock Falls, IL, USA
e-mail: peter.toth@cghmc.com

In the United States, the American Heart Association estimates that: [1] CVD accounted for 840,678 deaths in the US in 2016, equal to approximately 1 of every 3 deaths [2]. CVD mortality exceeded all forms of cancer and chronic lower respiratory disease combined [3]. Between 2013 and 2016, 121.5 million American adults were afflicted with some form of CVD. [4] Between 2014 and 2015, direct and indirect costs of CVD and stroke amounted to $351.2 billion ($213.8 billion in direct costs and $137.4 billion in lost productivity/mortality) [5]. In 2016, CAD was the leading cause (43.2%) of deaths attributable to cardiovascular disease in the US, followed by stroke (16.9%), HTN (9.8%), heart failure (9.3%), diseases of the arteries (3.0%), and other cardiovascular diseases (17.7%) [6]. CVD and stroke accounted for 14% of total health expenditures in 2014–2015. This is more than any major diagnostic group [7]. In addition, total direct medical costs of CVD are estimated to increase to $749 billion in 2035, according to a 2016 study [5].

This chapter focuses on cardiovascular epidemiology. Epidemiology quantifies the distribution and determinants of health and disease. More specifically, epidemiologic investigation evaluates associations between exposures to specific genetic, environmental, and behavioral features and the risk for developing disease or maintaining health. After seven decades of research conducted within large prospective longitudinal cohorts around the world, risk factors for the development of CVD are biologically plausible and have been firmly established. Prospective, double-blind, randomized clinical trials testing specific interventions to treat these risk factors have also established that they are either treatable or reversible, and that these actions reduce risk for CVD. Cardiovascular epidemiology has made possible the prevention of some types of CVD events in the primordial, primary, and secondary prevention settings.

Global Perspective of Cardiovascular Disease

Subsequent to World War II, it became clear that efforts to reduce the incidence of CVD were urgently needed. In the United States the Framingham Heart Study (FSH) was initiated in 1948 with the inclusion of 5209 men and women in the original cohort that was free of CVD at baseline [6, 7]. Being a prospective, longitudinal cohort observed over many years, the temporal relationship between numerous risk factors and the incidence (new cases of specific forms of CVD within a defined time frame) as well as causation of disease could be established in a study such as the FHS. The FHS established dyslipidemia, hypertension, diabetes, smoking, and other genetic and behavioral features as risk factors for the development of CVD. In subsequent decades the FHS also evolved an Offspring cohort, a Third-Generation cohort, and a Spouses cohort, all which continue to yield novel insight into the genesis of CVD.

The Seven Countries Study lent support to many of the most important conclusions reached by the FHS [8, 9]. In the US numerous other cohorts exploring features that predispose to CVD were also introduced, including the Cardiovascular Health Study, [10] the Atherosclerosis Risk in Communities Study (ARIC), [11] the Multiethnic Study of Atherosclerosis (MESA), [12] Reasons for Geographic and Racial Differences in Stroke Study (REGARDS), [13] and the Jackson Heart Study

(JHS), [14] among others. Similar cohorts were recruited in Europe, [15, 16] South America, [17] Asia, [2, 18–20] India, [21] Africa, [22] and elsewhere [23, 24]. The INTERHEART Study evaluated CVD risk factors in 52 countries and affirmed that nearly 92% of risk for an MI is attributable to treatable/preventable risk factors and that risk factors behave similarly in peoples from around the world [25]. The pooling of data has allowed for the generation of global maps depicting the prevalence of specific forms of CVD, such as ischemic heart disease (IHD. (Fig. 1.1). It is

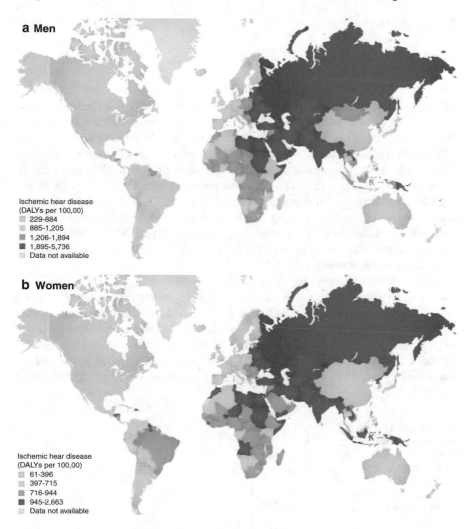

a Men

Ischemic hear disease
(DALYs per 100,00)
- 229-884
- 885-1,205
- 1,206-1,894
- 1,895-5,736
- Data not available

b Women

Ischemic hear disease
(DALYs per 100,00)
- 61-396
- 397-715
- 716-944
- 945-2,663
- Data not available

Fig. 1.1 The Global Distribution of Ischemic Heart Disease for both men and women, in DALYs, in 2011. (**a**)l Men (**b**) lWomen. Data are age-standardized per 100,000 of the population. Abbreviation: DALYs, disability-adjusted life years. (Reproduced, with permission from the publisher, from Mendis, S., Puska, P. & Norrving, B. (Eds) Global Atlas on Cardiovascular Disease Prevention and Control. Geneva, World Health Organization, 2011 (Figures 19 & 20, Page12 http://whqlibdoc.who.int.proxy2.cl.msu.edu/publications/2011/9789241564373_eng.pdf?ua=1, accessed 29 December 2019)

easily discerned that IHD is widely prevalent in all nations and continents and that Eastern Europe, the Middle East, the Indian Subcontinent, and Northern Africa are particularly impacted by IHD.

Risk Factors for Atherosclerotic Disease

Dyslipidemia

Low-Density Lipoprotein

After nearly 100 years of experimental investigation, low-density lipoprotein cholesterol (LDL-C) is indisputably established as atherogenic [26]. LDL particles are the most abundant in serum and are scavenged in the subendothelial space by activated macrophages [27]. Lipid-laden macrophages are an important substrate for atheromatous plaque formation and provide pro-inflammatory stimuli to propagate plaque and ultimately render it unstable and prone to rupture, leading to the development of acute tissue ischemia in affected vascular territories [27–29]. There is a log-linear relationship between LDL-C and risk for CAD. (Fig. 1.2.) There is unequivocal evidence that lowering LDL-C with statins (3'-hydroxymethyl-glutaryl coenzyme A inhibitors) [30] and other drugs such as ezetimibe [31] and proprotein convertase/subtilisin kexin type-9 inhibitors [32, 33] beneficially impact risk for acute cardiovascular events (Fig. 1.3).

A relatively novel means by which to view the relationship between LDL-C and risk for CAD-related events is by assessing life years of exposure to specific serum levels of this lipoprotein [34]. The higher the level and the longer the exposure, the higher the risk for developing CHD. By lowering LDL-C earlier and more and more aggressively, the age at which an acute CV event may be expected to occur is extended to older and older ages (Fig. 1.4) [34, 35]. Hence, time is of the essence since limiting exposure to LDL-C is akin to limiting exposure to an established

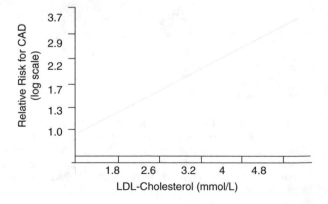

Fig. 1.2 Log-Linear relationship between LDL-C and Relative Risk for Coronary Artery Disease. (Reproduced with permission from Grundy et al. Circulation 2004; 110: 227–239)

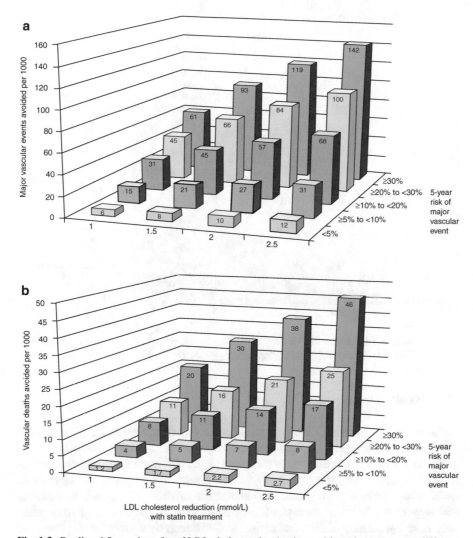

Fig. 1.3 Predicted 5-year benefits of LDL cholesterol reductions with statin treatment at different levels of risk. (**a**) Major vascular events and (**b**) vascular deaths. Lifetable estimates using major vascular event risk or vascular death risk in the respective risk categories and overall treatment effects per 1.0 mmol/L (38 mg/dL) reduction in LDL cholesterol with statin therapy. (Reproduced from Cholesterol Treatment Trialists, C., et al. (2012). "The effects of lowering LDL cholesterol with statin therapy in people at low risk of vascular disease: meta-analysis of individual data from 27 randomised trials." Lancet (London, England) **380**(9841): 581–590. This article is open access and free to read and use)

vascular toxin. Thus, when it comes to LDL-C and CVD risk reduction, lower is better, but lowest is best. Guidelines for the management of dyslipidemia continue to emphasize that LDL-C is the primary target of therapy for patients with dyslipidemia [36, 37].

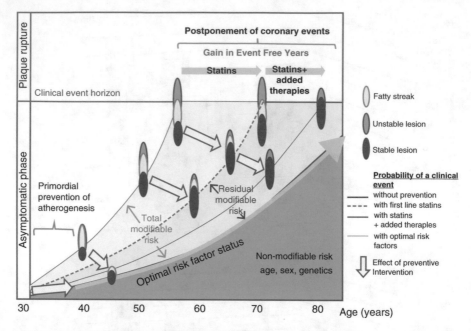

Fig. 1.4 Disease Trajectories in Coronary Heart Disease Prevention. (Reproduced with permission from Packard, C. J., et al. Vascular Pharmacology 215; 71: 37–39)

High-Density Lipoprotein

High-density lipoprotein (HDL) is still incompletely characterized and understood [38]. It is characterized by a lipidome and proteome of enormous complexity, and can bind to a variety of cell surface receptors [39]. HDL particles drive reverse cholesterol transport (i.e., the process by which cholesterol is extracted from lipid-enriched macrophages in the subendothelial space and transported back to the liver) and appear to have a variety of antiatherogenic properties, including anti-inflammatory, antithrombotic, and anti-oxidative effects by virtue of their proteomic constituents [40, 41]. Perhaps for these reasons virtually all prospective longitudinal cohorts have shown that HDL-cholesterol (HDL-C) is protective or a "negative risk factor" when its level in serum is elevated [42, 43]. It is an important component of most 10 year and lifetime risk calculators [44–46]. However, current guidelines recommend against making HDL-C a therapeutic target because prospective, randomized clinical trials with agents that raise HDL-C have failed to demonstrate any CV benefit [47–50]. More recent analyses suggest that HDL particles are likely not as protective as once thought [51, 52]. HDL-C tends to decrease in patients with insulin resistance, metabolic syndrome, obesity, chronic kidney disease, and inflammatory disease [53, 54].

Triglycerides

Triglycerides constitute an enormously important storage form of energy for systemic tissues. Because triglycerides are not soluble in an aqueous phase, triglycerides are exported from the liver within very low-density lipoprotein (VLDL) particles. Free fatty acid is liberated from triglycerides by lipoprotein lipase. Lipoprotein lipase progressively delipidates VLDL to form, in succession, intermediate-density lipoprotein (IDL) and then LDL. In the setting of insulin resistance or when there are genetic polymorphisms leading to reduced lipoprotein lipase activity (increased apoprotein CIII, reduced apoprotein CII, reduced expression of lipoprotein lipase, etc.), small VLDLs and IDLs accumulate because they are inadequately lipolyzed. Small VLDLs and IDLs together comprise remnant lipoproteins, which are triglyceride rich lipoproteins. In patients with hypertriglyceridemia, remnant lipoproteins are elevated in serum.

A variety of genetic polymorphisms associated with hypertriglyceridemia correlate with increased risk for CV events, increased coronary calcium burden, and accelerated atherogenesis [55]. Hypertriglyceridemia is recognized as an important risk factor and is a defining feature of the metabolic syndrome [56, 57]. Serum levels that exceed 150 mg/dL are considered abnormal in the fasting state. Hypertriglyceridemia correlates with increased risk for acute coronary syndromes, health care costs, renal disease, and heart failure [58–61]. Triglyceride rich lipoproteins strongly correlate with increased risk for CVD events [62–65] and have been shown to be pro-inflammatory [66]. The treatment of high risk hypertriglyceridemic patients with eicosapentaenoic acid has been shown to reduce risk for all major CV endpoints [67].

Hypertension

The World Health Organization Reports that: [1] Worldwide, hypertension (HTN) causes 7.5 million deaths, or approximately 12.8% of the total of all annual deaths [2] HTN is responsible for 57 million disability-adjusted life years (DALYS) or 3.7% of total DALYS [3]. HTN is a major risk factor for CAD and cerebrovascular disease. [4] Blood pressure levels are positively and continuously related to the risk of stroke and CAD [5]. In some age groups, the risk of CVD doubles for each incremental increase of 20/10 mmHg of blood pressure, beginning as low as 115/75 mmHg [6]. In addition to CAD and cerebrovascular disease, poorly controlled blood pressure increases risk for heart failure, chronic kidney disease and end-stage renal disease (ESRD), peripheral vascular disease, as well as retinopathy and blindness [4].

HTN is widely prevalent throughout the world. It is generally accepted that a blood pressure > 140 mm Hg systolic and > 90 mm Hg diastolic constitutes HTN. For adults without HTN, prehypertension is defined by an untreated SBP of 120 to 139 mm Hg or untreated DBP of 80 to 89 mm Hg. The American Heart Association (AHA) notes that: [1] between 2011 and 2014, the prevalence of hypertension among US adults was 45.6% [2]. Meta-analyses demonstrate that pre-hypertension correlates with an increased risk for CVD, ESRD, and death. These risks are greater for people in the upper (130–139/85–89 mm Hg) versus lower (120–129/80–84 mm Hg) range of prehypertension [3]. In prospective follow-up of the MESA, REGARDS, and JHS cohorts, 63.0% of incident CVD events occurred in participants with systolic BP (SBP) <140 mm Hg and diastolic BP <90 mm Hg [4]. In the US, the estimated direct and indirect cost of HTN from 2014 to 2015 (annual average) was approximately $55.9 billion [6]. HTN was the fourth-leading risk factor for global disease burden in 1990, as quantified by DALYs, but became the number 1 risk factor in 2010 [68].

As demonstrated in the Multiple Risk Factor Intervention Trial (MRFIT) and other cohorts, risk for CVD increases continuously as both systolic and diastolic blood pressure rise; however, the relationship is substantially steeper for systolic blood pressure elevations [69, 70] (Fig. 1.5). Hypertension is polyfactorial and is strongly influenced by lifestyle, environmental, and genetic factors [71–73]. Guidelines for the diagnosis and management of HTN are available for different regions of the world, and generally state that blood pressure should be reduced to <140/90 mm Hg in patients with HTN [74–76]. It is highly established that blood pressure reduction reduces risk for CV events, mortality, left ventricular hypertrophy (LVH), heart failure, renal injury and proteinuria, and stroke (both hemorrhagic

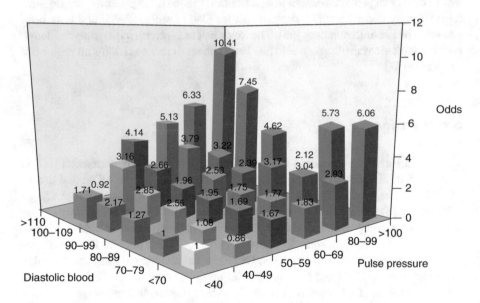

Fig. 1.5 Odds for the likelihood of a cardiovascular event with combined pulse pressure (PP) and mean arterial pressure (MAP). Data are adjusted for age, sex, total cholesterol, smoking, body mass index, diabetes, and secular trend. (Reproduced with permission from Franklin, S. S. and N. D. Wong. Hypertension and Cardiovascular Disease: Contributions of the Framingham Heart Study." Global Heart 2013; 8 [1]: 49–57)

and ischemic) [77, 78] and novel means for studying HTN are continuously being developed [79]. Blood pressure can be reduced by antagonizing the renin-angiotensin-aldosterone axis, inhibiting α- and β- adrenergic receptors, calcium channel blockade, diuretics, and nitrates, among other approaches. Despite widely recognized benefits of treating HTN, substantial disparities in the prevalence and treatment of HTN have been identified (Fig. 1.6). Based on a global analysis for 2010, 46.5% of adults with HTN knew they had the condition and only 36.9% were taking antihypertensive medication [80]. Despite widespread availability of antihypertensive medications, only 13.8% of hypertensive patients had their blood pressure controlled to guideline specified targets. These investigators further demonstrated that high-income countries had twice the rate of awareness (67.0% versus 37.9%) and treatment (55.6% versus 29.0%) and 4 times the rate of BP control in patients with HTN (28.4% versus 7.7%) when compared to low- and middle-income countries. These treatment and awareness disparities warrant urgent recognition and intervention.

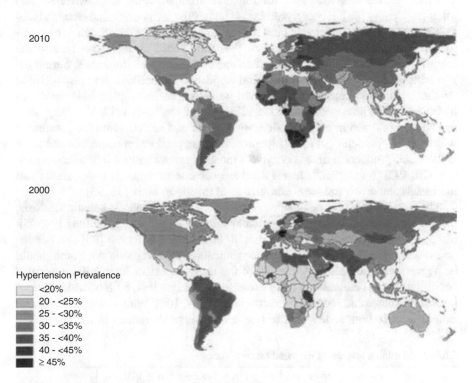

2010

2000

Hypertension Prevalence
- <20%
- 20 - <25%
- 25 - <30%
- 30 - <35%
- 35 - <40%
- 40 - <45%
- ≥ 45%

Fig. 1.6 Worldwide age- and sex-standardized prevalence of hypertension in adults 20 years and older by country. Top, Country-specific prevalence in 2010. Bottom, Country-specific prevalence in 2000. Maps are shaded according to prevalence, from light (lower prevalence) to dark (higher prevalence). (Reproduced with permission from Mills et al. Circulation. 2016;134: 441–450)

Metabolic Syndrome

Metabolic syndrome (MS) represents a constellation of CV risk factors defined by elevations in blood pressure, hypertriglyceridemia, hyperglycemia, obesity, and low HDL-C [81, 82]. (Table 1.1) Insulin resistance is etiologic for MS. [83] Insulin resistance typically develops in the setting of obesity [84]. In the insulin resistant state there is impairment in the transduction of the insulin receptor signal; this results in less nuclear transcription and cell surface expression of glucose transport proteins [85]. As this occurs the capacity to transport glucose from the extracellular milieu into the cytosol is progressively reduced. Hyperglycemia is a manifestation of less cellular glucose uptake.

Insulin resistance induces endothelial cell dysfunction, [86] which leads to reduced nitric oxide and prostacyclin production as well as increased blood pressure secondary to decreased vasodilatory inputs into the arterial wall. This is exacerbated by increased endothelin-1 production, a potent vasoconstrictor [87]. Endothelial dysfunction also increases risk for impaired microvascular responsiveness and microangiopathy [88]. Hyperglycemia potentiates the formation of advanced glyco-sylated end products which can bind to receptors that trigger development of a pro-oxidative and proinflammatory milieu [89, 90]. These changes can lead to the intensification of endothelial dysfunction and accelerated atherogenesis. Serum tri-glyceride levels rise because: [1] Visceral adipose tissue becomes less responsive to insulin, leading to persistent activation of hormone sensitive lipase and continuous hydrolysis of adipocyte triglyceride and release of free fatty acid. The fatty acids can be reassimilated into triglycerides by the liver and secreted into the circulation within VLDL particles [91] [2]. Lipoprotein lipase production decreases and there is increased production of this enzyme's most important natural inhibitor, apopro-tein CIII [92]. Serum HDL levels decrease because of reduced biosynthesis and increased catabolism and renal elimination of this lipoprotein [38, 93].

The metabolic syndrome increases risk for CVD, nonalcoholic hepatic steatosis, erectile dysfunction, polycystic ovarian syndrome, and diabetes mellitus [94, 95]. Metabolic syndrome also increases risk for both atrial fibrillation [96] and periph-eral vascular disease [97]. Individual components of the metabolic syndrome should be aggressively treated, [98] but two of the most important interventions for this condition should be increased daily exercise and weight loss, both of which relieve insulin resistance and reduce risk factor burden [99, 100]. With increased mechani-zation, urbanization, sedentary lifestyle, and adverse alterations in dietary habits,

Table 1.1 Defining features of the metabolic syndrome

Abdominal obesity (waist circumference $\geq$ 40 inches in men, and $\geq$ 35 inches in women)
Triglyceride level of 150 mg/dL or greater
HDL-C < 40 mg/dL in men or < 50 mg/dL in women
Systolic blood pressure 130 millimeters of mercury (mm Hg) or greater, *or* diastolic blood pressure of 85 mm Hg or greater
Fasting serum glucose of 100 mg/dL or greater

there is a worldwide epidemic of MS. [101, 102] In Europe the prevalence of MS is estimated to be 24.3 and 24.6% for men and women, respectively, and its prevalence increases with age [103]. In the United States, the prevalence of MS is approximately 23% and includes just over 50 million persons [104].

Diabetes Mellitus

Diabetes mellitus (DM) is a complex disorder whose principal diagnostic manifestation is the dysregulation of glucose metabolism resulting in hyperglycemia (blood glucose $\geq$126 mg/dL). Diabetes increases risk for CVD and its clinical sequelae (MI, stroke, mortality, heart failure) and microangiopathy (retinopathy with adult onset blindness, neuropathy and lower extremity amputation, nephropathy with ESRD and need for renal allografting or dialysis).

Diabetes is pathophysiologically devastating to the CV system because it is characterized by the "*ominous octet*," which includes: [105].

A. Decreased β-islet secretion of insulin. In the setting of DM there is increasing loss of β-islet cell mass over time, leading to progressive rises in glucose.
B. Increased α-islet secretion of glucagon. Glucagon stimulates hepatic glucose secretion, exacerbating the hyperglycemia of DM.
C. Reduced incretin effect. The incretins are secreted by the gut in response to glucose exposure. They include glucose-dependent insulinotropic polypeptide (GIP) and glucagon-like peptide-1 (GLP-1) and are secreted from K cells and L cells, respectively, in the gastrointestinal tract [106]. They both stimulate pancreatic insulin secretion.
D. Increased adipocyte lipolysis. This was discussed above and is the result of increased triglyceride lipolysis by hormone sensitive lipase visceral adipose tissue secondary to insulin resistance. Insulin resistant visceral adipose tissue is also an important source of adipokines that potentiate systemic inflammation [107].
E. Increased renal reabsorption of glucose by the sodium-glucose cotransport protein (SGLT2) along the proximal tubular epithelium [108]. This also augments the hyperglycemic state observed in DM.
F. Decreased glucose uptake by skeletal muscle. Insulin resistance is associated with reduced cell surface expression of such glucose transport proteins as glut2 and glut4 [109].
G. Increased hepatic glucose production. Insulin resistance is associated with increased activity of phosphoenolpyruvate carboxykinase activity, an enzyme responsible for converting oxaloacetate to phosphoenolpyruvate during gluconeogenesis [110].
H. Central nervous system neurotransmitter dysfunction. There is increased central sympathetic outflow which can lead to HTN, tachycardia, and potentiate hyperglycemia. In addition, this is associated with impaired sensing of satiety.

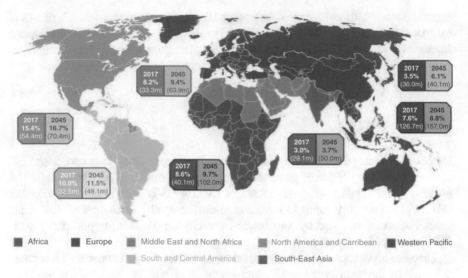

Fig. 1.7 Global Prevalence of impaired glucose tolerance (IGT) in 2017 and prevalence projected in 2045. Percentages are unadjusted regional prevalence estimates. Numbers in parentheses are the estimated number of persons affected by IGT in each region. (Reproduced with permission from Hostalek. Clinical diabetes and endocrinology. 2019;5:5)

Secondary to the global epidemic of obesity, the incidence of global diabetes is rising at shocking rates. In 2014 there was an estimated 382 million people with diabetes worldwide; this is projected to increase to 592 million by the year 2035 [111]. Estimates for the prevalence of impaired glucose tolerance (IGT or prediabetes; defined as two-hour glucose levels of 140 to 199 mg per dL (7.8 to 11.0 mmol) on the 75-g oral glucose tolerance test.) are shown in Fig. 1.7 [112]. These data portend a catastrophic rise in global incidence and prevalence of DM. In the US an estimated 26 million adults have diagnosed DM, 9.4 million adults have undiagnosed DM, and 91.8 million adults (37.6% of the population) have prediabetes [68]. In Europe in 2013 it was estimated that 56 million persons have DM with an overall prevalence of 8.5% of the population [113]. As diabetes progresses and hemoglobin a1c values increase, risk for CV events, all-cause mortality, and CVD mortality all increase continuously [114, 115] (Fig. 1.8). Controlling hemoglobin a1c levels especially below 7% is associated with less risk of microangiopathy [116, 117]. Controlling DM with GLP-1 receptor agonists and SGLT2 inhibitors has been shown to reduce risk for CV events [118–121].

Inflammation

It is now highly established that atherosclerosis is an inflammatory disease. There is considerable complexity and built-in redundancy with interconnecting networks of pro-inflammatory cells and biochemical signaling pathways of inflammation regulated by nuclear factor κB, [122] Krüppel-like factors, [123], and activator

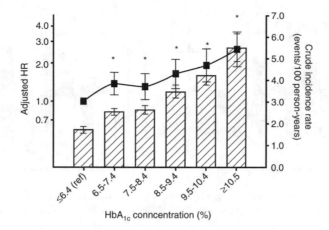

Fig. 1.8 Adjusted HRs (squares) and crude incidence rates (bars) for primary CV outcome events associated with HbA_{1c} concentrations at baseline. Error bars represent 95% CIs. *$p < 0.05$ for difference between reference group ($HbA_{1c} \leq 6.4\%$) and actual group. Adjusted analysis included sex, age, randomised treatment assignment, diabetes duration, history of arterial hypertension, history of congestive heart failure, history of cardiovascular disease, history of revascularization, ethnicity, tobacco use, systolic and diastolic blood pressure, heart rate, BMI, HDL-cholesterol concentration, LDL-cholesterol concentration, urine albumin/creatinine ratio and use of insulin, metformin, thiazolidinediones and sulfonylureas. (Reproduced with permission from Andersson, C., et al. Diabetologia 2012; 55 [9]: 2348–2355)

protein-1, [124] among others. In the setting of endothelial cell dysfunction, endothelial cells express a variety of cell adhesion molecules (intercellular adhesion molecule-1, vascular cell adhesion molecule-1, selectin P, and others) that promote the binding, rolling, and transmigration of inflammatory white cells into the subendothelial space [125]. The gap junctions holding endothelial cells together can become stressed and leaky, allowing for increased influx of circulating white cells and atherogenic lipoprotein particles [126]. Platelets, neutrophils, mast cells, macrophages, and T helper cells all participate in atherogenesis and can function as delivery vehicles of pro-inflammatory interleukins and cytokines that alter the histologic composition of the vessel wall and potentiate the creation of macrophage foam cells, fatty streaks, atheromatous plaques, and ultimately, unstable plaque that can rupture and lead to the formation of an acute cardiovascular events [127, 128].

C-Reactive protein (CRP) is a pentraxin molecule and a marker of systemic inflammation [129]. It may also directly induce a variety of proatherogenic phenomena and boost the inflammatory response [130]. Increased serum levels of CRP portend heightened risk for CVD, MI, stroke, and death in a variety of cohorts [131–133]. The measurement of CRP levels has been shown to refine 10-year risk prediction for CVD events [134, 135]. As CRP increases at any level of 10-year Framingham risk or any level of LDL-C, risk for CVD increases continuously [136] (Fig. 1.9). Although many inflammatory mediators can be measured, CRP is remarkably stable and can be accurately measured in commercial laboratories. One recent clinical trial showed that lowering systemic inflammatory tone using a monoclonal

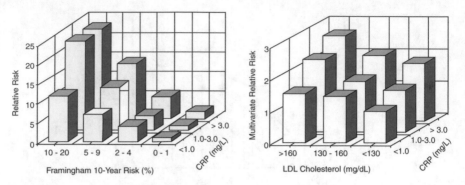

Fig. 1.9 Relationships between CRP, CVD risk, and Framingham 10-year risk (left) or LDL-C level (right). (Reproduced with permission from Ridker. Circulation. 2003; 107:363–369)

antibody directed against interleukin-1β is associated with significant reductions in risk for CVD events independent of lipid lowering [137].

Chronic Kidney Disease

Chronic kidney disease (CKD) is defined as a glomerular filtration rate (GFR) <60 mL/min/1.73 m²), albuminuria (defined ≥30 mg/d), or both. The prevalence of CKD increases with age, and because populations are aging worldwide, the global incidence of CKD is increasing. The current world prevalence of CKD is estimated to be 276 million persons and the majority of people with CKD have stage 3 [138]. DM and HTN are strong risk factors for CKD. Patients with CKD have a greatly magnified risk for developing CAD, stroke, arrhythmias, and congestive heart failure and the uremic state is accompanied by a variety of toxins that can accelerate the rate of progression of each of these disorders [139]. Albuminuria is a strong adverse prognostic indicator for CVD, renal failure, and mortality, and represents injury to renal podocytes and glomeruli [140, 141] (Fig. 1.10).

Cigarette Smoking

The World Health Organization estimates that there are approximately 1 billion smokers in the world [4]. Smoking is the number one cause of preventable death in the United States and throughout the world. It is estimated to account for 7.1 million deaths globally in 2016 [68]. In the US, approximately 17.5% of males and 13.5% of females are smokers [68]. Smoking increases risk for CVD, CAD, MI, stroke, mortality, and a variety of cancers, including lung and transitional cell cancers of the bladder. Compared to lifelong nonsmokers, men and women who smoke on

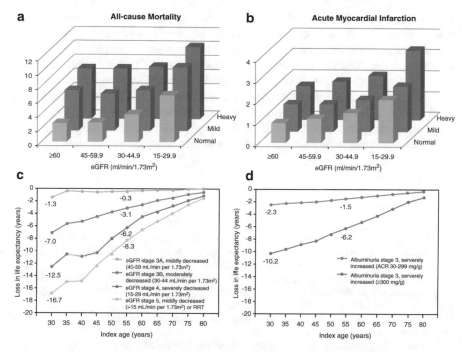

Fig. 1.10 Relationships between cardiac events and mortality from cardiovascular disease (CVD) by stage of chronic kidney disease (CKD). A and B, The adjusted relative rate of all-cause mortality (ACM) and acute myocardial infarction as a function of glomerular filtration rate and severity of albuminuria as assessed by albumin-to-creatinine ratio (ACR; normal, ACR <30 mg/g; mild, ACR 30–300 mg/g; or heavy, ACR >300 mg/g). C and D, Adjusted mortality resulting from CVD by CKD stage. Loss is compared with life expectancy in people with normal or mildly impaired kidney function (stage 1–2, eGFR ≥60 mL·min⁻¹/1.73 m²) and normal or mildly increased albuminuria (stage 1, ACR < 30 mg/g). RRT: renal replacement therapy. (Reproduced with permission from Tonelli et al. Circulation. 2016;133:518–536)

average lose 12 and 11 years of life, respectively [68]. A meta-analysis of 75 studies and including approximately 2.4 million persons showed a 25% higher risk for CHD in female smokers than in male smokers [142]. There is considerable urgency in developing and promoting programs to encourage men and women to engage in lifelong smoking cessation.

Conclusions

Significant progress has been made in recent decades in identifying risk factors for CVD and in developing safe and efficacious therapies for these disorders. Screening programs are in place in most nations, but more needs to be done. Significant progress has been made in reducing the clinical sequelae of CVD in many nations around the world, though important deficiencies persist [143]. The global population is aging making it essentially certain that more people will live to develop CVD. It is crucial that global efforts embrace primordial and primary prevention more fully so as to reduce the incidence of disease as well as the costs of treating established disease. It is also important that persons identified with risk factors remain adherent to therapies, as low adherence rates and low guideline directed goal attainment rates are the norm worldwide. There is an urgent need for newer and less costly interventions, and perhaps nutraceuticals will be developed that help to fill some of the gaps for treating risk factors in both the primary and secondary prevention settings.

References

1. Gheorghe A, Griffiths U, Murphy A, Legido-Quigley H, Lamptey P, Perel P. The economic burden of cardiovascular disease and hypertension in low- and middle-income countries: a systematic review. BMC Public Health. 2018;18:975.
2. Walker IF, Garbe F, Wright J, et al. The economic costs of cardiovascular disease, diabetes mellitus, and associated complications in South Asia: a systematic review. Value Health Reg Issues. 2018;15:12–26.
3. https://www.world-heart-federation.org/resources/cardiovascular-diseases-cvds-global-facts-figures/
4. https://www.who.int/en/news-room/fact-sheets/detail/cardiovascular-diseases-(cvds)
5. https://professional.heart.org/idc/groups/ahamah-public/@wcm/@sop/@smd/documents-downloadable/ucm_503396.pdf
6. Tsao CW, Vasan RS. Cohort profile: the Framingham Heart Study (FHS): overview of milestones in cardiovascular epidemiology. Int J Epidemiol. 2015;44:1800–13.
7. Mahmood SS, Levy D, Vasan RS, Wang TJ. The Framingham Heart Study and the epidemiology of cardiovascular disease: a historical perspective. Lancet. 2014;383:999–1008.
8. Pett KD, Willett WC, Vartiainen E, Katz DL. The seven countries study. Eur Heart J. 2017;38:3119–21.
9. Keys A, Menotti A, Aravanis C, et al. The seven countries study: 2,289 deaths in 15 years. Prev Med. 1984;13:141–54.
10. Fried LP, Borhani NO, Enright P, et al. The cardiovascular health study: design and rationale. Ann Epidemiol. 1991;1:263–76.
11. The ARIC Investigators. The Atherosclerosis Risk in Communities (ARIC) Study: design and objectives. Am J Epidemiol. 1989;129:687–702.
12. Bild DE, Bluemke DA, Burke GL, et al. Multi-ethnic study of atherosclerosis: objectives and design. Am J Epidemiol. 2002;156:871–81.
13. Howard VJ, Cushman M, Pulley L, et al. The reasons for geographic and racial differences in stroke study: objectives and design. Neuroepidemiology. 2005;25:135–43.
14. Wyatt SB, Akylbekova EL, Wofford MR, et al. Prevalence, awareness, treatment, and control of hypertension in the Jackson heart study. Hypertension. 2008;51:650–6.
15. Sivapalaratnam S, Boekholdt SM, Trip MD, et al. Family history of premature coronary heart disease and risk prediction in the EPIC-Norfolk prospective population study. Heart. 2010;96:1985–9.
16. Assmann G, Schulte H. The prospective cardiovascular Munster (PROCAM) study: prevalence of hyperlipidemia in persons with hypertension and/or diabetes mellitus and the relationship to coronary heart disease. Am Heart J. 1988;116:1713–24.
17. Aquino EML, Barreto SM, Bensenor IM, et al. Brazilian longitudinal study of adult health (ELSA-Brasil): objectives and design. Am J Epidemiol. 2012;175:315–24.

18. Shim JS, Song BM, Lee JH, et al. Cohort profile: the cardiovascular and metabolic diseases Etiology Research Center Cohort in Korea. Yonsei Med J. 2019;60:804–10.
19. Nojiri S, Daida H. Atherosclerotic cardiovascular risk in Japan. Jpn Clin Med. 2017;8:1179066017712713.
20. Weiwei C, Runlin G, Lisheng L, et al. Outline of the report on cardiovascular diseases in China, 2014. Eur Heart J Suppl. 2016;18:F2–F11.
21. Prabhakaran D, Jeemon P, Roy A. Cardiovascular diseases in India. Circulation. 2016;133:1605–20.
22. Kengne AP, Ntyintyane LM, Mayosi BM. A systematic overview of prospective cohort studies of cardiovascular disease in sub-Saharan Africa. Cardiovasc J Afr. 2012;23:103–12.
23. Morales LS, Flores YN, Leng M, Sportiche N, Gallegos-Carrillo K, Salmeron J. Risk factors for cardiovascular disease among Mexican-American adults in the United States and Mexico: a comparative study. Salud Publica Mex. 2014;56:197–205.
24. McAreavey D, Vidal JS, Aspelund T, et al. Midlife cardiovascular risk factors and late-life unrecognized and recognized myocardial infarction detect by cardiac magnetic resonance: ICELAND-MI, the AGES-Reykjavik study. J Am Heart Assoc. 2016;5:e002420.
25. Yusuf S, Hawken S, Ounpuu S, et al. Effect of potentially modifiable risk factors associated with myocardial infarction in 52 countries (the INTERHEART study): case-control study. Lancet. 2004;364:937–52.
26. Ference BA, Ginsberg HN, Graham I, et al. Low-density lipoproteins cause atherosclerotic cardiovascular disease. 1. Evidence from genetic, epidemiologic, and clinical studies. A consensus statement from the European Atherosclerosis Society Consensus Panel. Eur Heart J. 2017;38:2459–72.
27. Tabas I. Consequences and therapeutic implications of macrophage apoptosis in atherosclerosis: the importance of lesion stage and phagocytic efficiency. Arterioscler Thromb Vasc Biol. 2005;25:2255–64.
28. Tabas I, Seimon T, Timmins J, Li G, Lim W. Macrophage apoptosis in advanced atherosclerosis. Ann N Y Acad Sci. 2009;1173(Suppl 1):E40–5.
29. Libby P, Ridker PM, Hansson GK. Inflammation in atherosclerosis: from pathophysiology to practice. J Am Coll Cardiol. 2009;54:2129–38.
30. Baigent C, Blackwell L, Emberson J, et al. Efficacy and safety of more intensive lowering of LDL cholesterol: a meta-analysis of data from 170,000 participants in 26 randomised trials. Lancet. 2010;376:1670–81.
31. Cannon CP, Blazing MA, Giugliano RP, et al. Ezetimibe added to statin therapy after acute coronary syndromes. N Engl J Med. 2015;372:2387–97.
32. Sabatine MS, Giugliano RP, Keech AC, et al. Evolocumab and clinical outcomes in patients with cardiovascular disease. N Engl J Med. 2017;376.1713–22.
33. Schwartz GG, Steg PG, Szarek M, et al. Alirocumab and cardiovascular outcomes after acute coronary syndrome. N Engl J Med. 2018;379:2097–107.
34. Ference BA, Graham I, Tokgozoglu L, Catapano AL. Impact of Lipids on cardiovascular health. JACC Health Promotion Ser J Am Coll Cardiol. 2018;72:1141–56.
35. Packard CJ, Weintraub WS, Laufs U. New metrics needed to visualize the long-term impact of early LDL-C lowering on the cardiovascular disease trajectory. Vasc Pharmacol. 2015;71:37–9.
36. Grundy SM, Stone NJ, Bailey AL, et al. AHA/ACC/AACVPR/AAPA/ABC/ACPM/ADA/AGS/APhA/ASPC/NLA/PCNA guideline on the management of blood cholesterol: a report of the American College of Cardiology/American Heart Association Task Force on Clinical Practice Guidelines. Circulation, 2019. 2018;139:e1082–143.
37. Mach F, Baigent C, Catapano AL, et al. ESC/EAS guidelines for the management of dyslipidaemias: lipid modification to reduce cardiovascular risk: the task force for the management of dyslipidaemias of the European Society of Cardiology (ESC) and European Atherosclerosis Society (EAS). Eur Heart J. 2019:2019.

38. Toth PP, Barter PJ, Rosenson RS, et al. High-density lipoproteins: a consensus statement from the National Lipid Association. J Clin Lipidol. 2013;7:484–525.
39. Heinecke JW. The HDL proteome: a marker--and perhaps mediator–of coronary artery disease. J Lipid Res. 2009;50(Suppl):S167–71.
40. Brewer HB Jr, Remaley AT, Neufeld EB, Basso F, Joyce C. Regulation of plasma high-density lipoprotein levels by the ABCA1 transporter and the emerging role of high-density lipoprotein in the treatment of cardiovascular disease. Arterioscler Thromb Vasc Biol. 2004;24:1755–60.
41. Toth P. High-density lipoprotein: epidemiology, metabolism, and antiatherogenic effects. Dis Mon. 2001;47:365–416.
42. Castelli WP. Cholesterol and lipids in the risk of coronary artery disease–the Framingham Heart Study. Can J Cardiol. 1988;4(Suppl A):5a–10a.
43. Assmann G, Cullen P, Schulte H. The Munster Heart Study (PROCAM). Results of follow-up at 8 years. Eur Heart J. 1998;19(Suppl A):A2–A11.
44. Preiss D, Kristensen SL. The new pooled cohort equations risk calculator. Can J Cardiol. 2015;31:613–9.
45. Coleman RL, Stevens RJ, Retnakaran R, Holman RR. Framingham, SCORE, and DECODE risk equations do not provide reliable cardiovascular risk estimates in type 2 diabetes. Diabetes Care. 2007;30:1292–3.
46. Cook NR, Paynter NP, Eaton CB, et al. Comparison of the Framingham and Reynolds Risk scores for global cardiovascular risk prediction in the multiethnic Women's Health Initiative. Circulation. 2012;125:1748–56, s1–11
47. Boden WE, Probstfield JL, Anderson T, et al. Niacin in patients with low HDL cholesterol levels receiving intensive statin therapy. N Engl J Med. 2011;365:2255–67.
48. Landray MJ, Haynes R, Hopewell JC, et al. Effects of extended-release niacin with laropiprant in high-risk patients. N Engl J Med. 2014;371:203–12.
49. Schwartz GG, Olsson AG, Abt M, et al. Effects of Dalcetrapib in patients with a recent acute coronary syndrome. N Engl J Med. 2012;367:2089–99.
50. Bowman L, Hopewell JC, Chen F, et al. Effects of Anacetrapib in patients with atherosclerotic vascular disease. N Engl J Med. 2017;377:1217–27.
51. Voight BF, Peloso GM, Orho-Melander M, et al. Plasma HDL cholesterol and risk of myocardial infarction: a mendelian randomisation study. Lancet. 2012;380:572–80.
52. Agerholm-Larsen B, Nordestgaard BG, Steffensen R, Jensen G, Tybjaerg-Hansen A. Elevated HDL cholesterol is a risk factor for ischemic heart disease in white women when caused by a common mutation in the cholesteryl ester transfer protein gene. Circulation. 2000;101:1907–12.
53. Yamamoto S, Yancey PG, Ikizler TA, et al. Dysfunctional high-density lipoprotein in patients on chronic hemodialysis. J Am Coll Cardiol. 2012;60:2372–9.
54. Grundy SM. Atherogenic dyslipidemia associated with metabolic syndrome and insulin resistance. Clin Cornerstone. 2006;8(Suppl 1):S21–7.
55. Budoff M. Triglycerides and triglyceride-rich lipoproteins in the causal pathway of cardiovascular disease. Am J Cardiol. 2016;118:138–45.
56. Miller MSN, Ballantyne C, Bittner V, et al. Triglycerides and cardiovascular disease: a scientific statement from the American Heart Association. Circulation. 2011;123:2292–333.
57. Chapman MJ, Ginsberg HN, Amarenco P, et al. Triglyceride-rich lipoproteins and high-density lipoprotein cholesterol in patients at high risk of cardiovascular disease: evidence and guidance for management. Eur Heart J. 2011;32:1345–61.
58. Toth PP, Philip S, Hull M, Granowitz C. Elevated triglycerides (>/=150 mg/dL) and high triglycerides (200-499 mg/dL) are significant predictors of new heart failure diagnosis: a real-world analysis of high-risk statin-treated patients. Vasc Health Risk Manag. 2019;15:533–8.
59. Toth PP, Philip S, Hull M, Granowitz C. Elevated triglycerides (>/=150 mg/dL) and high triglycerides (200-499 mg/dL) are significant predictors of hospitalization for new-onset

kidney disease: a real-world analysis of high-risk statin-treated patients. Cardiorenal Med. 2019;9:400–7.

60. Toth PP, Philip S, Hull M, Granowitz C. Association of elevated triglycerides with increased cardiovascular risk and direct costs in statin-treated patients. Mayo Clin Proc. 2019;94:1670–80.

61. Toth PP, Granowitz C, Hull M, Liassou D, Anderson A, Philip S. High triglycerides are associated with increased cardiovascular events, medical costs, and resource use: a real-world administrative claims analysis of statin-treated patients with high residual cardiovascular risk. J Am Heart Assoc. 2018;7:e008740.

62. Nordestgaard BG, Varbo A. Triglycerides and cardiovascular disease. Lancet. 2014;384:626–35.

63. Varbo A, Benn M, Nordestgaard BG. Remnant cholesterol as a cause of ischemic heart disease: evidence, definition, measurement, atherogenicity, high risk patients, and present and future treatment. Pharmacol Ther. 2014;141:358–67.

64. Varbo A, Benn M, Tybjaerg-Hansen A, Jorgensen AB, Frikke-Schmidt R, Nordestgaard BG. Remnant cholesterol as a causal risk factor for ischemic heart disease. J Am Coll Cardiol. 2013;61:427–36.

65. Joshi PH, Khokhar AA, Massaro JM, et al. Remnant lipoprotein cholesterol and incident coronary heart disease: the Jackson heart and Framingham offspring cohort studies. J Am Heart Assoc. 2016;5

66. Varbo A, Benn M, Tybjaerg-Hansen A, Nordestgaard BG. Elevated remnant cholesterol causes both low-grade inflammation and ischemic heart disease, whereas elevated low-density lipoprotein cholesterol causes ischemic heart disease without inflammation. Circulation. 2013;128:1298–309.

67. Bhatt DL, Steg PG, Miller M, et al. Reduction in first and Total ischemic events with Icosapent ethyl across baseline triglyceride tertiles. J Am Coll Cardiol. 2019;74:1159–61.

68. Benjamin EJ, Muntner P, Alonso A, et al. Heart disease and stroke statistics; 2019 update: a report from the American Heart Association. Circulation. 2019;139:e56–e528.

69. Neaton JD, Blackburn H, Jacobs D, et al. Serum cholesterol level and mortality findings for men screened in the multiple risk factor intervention trial. Multiple risk factor intervention trial research group. Arch Intern Med. 1992;152:1490–500.

70. Franklin SS, Wong ND. Hypertension and cardiovascular disease: contributions of the Framingham Heart Study. 2013;8:49–57.

71. Schiffrin EL. Novel mechanisms of hypertension and vascular dysfunction. Nat Rev Nephrol. 2018;14:73–4.

72. Sedeek M, Hébert RL, Kennedy CR, Burns KD, Touyz RM. Molecular mechanisms of hypertension: role of Nox family NADPH oxidases. Curr Opin Nephrol Hypertens. 2009;18:122–7.

73. Safar ME, Boudier HS. Vascular development, pulse pressure, and the mechanisms of hypertension. Hypertension. 2005;46:205–9.

74. Whelton PK, Carey RM, Aronow WS, et al. ACC/AHA/AAPA/ABC/ACPM/AGS/APhA/ASH/ASPC/NMA/PCNA guideline for the prevention, detection, evaluation, and management of high blood pressure in adults: a report of the American College of Cardiology/American Heart Association Task Force on Clinical Practice Guidelines. Hypertension 2018. 2017;71:e13–e115.

75. Williams B, Mancia G, Spiering W, et al. 2018 ESC/ESH guidelines for the management of arterial hypertension: The Task Force for the management of arterial hypertension of the European Society of Cardiology (ESC) and the European Society of Hypertension (ESH). Eur Heart J. 2018;39:3021–104.

76. Nerenberg KA, Zarnke KB, Leung AA, et al. Hypertension Canada's 2018 guidelines for diagnosis, risk assessment, prevention, and treatment of hypertension in adults and children. Can J Cardiol. 2018;34:506–25.

77. Jennings GLR. Recent clinical trials of hypertension management. Hypertension. 2013;62:3–7.

78. Sever P. Will the recent hypertension trials change the guidelines? J Renin Angiotensin Aldosterone Syst JRAAS. 2017;18:1470320317710891.
79. Dzau VJ, Balatbat CA. Future of hypertension. Hypertension. 2019;74:450–7.
80. Mills KT, Bundy JD, Kelly TN, et al. Global disparities of hypertension prevalence and control: a systematic analysis of population-based studies from 90 countries. Circulation. 2016;134:441–50.
81. Grundy SM. Does the metabolic syndrome exist? Diabetes Care. 2006;29:1689–92. discussion 1693-6
82. Grundy SM. Metabolic syndrome: connecting and reconciling cardiovascular and diabetes worlds. J Am Coll Cardiol. 2006;47:1093–100.
83. Roberts CK, Hevener AL, Barnard RJ. Metabolic syndrome and insulin resistance: underlying causes and modification by exercise training. In: Comprehensive physiology, vol. 3; 2013. p. 1–58.
84. Kahn BB, Flier JS. Obesity and insulin resistance. J Clin Invest. 2000;106:473–81.
85. Watson RT, Pessin JE. Intracellular organization of insulin signaling and GLUT4 translocation. Recent Prog Horm Res. 2001;56:175–93.
86. Lteif AA, Han K, Mather KJ. Obesity, insulin resistance, and the metabolic syndrome. Circulation. 2005;112:32–8.
87. Rocha NG, Templeton DL, Greiner JJ, Stauffer BL, DeSouza CA. Metabolic syndrome and endothelin-1 mediated vasoconstrictor tone in overweight/obese adults. Metabolism. 2014;63:951–6.
88. Sorrentino FS, Matteini S, Bonifazzi C, Sebastiani A, Parmeggiani F. Diabetic retinopathy and endothelin system: microangiopathy versus endothelial dysfunction. Eye. 2018;32:1157–63.
89. Rhee SY, Kim YS. The role of advanced glycation end products in diabetic vascular complications. Diabetes Metab J. 2018;42:188–95.
90. Singh VP, Bali A, Singh N, Jaggi AS. Advanced glycation end products and diabetic complications. Korean J Physiol Pharmacol. 2014;18(1):14.
91. Costabile G, Annuzzi G, Di Marino L, et al. Fasting and post-prandial adipose tissue lipoprotein lipase and hormone-sensitive lipase in obesity and type 2 diabetes. J Endocrinol Investig. 2011;34:e110–4.
92. Juntti-Berggren L, Berggren PO. Apolipoprotein CIII is a new player in diabetes. Curr Opin Lipidol. 2017;28:27–31.
93. Rashid S, Watanabe T, Sakaue T, Lewis GF. Mechanisms of HDL lowering in insulin resistant, hypertriglyceridemic states: the combined effect of HDL triglyceride enrichment and elevated hepatic lipase activity. Clin Biochem. 2003;36:421–9.
94. Ballantyne CM, Hoogeveen RC, McNeill AM, et al. Metabolic syndrome risk for cardiovascular disease and diabetes in the ARIC study. Int J Obes. 2008;32(Suppl 2):S21–4.
95. Dekker JM, Girman C, Rhodes T, et al. Metabolic syndrome and 10-year cardiovascular disease risk in the Hoorn study. Circulation. 2005;112:666–73.
96. Kumar P, Gehi AK. Atrial fibrillation and metabolic syndrome: understanding the connection. J Atrial Fibrillation. 2012;5:647.
97. Whayne TF Jr. Metabolic syndrome, peripheral vascular disease and coronary artery disease: a concise review. Int J Angiol. 2010;19:e96–9.
98. Cornier MA, Dabelea D, Hernandez TL, et al. The metabolic syndrome. Endocr Rev. 2008;29:777–822.
99. Golbidi S, Mesdaghinia A, Laher I. Exercise in the metabolic syndrome. Oxidative Med Cell Longev. 2012;2012:349710.
100. Pitsavos C, Panagiotakos D, Weinem M, Stefanadis C. Diet, exercise and the metabolic syndrome. Rev Diabet Stud: RDS. 2006;3:118–26.
101. Saklayen MG. The global epidemic of the metabolic syndrome. Curr Hypertens Rep. 2018;20:12.
102. Gurka MJ, Filipp SL, DeBoer MD. Geographical variation in the prevalence of obesity, metabolic syndrome, and diabetes among US adults. Nutr Diabetes. 2018;8:14.

103. Scuteri A, Laurent S, Cucca F, et al. Metabolic syndrome across Europe: different clusters of risk factors. Eur J Prev Cardiol. 2015;22:486–91.
104. Palmer MK, Trends in Lipids TPP. Obesity, metabolic syndrome, and diabetes mellitus in the United States: an NHANES analysis (2003-2004 to 2013-2014). Obesity (Silver Spring). 2019;27:309–14.
105. DeFronzo RA. From the triumvirate to the ominous octet: a new paradigm for the treatment of type 2 diabetes mellitus. Diabetes. 2009;58:773–95.
106. Nauck MA, Meier JJ. Incretin hormones: their role in health and disease. Diabetes Obes Metab. 2018;20(Suppl 1):5–21.
107. Fontana L, Eagon JC, Trujillo ME, Scherer PE, Klein S. Visceral fat Adipokine secretion is associated with systemic inflammation in obese humans. Diabetes. 2007;56:1010–3.
108. Hsia DS, Grove O, Cefalu WT. An update on sodium-glucose co-transporter-2 inhibitors for the treatment of diabetes mellitus. Curr Opin Endocrinol Diabetes Obes. 2017;24:73–9.
109. Klip A, McGraw TE, James DE. Thirty sweet years of GLUT4. J Biol Chem. 2019;294:11369–81.
110. Sun Y, Liu S, Ferguson S, et al. Phosphoenolpyruvate carboxykinase overexpression selectively attenuates insulin Signaling and hepatic insulin sensitivity in transgenic mice. J Biol Chem. 2002;277:23301–7.
111. Leon BM, Maddox TM. Diabetes and cardiovascular disease: epidemiology, biological mechanisms, treatment recommendations and future research. World J Diabetes. 2015;6:1246–58.
112. Hostalek U. Global epidemiology of prediabetes – present and future perspectives. Clin Diabet Endocrinol. 2019;5:5.
113. Tamayo T, Rosenbauer J, Wild SH, et al. Diabetes in Europe: an update. Diabetes Res Clin Pract. 2014;103:206–17.
114. Lu J, Wang W, Li M, et al. Associations of hemoglobin A_{1c} with cardiovascular disease and mortality in Chinese adults with diabetes. J Am Coll Cardiol. 2018;72:3224–5.
115. Andersson C, Van Gaal L, Caterson ID, et al. Relationship between HbA1c levels and risk of cardiovascular adverse outcomes and all-cause mortality in overweight and obese cardiovascular high-risk women and men with type 2 diabetes. Diabetologia. 2012;55:2348–55.
116. Kohner EM. Microvascular disease: what does the UKPDS tell us about diabetic retinopathy? Diabet Med. 2008;25(Suppl 2):20–4.
117. Implications of the United Kingdom prospective diabetes study. Diabetes Care. 2002;25:s28–32.
118. Marso SP, Daniels GH, Brown-Frandsen K, et al. Liraglutide and cardiovascular outcomes in type 2 diabetes. N Engl J Med. 2016;375:311–22.
119. Marso SP, Bain SC, Consoli A, et al. Semaglutide and cardiovascular outcomes in patients with type 2 diabetes. N Engl J Med. 2016;375:1834–44.
120. Gerstein HC, Colhoun HM, Dagenais GR, et al. Dulaglutide and cardiovascular outcomes in type 2 diabetes (REWIND): a double-blind, randomised placebo-controlled trial. Lancet. 2019;394:121–30.
121. Zinman B, Wanner C, Lachin JM, et al. Empagliflozin, cardiovascular outcomes, and mortality in type 2 diabetes. N Engl J Med. 2015;373:2117–28.
122. MPJd W, Kanters E, Kraal G, Hofker MH. Nuclear factor kappaB signaling in atherogenesis. Arterioscler Thromb Vasc Biol. 2005;25:904–14.
123. Jain MK, Sangwung P, Hamik A. Regulation of an inflammatory disease: Kruppel-like factors and atherosclerosis. Arterioscler Thromb Vasc Biol. 2014;34:499–508.
124. Meijer CA, Le Haen PA, van Dijk RA, et al. Activator protein-1 (AP-1) signalling in human atherosclerosis: results of a systematic evaluation and intervention study. Clin Sci (Lond). 2012;122:421–8.
125. Galkina E, Ley K. Vascular adhesion molecules in atherosclerosis. Arterioscler Thromb Vasc Biol. 2007;27:2292–301.
126. Figueroa XF, Duling BR. Gap junctions in the control of vascular function. Antioxid Redox Signal. 2009;11:251–66.

127. Libby P, Pasterkamp G. Requiem for the 'vulnerable plaque'. Eur Heart J. 2015;36:2984–7.
128. Libby P, Nahrendorf M, Swirski FK. Leukocytes link local and systemic inflammation in ischemic cardiovascular disease: an expanded "Cardiovascular Continuum". J Am Coll Cardiol. 2016;67:1091–103.
129. Fonseca FA, Izar MC. High-sensitivity C-reactive protein and cardiovascular disease across countries and ethnicities. Clinics (Sao Paulo, Brazil). 2016;71:235–42.
130. Ridker PM, Bassuk SS, Toth PP. C-reactive protein and risk of cardiovascular disease: evidence and clinical application. Curr Atheroscleros Rep. 2003;5:341–9.
131. Ridker PM, Danielson E, Fonseca FAH, et al. Rosuvastatin to prevent vascular events in men and women with elevated C-reactive protein. N Engl J Med. 2008;359:2195–207.
132. Bohula EA, Giugliano RP, Cannon CP, et al. Achievement of dual low-density lipoprotein cholesterol and high-sensitivity C-reactive protein targets more frequent with the addition of ezetimibe to simvastatin and associated with better outcomes in IMPROVE-IT. Circulation. 2015;132:1224–33.
133. Ridker PM, Cannon CP, Morrow D, et al. C-reactive protein levels and outcomes after statin therapy. N Engl J Med. 2005;352:20–8.
134. Albert MA, Ridker PM. C-reactive protein as a risk predictor. Circulation. 2006;114:e67–74.
135. Wilson PW, Pencina M, Jacques P, Selhub J, D'Agostino R Sr, O'Donnell CJ. C-reactive protein and reclassification of cardiovascular risk in the Framingham Heart Study. Circ Cardiovasc Qual Outcomes. 2008;1:92–7.
136. Ridker PM. Clinical application of C-reactive protein for cardiovascular disease detection and prevention. Circulation. 2003;107:363–9.
137. Ridker PM, Everett BM, Thuren T, et al. Antiinflammatory therapy with canakinumab for atherosclerotic disease. N Engl J Med. 2017;377:1119–31.
138. Hill NR, Fatoba ST, Oke JL, et al. Global prevalence of chronic kidney disease – a systematic review and meta-analysis. PLoS One. 2016;11:e0158765.
139. Tonelli M, Karumanchi SA, Thadhani R. Epidemiology and mechanisms of Uremia-related cardiovascular disease. Circulation. 2016;133:518–36.
140. Nauta FL, Scheven L, Meijer E, et al. Glomerular and tubular damage markers in individuals with progressive albuminuria. Clin J Am Soc Nephrol. 2013;8:1106–14.
141. Abbate M, Zoja C, Remuzzi G. How does proteinuria cause progressive renal damage? J Am Soc Nephrol. 2006;17:2974–84.
142. Huxley RR, Woodward M. Cigarette smoking as a risk factor for coronary heart disease in women compared with men: a systematic review and meta-analysis of prospective cohort studies. Lancet. 2011;378:1297–305.
143. Barquera S, Pedroza-Tobías A, Medina C, et al. Global overview of the epidemiology of atherosclerotic cardiovascular disease. Arch Med Res. 2015;46:328–38.

Chapter 2
A Brief Historical Perspective on the Use of Natural Compounds Influencing Cardiovascular Health

Francesco M. Galassi and Elena Varotto

All human history attests
That happiness for man, – the hungry sinner! -
Since Eve ate apples, much depends on dinner.

Lord George Gordon Byron (1788–1824)

Nutraceutics first emerged as a scientific branch of medicine in 1989 owing to the work of physician Stephen L. DeFelice (born 1936), who described a nutraceutical as a "food or part of a food that provides medical or health benefits, including the prevention and/or treatment of a disease" [1]. Today more refined definitions are available such as that provided by *Health Canada*: "a product prepared from foods, but sold in the form of pills, or powder (potions) or in other medicinal forms, not usually associated with foods" [1].

Over a decade after DeFelice coined the term, in 2004, this new discipline had experienced a major cultural and scientific expansion, testified by the introduction of the headword "Nutraceutical", both as a noun and an adjective, in the *Oxford English Dictionary* [2]. However, the recent success of nutraceutical products should not lead one to believe that the importance of natural dietary substances is but a recent discovery. Despite the understandable lack of a full physiopathological

F. M. Galassi (✉)
Archaeology, College of Humanities, Arts and Social Sciences, Flinders University, Adelaide, SA, Australia

FAPAB Research Center, Avola, Siracusa, Sicily, Italy
e-mail: francescom.galassi@flinders.edu.au

E. Varotto
Archaeology, College of Humanities, Arts and Social Sciences, Flinders University, Adelaide, SA, Australia

FAPAB Research Center, Avola, Siracusa, Sicily, Italy

Department of Humanities (DISUM), University of Catania, Catania, Sicily, Italy

comprehension of the phenomena and changes brought about by foods on the human organism, there is a solid body of historical evidence supporting the notion that ancient civilizations had at least achieved some empirical knowledge of the potential beneficial effects of certain foodstuffs.

Nonetheless, any attempt at such a retrospective analysis should take into account the fact that in the past–especially before the clinical and pharmaceutical revolutions of the 19th and 20th centuries–the distinction between food and drugs was not as sharp as we would conceive it today. For instance, in the ancient Greek language the very word φάρμακον (/phármakon/, "drug") had an ambivalent meaning, it being used to indicate a range of substances from a healing remedy to a poison [3]. In addition, in ancient societies φάρμακον often consisted of food and officinal herbs. Some of the earliest examples of nutraceuticals used by ancient societies are represented by a series of plants (including yarrow, cornflower, St. Barnaby's thistle, ragwort, grape hyacinth, joint pine, etc.) found in Shanidar Cave (Iraq), which were probably used by its Neanderthalian inhabitants, who may have utilized them for both medical and ritual purposes [4]. Another classical example is that of the sweet flag (*Acorus calamus*), which due to its carminative, antidiarrhoic and appetite-stimulating properties, was common in ancient India, China and Egypt, being even found in the tomb of pharaoh Tutankhamun (discovered by Howard Carter in 1922) [5].

As part of the vast spectrum of chronic diseases, cardiovascular pathologies represent a major nosological category ranking first in Western and Westernized countries nowadays in terms of mortality rates. Despite their being second to infectious diseases in the past, they have always been present in the human species, as established through the scientific study of mummies [6–8].

In our world, beside the prescription of traditional chemical pharmaceutical agents, nutraceutical components are proving a valuable and effective tool in the prevention of cardiovascular diseases in high-risk healthy subjects.

One of these products is **red yeast rice** (*Monascus purpureus*) which contains monocolin K, a molecule structurally analogous to lovastatin and capable of inhibiting the hepatic synthesis of cholesterol. Red yeast has been known since time immemorial, arising within the ancient Indian and Chinese civilizations [9].

Another substance is **dietary fibre** which can inhibit intestinal absorption of cholesterol and its fecal excretion. Although the term was coined only in 1953 by Dr. Eben Hipsley, its properties had already long been grasped, with some observations dating back to the classical world [10].

Dark chocolate, when regularly consumed, has been linked to a lower incidence of cardiovascular pathologies, probably as a result of the action of flavan-3-ols [11]. The history of chocolate is a long one and originates in pre-Columbian Mexico. Here seeds of the cacao tree (*Theobroma cacao*) were regarded as holy and a sort of gift from the god Quetzalcoatl, capable of proving beneficial to the health of those who drank a bitter foamy beverage made out of them, *xocoatl*, from whose phonetic adaptation the very word "chocolate" stems. Noticed but not given too much importance by Columbus during his voyages, chocolate started to become a part of European diet in the last decades of the sixteenth century AD. With an enhanced status during the following centuries, its reputation has often been that of a regrettable pleasure, although in recent years its positive effects have been stressed in the medical literature [12].

Strawberries (*Fragaria* × *ananassa*) have been described in some studies to exert an antioxidant effect and to be able to decrease cardiovascular risk factors [13], and some studies have linked them to uric acid reduction [14].

A historical example of their preventive/therapeutical use is offered by the case of the great Swedish taxonomist Carl Linnaeus (1707–1778). As reported in Dietrich Heinrich Stöver's *Leben des Ritters Carl von Linné* [15] – a passage also commented upon in 1899 by the Victorian polymath Francis Galton (1822–1911) in a famous letter to the journal *Nature* [16] – Linnaeus suffered from gout ("Podagra"), a chronic condition that was common amongst the upper classes in the past [17, 18], but he managed to control its attacks by eating strawberries. Interestingly, Linnaeus ultimately died of cerebrovascular disease, for whose development gout is a known risk factor [19, 20], only much later, hence some preventive cardiovascular role played by strawberries can be reasonably postulated.

Garlic (*Allium sativum L.*) shows an interesting profile as a cardiovascular nutraceutical due to its anti-thrombotic and lipid-lowering properties [21]. This vegetable has been known since antiquity and held in great esteem: in Greece and Rome athletes and soldiers allegedly ate it in order to increase their physical strength and courage, as well as it was considered a remedy against several infectious and other clinical conditions [22].

Finally, the **Mediterranean diet**, whose beneficial effects are attested in the prevention of cardiovascular diseases [23], is firmly based on a long culinary tradition whose origins can be found in ancient Egypt and gradually moulded by successive civilizations arriving onto the historical stage, including the Greeks, Romans and Arabs. One of its key aspects is the presence of vegetables, such as mushrooms, olives (with their oil), and cereals, which have traditionally been able to feed the poorer classes, fish and little meat. After the discovery of the Americas, more products came to enrich the old Mediterranean diet, including tomatoes [24].

Although the scant information retrieved from the perusal of the available historical sources does not allow us to describe an exclusively informed and prevention-oriented prescription of certain foods and substances in the past to an extent even slightly comparable to the present situation, it can be reasonably postulated that the beneficial effects derived from the intake of certain products had been observed by ancient civilizations.

References

1. Kalra EK. Nutraceutical-definition and introduction. AAPS PharmSci. 2003;5(3):27–8.
2. https://public.ucd.com/updates/new-words-list-march-2004/
3. Liddell HG, Scott R. A Greek-English Lexicon. Oxford: Clarendon Press; 1940, sub voce φάρμακον: http://www.perseus.tufts.edu/hopper/text?doc=Perseus%3Atext%3A1999.04.005 7%3Aentry%3Dfa%2Frmakon

4. Shipley GP, Kindscher K. Evidence for the paleoethnobotany of the Neanderthal: a review of the literature. Scientifica (Cairo). 2016;2016:8927654.
5. Rudgley R. The encyclopedia of psychoactive substances: Macmillan; 2014. p. 3.
6. Galassi FM, Habicht ME, Rühli FJ, De Carolis S. A unique case of stroke and upper limb paralysis in a mid-18th century natural mummy. Circ Res. 2017;121(4):338–440.
7. Galassi FM, Borghi C, Ballestriero R, Habicht ME, Henneberg M, Rühli FJ. Palaeopathology of the earlobe crease (Frank's sign): new insights from Renaissance art. Int J Cardiol. 2017;236:82–4.
8. Allam AH, Mandour Ali MA, Wann LS, Thompson RC, Sutherland ML, Sutherland JD, Frohlich B, Michalik DE, Zink A, Lombardi GP, Watson L, Cox SL, Finch CE, Miyamoto MI, Sallam SL, Narula J, Thomas GS. Atherosclerosis in ancient and modern Egyptians: the Horus study. Glob Heart. 2014;9(2):197–202.
9. Ma J, Li Y, Ye Q, Li J, Hua Y, Ju D, Zhang D, Cooper R, Chang M. Constituents of red yeast rice, a traditional Chinese food and medicine. J Agric Food Chem. 2000;48(11):5220–5.
10. Hipsley EH. Dietary "fibre" and pregnancy toxaemia. Br Med J. 1953;2(4833):420–2.
11. Duttaroy AK. Nutraceuticals and human blood platelet function: applications in cardiovascular health: Wiley; 2018. p. 183–5.
12. Lippi D. Chocolate and medicine: dangerous liaisons? Nutrition. 2009;25(11–12):1100–3.
13. Basu A, Fu Dong X, Wilkinson M, Simmons B, Wu M, Betts NM, Du M, Lyons TJ. Strawberries decrease atherosclerotic markers in subjects with metabolic syndrome. Nutr Res. 2010;30(7):462–9.
14. Chen PE, Liu CY, Chien WH, Chien CW, Tung TH. Effectiveness of cherries in reducing uric acid and gout: a systematic review. Evid Based Complement Alternat Med. 2019;2019:9896757.
15. Stöver DH. Leben des Ritters Carl von Linné. Hoffmann: Hamburg; 1792. p. 356–7.
16. Galton F. Strawberry cure for gout. Nature. 1899;60:125.
17. Schleifring JH, Galassi FM, Habicht ME, Rühli FJ. Autopsing history: the mummy of Charlemagne (c. 747–814 AD), father of Europe. Econ Hum Biol. 2019;32:11–7.
18. Fornaciari A, Giuffra V, Armocida E, Caramella D, Rühli FJ, Galassi FM. Gout in Duke Federico of Montefeltro (1422–1482): a new pearl of the Italian Renaissance. Clin Exp Rheumatol. 2018;36(1):15–20.
19. Singh JA, Ramachandaran R, Yu S, Yang S, Xie F, Yun H, Zhang J, Curtis JR. Is gout a risk equivalent to diabetes for stroke and myocardial infarction? A retrospective claims database study. Arthritis Res Ther. 2017;19(1):228.
20. Galassi FM, Borghi C. A brief history of uric acid: from gout to cardiovascular risk factor. Eur J Intern Med. 2015;26(5):373.
21. Bhagyalakshmi N, Thimmaraju R, Venkatachalam L, Murthy KN, Sreedhar RV. Nutraceutical applications of garlic and the intervention of biotechnology. Crit Rev Food Sci Nutr. 2005;45(7–8):607–21.
22. Rivlin RS. Historical perspective on the use of garlic. J Nutr. 2001;131(3):951S–4S.
23. Bonaccio M, Iacoviello L, de Gaetano G, Investigators M-S. The Mediterranean diet: the reasons for a success. Thromb Res. 2012;129(3):401–4.
24. Altomare R, Cacciabaudo F, Damiano G, Palumbo VD, Gioviale MC, Bellavia M, Tomasello G, Lo Monte AI. The Mediterranean Diet: A History of Health. Iran J Public Health. 2013;42(5):449–57.

Chapter 3
Nutraceuticals: Scientific and Legal Definitions around the World

Orlando Petrini

Introduction

Nutraceuticals are substances that are food or part of a food and provide health benefits by preventing or treating a disease. The term "nutraceutical" was coined by S. DeFelice in the early 80s [1, 2] and it was quickly adopted by the dietary supplements community. According to DeFelice's definition, nutraceuticals may range from "isolated nutrients, dietary supplements and specific diets to genetically engineered designer foods, herbal products, and processed foods such as cereals, soups and beverages [..] this definition applies to all categories of foods and parts of food, ranging from dietary supplements such as folic acid, used for the prevention of spina bifida, to chicken soup, taken to lessen the discomfort of the common cold. This definition also includes a bioengineered designer vegetable food, rich in antioxidant ingredients, and a stimulant functional food or pharmafood." [2]. Thus, the term nutraceutical refers to a large number of substance classes belonging to categories already subjected to distinct regulations (Table 3.1). This is also one of the reasons why most regulatory authorities do not consider nutraceuticals a well-defined, homogeneous product group with own distinct regulations.

The nutraceutical market is expanding and presently includes functional food (e.g., probiotics, omega-3 fatty acids, ionized salts, branded wheat flour), functional drinks (dairy and non-carbonated drinks, fruit and vegetable juices and drinks, herbal teas, sports and energy drinks), dietary supplements (proteins and peptides, vitamins, minerals), herbals (including algae, fungi and phytochemicals), fatty acids and fiber, as well as some specific personal care products. The global nutraceutical

O. Petrini (✉)
POLE Pharma Consulting, Breganzona, Switzerland

Laboratory of Applied Microbiology, Department of Environment, Constructions and Design, University of Applied Sciences of Southern Switzerland – SUPSI, Bellinzona, Switzerland
e-mail: orlando@poleconsult.com

© Springer Nature Switzerland AG 2021
A. F.G. Cicero, M. Rizzo (eds.), *Nutraceuticals and Cardiovascular Disease*, Contemporary Cardiology, https://doi.org/10.1007/978-3-030-62632-7_3

Table 3.1 Categories of nutraceuticals

Food supplement (Dietary supplement)	A product used to supplement the normal diet and aiming at enhancing health. It may contain vitamins, minerals, amino acids and be administered single or combined in dosed formulations, such as capsules, tablets, pills, sachets of powder, ampoules of liquids, drop dispensing bottles or other pharmaceutical formulations [3, 4].
Functional food[a]	A food or ingredient with a nutritive value and additionally a positive impact on health, physical performance or state of mind [5–7]
Botanicals (Herbals, phytochemicals)[b]	Preparations derived from plants, algae, fungi or lichens. Examples include hawthorn (*Crataegus*), garlic (*Allium*), St. John's Wort (*Hypericum*) or ginseng (*Panax ginseng*).
Superfoods, Ultraceuticals	A purely marketing term for food (mostly botanicals but some fish and dairy products are also included) purportedly conferring health benefits resulting from an exceptional nutrient content. These terms should be avoided as they do not carry any scientific meaning.

[a]In some countries included in the food supplement category
[b]no regulatory status in most countries

market has increased exponentially in value in the last decade and it is expected to reach $302,300 million by 2022, up from $184,092 million in 2015, with a compound annual growth rate of approximately 7% [8].

DeFelice [2] subdivided nutraceuticals in "potential nutraceuticals", i.e. substances that may potentially provide a particular health or benefit, and "established nutraceuticals", for which sufficient clinical data are available to support a health claim. Health claims are at the core of most marketing activities, but they need to be substantiated by sound scientific research and clinical studies to be authorized by regulatory authorities. This has spurred both academy and industry to start research efforts aiming at proving the efficacy of specific nutraceuticals and to obtain suitable health claims. Thus, after 1990 the number of publications reporting research on nutraceutical products has increased exponentially, as reflected also by a search in PubMed using (in different combinations) the search strings "dietary supplement", "nutraceuticals", "cardiovascular", and "heart". For instance, more than 4000 articles published in 2018 were devoted to nutraceuticals in general, and approximately 350 of them referred to cardiovascular topics (Fig. 3.1). Within this last group, however, only less than one third (104) reported results from clinical trials, regardless of study design and quality.

There is general consensus on the importance of a balanced diet to promote health, but disagreement on the use of supplementation in the general population [9]. Even the usefulness of well-established supplements such as vitamin C, vitamin D and minerals for people in healthy conditions is controversial [10–13] and some authors have even questioned the utility of multivitamin and mineral supplementation to reduce the risk of chronic and acute diseases [14, 15]. The contradictory and often inconsistent findings in clinical trials, systematic reviews and meta-analyses do not help regulatory bodies to take informed and evidence-based decisions and add to the already confused regulatory status of nutraceutical products.

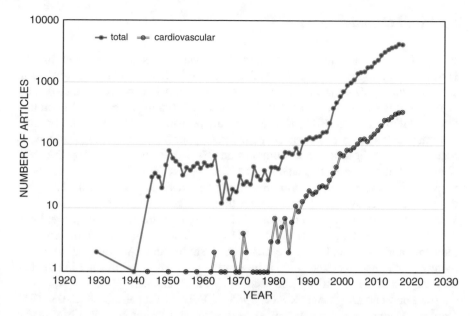

Fig. 3.1 Number of publications referring to nutraceuticals, 1930–2018

The scope of this chapter is to briefly review the regulatory status of nutraceuticals in selected countries. It does not attempt to address details related to marketing applications in specific countries, but to provide a general framework to understand current regulations of nutraceuticals, with a focus on USA and Canada, Europe, Australia and New Zealand, and Japan.

Regulatory Situation

The perceived toxicity of some pharmaceuticals as well as their costs are two of the main factors driving a fundamental shift from pharmaceutical products towards the use of dietary supplements and functional foods. While the amount of marketed dietary supplement products is very large, the acceptance of nutraceuticals by regulatory authorities depends on the scientific support provided for the efficacy and safety claims that companies or academic researchers are requesting for their products. These aspects are addressed in most countries by policies that regulate their marketing applications, with regulatory bodies expecting health claims to be supported by extensive research and appropriate quality controls to ensure human safety, and to adhere to the health food standards set by the Rome-based Codex Alimentarius [16], jointly established by the Food and Agriculture Organization (FAO) and the World Health Organization (WHO), which has become a reference and a unique opportunity to harmonize food standards and trade globally.

USA and Canada

In the U.S., dietary supplements and functional foods are regulated by the U.S. Dietary Supplement Health and Education Act (DSHEA) [17] established in 1994. Under this Act, the manufacturer is solely responsible to ensure that a dietary supplement is safe before putting it on the market. It is then the federal Food and Drug Administration's (FDA) task to monitor post-marketing safety and product information (labeling, claims, package insert, supporting literature). Advertising is regulated by the Federal Trade Commission (FTC) [18] and labeling by the 1990 Nutrition Labeling and Education Act (NLEA) that in the meantime has been repeatedly amended [19]. No prior government approval is needed for the label, but the label must carry a disclaimer stating that the claim has not been reviewed by FDA, and that the product is not intended to diagnose, treat, cure, or prevent any disease. It is important to note that the FDA's guidance documents on dietary supplements and functional food are not legally enforceable. A modification of the dietary supplement labeling guide is presently under consideration, aiming to clarify the types of claims that may be used under the DSHA Act.

The Food and Drugs Act (R.S.C., 1985, c. F-27, last amended on 23-05-2018) regulates Dietary Supplements, called Natural Health Products (NHP) in Canada. The NHP Regulation came into effect in 2004 and defines NHP as products containing vitamins and minerals, herbal remedies, homeopathic medicines, traditional medicines such as traditional Chinese medicines (TCM) products, probiotics, and other products like amino acids and essential fatty acids [20]. NHPs must be safe to use and can be sold as over-the-counter (OTC) products. Although Canada and the U.S. have fundamentally similar regulations, there is no mutual recognition agreement (MRA) between the two countries to facilitate trade. Barriers to MRA are set by the different regulatory regimes in the two countries, some of the Canada's NHPs being classified as dietary substances and others as OTC or homeopathic medicines in the U.S.

Europe

Risk management is the overarching principle of the dietary supplement regulation also in the EU [21, 22]. In Europe, nutraceuticals are regulated by the EU Directive 2002/46/EC [3]. As in the US and Canada, the main thrust of the regulations governing dietary supplements and functional food is consumer safety. This aspect is under the control of the European Food Safety Authority (EFSA), funded in 2002 by the EU with the mandate to be a source for scientific advice and assessment of risks linked with the food chain [23]. EFSA has to answer requests for scientific advice from the European Commission, the European Parliament and the EU Member States (MS).

Health claims substantiation must be provided but there is no separate regulatory framework for nutraceuticals or functional foods in the EU food laws. Nutrition or health claims are subjected to a pre-marketing approval set out in Regulation

1924/2006 [24], which covers the labeling as well as presentation and advertising of foodstuffs. The Regulation (EU) 2015/2283 [25], which replaced regulation EC 258/97 on novel foods [26], lays down the authorization procedure required for foods or food ingredients that are novel in the diet of EU consumers. Novel foods may be included in the Union list if the food does not pose a safety risk to human health, its intended use does not mislead the consumer, especially when the food is intended to replace another food and there is a significant change in the nutritional value, and, where the food is intended to replace another food, it does not differ from that food in such a way that its normal consumption would be nutritionally disadvantageous for the consumer (EU 2015/2283, Art. 7). Basically, the food regulations are counterparts of the governing drug regulations, with categories that are similar to those applied to prescription and OTC drugs as well as herbal medicinal products (HMP).

The EU legislation has also established a legal framework (Regulation (EU) No 609/2013) for a category of products defined as "Foods for Special Medical Purposes", specially processed or formulated and intended for the dietary management of patients, including infants, and to be used under medical supervision [27]. This law has replaced Directive 2009/39/EC [28], which regulated infant formulae, baby foods, foods for weight reduction, and food for special medical purposes.

A difference exists in the regulatory classification of botanicals in the EU as opposed to other countries, notably the U.S. and Canada. In the U.S. and Canada botanicals are classified as dietary supplements, although the FDA foresees the possibility to apply for the medical use of botanicals if an acceptable clinical development can be presented to substantiate a proposed indication. In the EU some botanicals (exclusively traditional herbal medicinal plants according to Directive 2004/24/EC, [29]) can be included in food supplements for nutritional or physiological purposes. The medical use of botanicals is regulated in the EU by Directives 2001/83/EC (well-established herbal medicinal products) [30] and 2004/24/EC (traditional herbal medicinal products), but national regulations still differ considerably. Theoretically, products lawfully marketed in a MS could be sold in other MS with no additional regulatory hurdles, but practically several MS have separate marketing authorization procedures in place and the MS have the competence to decide case by case whether or not a given botanical should be considered a HMP. In general, a botanical claimed to have therapeutic or preventive effects cannot be marketed as a food supplement, but registration of a botanical species as medicinal product does not preclude authorization of the same species (at different concentrations or in specific galenical forms) as a food supplement.

Australia and New Zealand

Since 2003, Australia and New Zealand have established a single, bi-national agency to regulate therapeutic products, including medical devices, prescription, over-the-counter and complementary medicines, replacing the Australian Therapeutic Goods Act and the New Zealand Medsafe. In Australia and New

Zealand, dietary supplement (referred to as "complementary medicines") are regulated by the Australia New Zealand Food Standards Code (Schedule 4 – Nutrition, health and related claims, [31]), under the scope of the Therapeutic Goods Act 1989; the code sets the conditions for nutrition content claims (S4–3), for permitted high level health claims (S4–4), as well as for general level health claims (S4–5). The Australian Government provides useful details on complementary medicines in a dedicated web page [32]. While medicinal products are regulated at the federal level, complementary medicines, i.e. dietary supplements and foods with health claims, are regulated at the state level. In New Zealand, dietary supplements are also regulated by the Natural Health and Supplementary Products Bill [33].

Japan

Japan has no clear definition of dietary supplements [34], but "Food with Health Claims" are an integral part of the Japanese system for health foods. They can be divided in two categories, i.e. "Food with Nutrient Function Claims" (FNFC) for vitamins and minerals and "Food for Specified Health Uses" (FoSHU) for other products. The first FoSHUs included hypoallergenic rice and low phosphorous milk [35], but these were later transferred to a different category ("food for illness"). In the meantime, more than 1000 FoSHU products are on the Japanese market and include foods for which health claims are allowed [35]. Probiotics (mainly *Lactobacillus* spp. and *Bifidobacterium* spp.) have a special place among FoSHU: some of them are routinely used in hospitals to treat gastrointestinal disorders and as such they are considered medicines; as food they are not subjected to any restriction but efficacy claims are not allowed on the labeling [36].

FoSHU approval is a complex process, and evidence-based data on efficacy and safety need to be provided for the product to be allowed health claims on the label [37]. In 2015 a new category ("food with function claims") was introduced in the hope to ease the strict FoSHU rules. The regulations for this category only require bibliographic references to support the product's effects, and production under strict quality control systems. No government approval is needed for the label: this is almost identical with the requirements for structure-function claims on dietary supplements in the U.S.

Other Countries

In Brazil, the health authority institute ANVISA (Agência Nacional de Vigilância Sanitaria) regulates the market authorization of dietary supplements, which include novel foods and novel ingredients, food with functional or health properties claims, food for infants and young children, and other categories less relevant to the scope of this review [38].

In China, health food (further divided into nutrition supplement and functional health food) is defined as having specific health functions or being intended to supply vitamins and (or) minerals. Health food may target specific populations but may not be used to cure or prevent disease [39, 40].

India contemplates nutraceuticals, along with food or health supplements, foods for special dietary uses, foods for special medical purpose, functional foods and novel food in its food safety and standards regulation of 2016 [41]. Brazil, China, and India foresee the use of health claims in their regulations.

Dietary supplements ("Biologically Active Supplements": BAS) need to be registered before being marketed in Russia. The major BAS categories aim at immune system enhancement, improving overall health and preventing disease. According to Art. 24 (TP TC 021/2011) of the Technical Regulations "About Safety of Foods", BASs may include mono- and polysaturated acids, minerals, some amino acids as well as mono and disaccharides, fibers, some microorganisms, vitamins, and also probiotic microorganisms intended for consumption with food or inclusion in products aiming at enriching the diet.

A complete review of dietary supplement regulations in several other countries is presented by Malla [42]. Detailed chapters on dietary supplement regulations world-wide are also included in Bagchi [21], but regulations are evolving rather quickly and the information presented in these reviews is likely to be superseded quite rapidly.

Nutrition and Health Claims

In the EU, nutrition and health claims are regulated by Regulation (EC) No 1924/2006 of the European Parliament and of the Council of 20 December 2006 on nutrition and health claims made on foods [43]. The EU definitions are similar to, albeit not identical with those used in other countries and for the sake of this review they can be safely used to characterize nutrition and health-related labeling claims for dietary supplements and functional foods world-wide.

In the EU, a nutrition claim is used to describe particular nutritional properties due to the energy provided by the food or the supplement as well as the beneficial properties due to the food or supplement content; in this respect, the U.S. authorities presently require more detailed information than the EU [44].

A health claim suggests or implies a relationship between a given product/substance and health, whilst a reduction of disease risk claim implies a significant reduction of a risk factor in the development of a specific disease. A special category is represented by structure/function claims, which describe how a nutrient affects the normal structure or the function in the body.

The EU and U.S., but also other regulatory authorities, require sound scientific data to support the claims made, as a decision-making aid to the consumers and physicians [45]. EFSA has provided a scientific guidance on health claim applications, with detailed information on the documentation to be submitted to

Table 3.2 Levels of clinical and scientific evidence

Level	Type of Evidence
Ia	Meta-analysis of randomized controlled trials
Ib	At least one randomised controlled trial
IIa	At least one well-designed controlled study without randomization
IIb	At least one other type of well-designed quasi-experimental study
III	Well-designed non experimental descriptive studies, such as comparative studies, correlation studies, case-control studies
IV	Expert committee reports or opinions and/or clinical experiences of respected authorities

Adapted from Atkins et al. [47] and U.S. Agency for Health Care Policy and Research [48]

substantiate them [46]. Overall, authorities in the EU, the US and, perhaps to a lesser extent in other countries, require a high standard of evidence that often corresponds to the highest evidence levels proposed by the U.S. Agency for Health Care Policy and Research (AHCPR, now US Agency for Healthcare Research and Quality) (Table 3.2).

In fact, out of 2337 total entries present in the EU Register of nutrition and health claims made on foods [49], only 261 have been accepted and for 6 protection of proprietary data has been granted.

There is no doubt that studies with nutraceuticals and botanicals need to adhere to the highest possible standards and this has been pointed out elsewhere [50–52]. However, the inherent problems linked to testing products that may be already present, albeit in small amounts, in the human body, as well as the need to use surrogate endpoints especially when preventive effects are tested, should not be underestimated and taken into consideration in the evaluation of health claims applications. An approach that is scientifically rigorous and appropriate for drug products may be too stringent for nutraceuticals and eventually even confusing to consumers. Hasler [45] pointed out that "the road to health claim approval is lengthy, expensive, and, as recent evidence would suggest, not particularly useful. The FDA requires an overwhelming body of evidence for a significant scientific agreement, unqualified health claim, and qualified health claims with less evidence are very wordy and confusing to consumers". In the same publication she proposes a scientific ranking and wording that closely resembles that recommended by the European Medicines Agency (EMA) Committee on Herbal Medicinal Product (HMPC) for the preparation of EU Herbal monographs [53] and that could be a useful means of evaluating health claims for nutraceuticals as well.

Nutraceuticals and Cardiovascular Diseases: A Regulatory Overview

Research has shown that several nutraceuticals are endowed with potentially useful cardiovascular effects. In a recent review, a large number of nutraceuticals has been shown to have clinically detectable blood pressure-lowering effects [54], and the lipid-lowering action of soluble fibers, phytosterols, soy proteins, omega 3 polyunsaturated fatty acids, red rice, policosanols, berberine and garlic extracts has also been demonstrated [55]. The HMPC has included *Crataegus* spp. among the traditional herbal medicinal products used to relieve symptoms of temporary nervous cardiac complaints [55], and several chapters in this book deal with the positive effects of nutraceuticals on dyslipidemia management, hypertension, heart function, and other dysfunctions directly or indirectly linked to cardiovascular functions. Overall, the efficacy of nutraceuticals in preventing or having therapeutic effects on cardiovascular diseases seems established.

So far, however, EFSA has authorized 5 health claims (homocysteine metabolism, blood cholesterol levels, blood pressure control, endothelium-dependent vasodilation, and cardiac function) in the cardiovascular field for only 26 different nutrient substances, food, or food categories (Table 3.3) and one wonders why several of the substances with positive scientific reviews [54–60] have not been included in the EU Register. Reasons put forward by the Regulators include the lack of multicenter, randomized clinical trials that study the long-term efficacy of the products on large at risk populations using morbidity and mortality as endpoints, the acknowledged lack of studies on special populations such as children, the elderly, patients with impaired liver or renal functions, as well as high-risk and polymedicated patients, or the absence of long-term safety data and crucial safety aspects that have often been neglected in the studies so far published.

Table 3.3 Authorized health claims for cardiovascular protection. Conditions and restrictions of use of the claim can be looked up in the EU Register on nutrition and health claims

Claim type	Substance	Claim	Health relationship	Reference*
Homocysteine metabolism				
Art.13(1)	Betaine	Contributes to normal homocysteine metabolism	Contribution to normal homocysteine metabolism	2011;9(4):2052
Art.13(1)	Choline	Contributes to normal homocysteine metabolism	Contribution to normal homocysteine metabolism	2011;9(4):2056
Art.13(1)	Folate	Contributes to normal homocysteine metabolism	Homocysteine metabolism	2009;7(9):1213
Art.13(1)	Vitamin B6	Contributes to normal homocysteine metabolism	Contribution to normal homocysteine metabolism	2010;8(10):1759
Blood cholesterol levels				
Art.13(1)	Alpha-linolenic acid (ALA)	Contributes to the maintenance of normal blood cholesterol levels	Maintenance of normal blood cholesterol concentrations	2009;7(9):1252

(continued)

Table 3.3 (continued)

Claim type	Substance	Claim	Health relationship	Reference*
Art.13(1)	Beta-glucans	Contributes to the maintenance of normal blood cholesterol levels	Maintenance of normal blood cholesterol concentrations	2009;7(9):1254
Art.13(1)	Chitosan	Contributes to the maintenance of normal blood cholesterol levels	Maintenance of normal blood LDL-cholesterol concentrations	2011;9(6):2214
Art.13(1)	Glucomannan (konjac mannan)	Contributes to the maintenance of normal blood cholesterol levels	Maintenance of normal blood cholesterol concentrations	2009;7(9):1258
Art.13(1)	Guar gum	Contributes to the maintenance of normal blood cholesterol levels	Maintenance of normal blood cholesterol concentrations	2010;8(2):1464
Art.13(1)	Hydroxypropyl methylcellulose (HPMC)	Contributes to the maintenance of normal blood cholesterol levels	Maintenance of normal blood cholesterol concentrations	2010;8(10):1739
Art.13(1)	Linoleic acid	Contributes to the maintenance of normal blood cholesterol levels	Maintenance of normal blood cholesterol concentrations	2009;7(9):1276
Art.13(1)	*Monascus purpureus* (red yeast rice: Monacolin K)	Contributes to the maintenance of normal blood cholesterol levels	Maintenance of normal blood LDL-cholesterol concentrations	2011;9(7):2304
Art.13(1)	Pectin	Contributes to the maintenance of normal blood cholesterol levels	Maintenance of normal blood cholesterol concentrations	2010;8(10):1747
Art.14(1) (a)	Barley beta-glucans	Barley beta-glucans has been shown to lower/reduce blood cholesterol. high cholesterol is a risk factor in the development of coronary heart disease		Q-2011-00799
Art.14(1) (a)	Oat beta-glucan	Oat beta-glucan has been shown to lower/reduce blood cholesterol. high cholesterol is a risk factor in the development of coronary heart disease		Q-2008-681

Table 3.3 (continued)

Claim type	Substance	Claim	Health relationship	Reference*
Art.14(1) (a)	Plant sterols/plant stanol esters	Plant sterols and plant stanol esters have been shown to lower/reduce blood cholesterol. high cholesterol is a risk factor in the development of coronary heart disease.		Q-2008-118; Q-2008-779
Art.14(1) (a)	Plant sterols: Sterols extracted from plants, free or esterified with food grade fatty acids.	Plant sterols have been shown to lower/reduce blood cholesterol. high cholesterol is a risk factor in the development of coronary heart disease.		Q-2008-085
Art.13(1)	Foods with a low or reduced content of saturated fatty acids	Reducing consumption of saturated fat contributes to the maintenance of normal blood cholesterol levels	Maintenance of normal blood LDL-cholesterol concentrations	2011;9(4):2062
Art.13(1)	Oleic acid	Replacing saturated fats in the diet with unsaturated fats contributes to the maintenance of normal blood cholesterol levels. Oleic acid is an unsaturated fat.	Maintenance of normal blood LDL-cholesterol concentrations	2011;9(4):2043
Art.13(1)	Monounsaturated and/or polyunsaturated fatty acids	Replacing saturated fats with unsaturated fats in the diet contributes to the maintenance of normal blood cholesterol levels [MUFA and PUFA are unsaturated fats]	Replacement of mixtures of saturated fatty acids (SFAs) as present in foods or diets with mixtures of polyunsaturated fatty acids (PUFAs) and maintenance of normal blood LDL-cholesterol concentrations	2011;9(4):2069
Art.14(1) (a)	Monounsaturated and/or polyunsaturated fatty acids	Replacing saturated fats with unsaturated fats in the diet has been shown to lower/reduce blood cholesterol. high cholesterol is a risk factor in the development of coronary heart disease		Q-2009-00458

(continued)

Table 3.3 (continued)

Claim type	Substance	Claim	Health relationship	Reference*
Blood pressure control				
Art.13(1)	Foods with a low or reduced content of sodium	Reducing consumption of sodium contributes to the maintenance of normal blood pressure	Maintenance of normal blood pressure	2011;9(6):2237
Art.13(1)	Docosahexaenoic acid and eicosapentaenoic acid (DHA/EPA)	Contributes to the maintenance of normal blood pressure	Maintenance of normal blood pressure	2009; 7(9); 1263
Art.13(1)	Potassium	Contributes to the maintenance of normal blood pressure	Blood pressure	2010;8(2):1469
Others				
Art.13(1)	Walnuts	Contributes to the improvement of the elasticity of blood vessels	Improvement of endothelium-dependent vasodilation	2011;9(4):2074
Art.13(1)	Thiamine	Contributes to the normal function of the heart	Cardiac function	2009;7(9):1222

* EFSA Journal citation

Conclusions

The nutraceuticals market is expanding very rapidly, with consumers increasingly convinced of the utility of nutraceuticals to prevent diseases or improve health conditions. While many nutraceuticals have been proven safe and effective in preclinical and clinical trials, there is still a plethora of products on the market with unsubstantiated claims. Rightfully, this has led health authorities around the world to enforce regulatory constraints to check efficacy and safety claims, which must be supported by extensive preclinical and clinical research and rigorous quality control programs. Europe, the U.S., Canada, Australia/New Zealand, and Japan have been at the forefront of the initiative aiming at introducing strict controls and checks on permissible health claims. World-wide, this initiative has been widely accepted and many other countries have introduced legislations aiming at regulating the introduction of nutraceuticals on the market. Presently, however, there is often a perceived gap between the efficacy and safety evaluations provided by scientists and those resulting from the application of the existing guidelines. Thus, there is a need for scientists and regulators to agree on a common set of rules to be applied while evaluating health claims and efficacy data, in particular with regards to the choice of patient populations and study designs, objectives and endpoints, sample size, and handling of confounding factors [51]. There are also other issues linked to the data collection, such as the product composition standardization, the choice of surrogate endpoints, the use of adequately powered sample sizes, the limited generalizability of some outcomes, as well as the sometimes limited believability of industry-sponsored research [52]. A continuous dialogue between science, business and regulatory bodies will have positive effects on the development and marketing of nutraceuticals that will benefit at the same time health authorities, manufacturers and consumers.

References

1. Baker, S. An interview with Dr. Stephen DeFelice. https://www.nutraceuticalsworld.com/contents/view_health-e-insights/2011-10-28/an-interview-with-dr-stephen-defelice. Last accessed: 7 June 2019.
2. DeFelice SL. The nutraceutical revolution: its impact on food industry R&D. Trends Food Sci Technol. 1995;6:59–61.
3. European Commission. Directive 2002/46/EC of the European Parliament and of the Council of 10 June 2002 on the approximation of the laws of the Member States relating to food supplements. https://eur-lex.europa.eu/legal-content/EN/TXT/PDF/?uri=CELEX:32002L0046&from=EN. Last accessed: 7 June 2019.
4. U.S. Food and Drug Administration. Dietary Supplement Health and Education Act of 1994, Public Law 103–417, 103rd Congress. https://ods.od.nih.gov/About/DSHEA_Wording.aspx. Last accessed: 7 June 2019.
5. European Commission Concerted Action on Functional Food Science in Europe (FUFOSE). Scientific concepts of functional foods in Europe: consensus document. Br J Nutr. 1999;81:s1–s27.
6. Hardy G. Nutraceuticals and functional foods: introduction and meaning. Nutrition. 2000;16:688–9.
7. Roberfroid MB. A European consensus of scientific concepts of functional foods. Nutrition. 2000;16:689–91.
8. Prasad, E. Nutraceutical market by type – global opportunity analysis and industry forecast 2014–2022. https://www.alliedmarketresearch.com/nutraceuticals-market. Last accessed: 7 June 2019.
9. Aronson JK. Defining 'nutraceuticals': neither nutritious nor pharmaceutical. Br J Clin Pharmacol. 2017 Jan;83:8–19.
10. Ashor AW, Siervo M, Lara J, Oggioni C, Afshar S, Mathers JC. Effect of vitamin C and vitamin E supplementation on endothelial function: a systematic review and meta-analysis of randomised controlled trials. Br J Nutr. 2015 Apr 28;113:1182–94.
11. Ashor AW, Brown R, Keenan PD, Willis ND, Siervo M, Mathers JC. Limited evidence for a beneficial effect of vitamin C supplementation on biomarkers of cardiovascular diseases: an umbrella review of systematic reviews and meta-analyses. Nutr Res. 2019;01(61):1–12.
12. Autier P, Mullie P, Macacu A, et al. Effect of vitamin D supplementation on non-skeletal disorders: a systematic review of meta-analyses and randomised trials. Lancet Diabetes Endocrinol. 2017;5(12):986–1004.
13. Bajnok L. Vitamin D and calcium in the mirror of clinical evidence. Orv Hetil. 2016 Jul;157:1242–7.
14. Angelo G, Drake VJ, Frei B. Efficacy of multivitamin/mineral supplementation to reduce chronic disease risk: a critical review of the evidence from observational studies and randomized controlled trials. Crit Rev Food Sci Nutr. 2015;55:1968–91.
15. Takagi H, Umemoto T, Alice A LIOCEG. Vitamins and abdominal aortic aneurysm. Int Angiol. 2017 Feb;36:21–30.

16. Food and Agriculture Organization. Codex Alimentarius. http://www.fao.org/3/y7867e/y7867e01.htm. Last accessed: 17 June 2019.

17. U.S. Food and Drug Administration. Dietary supplements guidance documents & regulatory information. https://www.fda.gov/food/guidance-documents-regulatory-information-topic-food-and-dietary-supplements/dietary-supplements-guidance-documents-regulatory-information. Last accessed: 7 June 2019.

18. Federal Trade Commission. Frequently Asked Questions (FAQ). https://ods.od.nih.gov/Health_Information/ODS_Frequently_Asked_Questions.aspx. Last accessed: 17 June 2019.

19. U.S. Food and Drug Administration. Dietary supplement labeling guide. https://www.fda.gov/food/dietary-supplements-guidance-documents-regulatory-information/dietary-supplement-labeling-guide. Last accessed: 17 June 2019.

20. Government of Canada. Natural health products. https://www.canada.ca/en/health-canada/services/drugs-health-products/natural-non-prescription.html. Last accessed: 17 June 2019.

21. Bagchi D. Nutraceutical and functional food regulations in the United States and around the world: Academic Press; 2014. p. 592.

22. Coppens P, da Silva MF, Pettman S. European regulations on nutraceuticals, dietary supplements and functional foods: a framework based on safety. Toxicology. 2006 Apr 3;221:59–74.

23. European Food Safety Authority. About EFSA. https://www.efsa.europa.eu/en/aboutefsa. Last accessed: 17 June 2019.

24. European Commission. Regulation (EC) No 1924/2006 of the European Parliament and of the Council of 20 December 2006 on nutrition and health claims made on foods. https://eur-lex.europa.eu/legal-content/en/ALL/?uri=CELEX%3A32006R1924. Last accessed: 17 June 2019.

25. European Commission. Regulation (EU) 2015/2283 of the European Parliament and of the Council of 25 November 2015 on novel foods, amending Regulation (EU) No 1169/2011 of the European Parliament and of the Council and repealing Regulation (EC) No 258/97 of the European Parliament and of the Council and Commission Regulation (EC) No 1852/2001 (Text with EEA relevance). https://eur-lex.europa.eu/legal-content/en/TXT/?uri=CELEX:32015R2283. Last accessed: 17 June 2019.

26. European Commission. Regulation (EC) No 258/97 of the European Parliament and of the Council of 27 January 1997 concerning novel foods and novel food ingredients. https://eur-lex.europa.eu/legal-content/EN/TXT/?uri=CELEX:31997R0258. Last accessed: 17 June 2019.

27. European Commission. Regulation (EU) No 609/2013 of the European Parliament and of the Council of 12 June 2013 on food intended for infants and young children, food for special medical purposes, and total diet replacement for weight control and repealing Council Directive 92/52/EEC, Commission Directives 96/8/EC, 1999/21/EC, 2006/125/EC and 2006/141/EC, Directive 2009/39/EC of the European Parliament and of the Council and Commission Regulations (EC) No 41/2009 and (EC) No 953/2009 Text with EEA relevance. https://eur-lex.europa.eu/legal-content/en/TXT/?uri=CELEX:32013R0609. Last accessed: 17 June 2019.

28. European Commission. Directive 2009/39/EC of the European Parliament and of the Council of 6 May 2009 on foodstuffs intended for particular nutritional uses (recast) (Text with EEA relevance). https://eur-lex.europa.eu/legal-content/en/TXT/?uri=CELEX:32009L0039. Last accessed: 17 June 2019.

29. European Commission. Directive 2004/24/EC of the European Parliament and of the Council of 31 March 2004 amending, as regards traditional herbal medicinal products, Directive 2001/83/EC on the Community code relating to medicinal products for human use. 2004.

30. European Commission. Directive 2001/83/EC of the European Parliament and of the Council of 6 November 2001 on the Community code relating to medicinal products for human use. 2001.

31. Federal Register of Legislation, Australian Government. Australia New Zealand Food Standards Code – Schedule 4 – Nutrition, health and related claims. https://www.legislation.gov.au/Details/F2017C00711. Last accessed: 7 June 2019.

32. Department of Health, Australian Government. Complementary medicine interface issues. https://www.tga.gov.au/complementary-medicine-interface-issues. Last accessed: 17 June 2019.
33. Parliamentary Counsel Office. Natural health and supplementary products bill. http://www.legislation.govt.nz/bill/government/2011/0324/latest/DLM3984610.html. Last accessed: 17 June 2019.
34. Chiba T, Sato Y, Kobayashi E, Ide K, Yamada H, Umegaki K. Behaviors of consumers, physicians and pharmacists in response to adverse events associated with dietary supplement use. Nutr J. 2017;16:18.
35. Shimizu M. History and current status of functional food regulations in Japan. Academic Press. 2014:592.
36. Amagase H. Current marketplace for probiotics: a Japanese perspective. Clin Infect Dis. 2008 Feb 1;46(Suppl 2):S73–5. discussion S144.
37. Consumer Affairs Agency. Food labelling. https://www.caa.go.jp/en/policy/food_labeling/. Last accessed: 17 June 2019.
38. Agency BHR. Food. http://portal.anvisa.gov.br/food. Last accessed: 17 June 2019.
39. Chemical Inspection and Regulation Service. China health food registration and filing. http://www.cirs-reach.com/news-and-articles/health-food-registration-and-filing.html. Last accessed: 18 June 2019.
40. Chemical Inspection and Regulation Service (CIRS). Interpretation on China health food registration application service guideline. http://www.cirs-reach.com/news-and-articles/requirement-for-china-health-food-registration-dossier.html. Last accessed: 07 June 2019.
41. Ministry of Health and Family Welfare, Government of India. Food safety and standards (Food or health supplements, nutraceuticals, foods for special dietary uses, foods for special medical purpose, functional foods and novel food) regulations, 2016. https://archive.fssai.gov.in/home/fss-legislation/fss-regulations.html. Last accessed: 18 June 2019.
42. Malla S, Hobbs JE, Kofi Sogah E. Functional foods and natural health products regulations In Canada and around the world: a summary. 2013. p. 132.
43. European Commission. Regulation (EC) No 1924/2006 of the European Parliament and of the Council of 20 December 2006 on nutrition and health claims made on foods. https://eur-lex.europa.eu/legal-content/EN/TXT/HTML/?uri=CELEX:32006R1924&from=en. Last accessed: 18 June 2019.
44. Agarwal S, Hordvik S, Morar S. Nutrition and health-related labeling claims for functional foods and dietary supplements in the United States. In: Bagchi D, editor. Nutraceutical and functional food regulations in the United States and around the world: Academic Press; 2014. p. 592.
45. Hasler CM. Health claims in the United States: an aid to the public or a source of confusion. J Nutr. 2008 Jun;138:1216S–20S.
46. European Food Safety Authority. General scientific guidance for stakeholders on health claim applications. EFSA J. 14:4367.
47. Atkins D, Best D, Briss PA, et al. Grading quality of evidence and strength of recommendations. BMJ. 2004;328:1490–2004.
48. Agency for Health Care Policy and Research. Acute pain management: operative or medical procedures and trauma. Rockville, MD: 1993:107.
49. European Commission. EU Register of nutrition and health claims made on foods. http://cc.europa.eu/food/safety/labelling_nutrition/claims/register/public/?event=register.home&CFID=15635509&CFTOKEN=e8ea0c8bfacf40b4-CAA913C9-DE97-0553-CBB-B436489A15B60. Last accessed: 17 June 2019.
50. Petrini O, Prasad C, Cicero AFG. Clinical studies with botanicals and how to carry them out: the European Union perspective. Curr Top Nutraceutical Res. 2017;15:57–62.
51. Cicero AFG, Petrini O, Prasad C. Clinical studies with nutraceuticals and how to carry them out. Curr Top Nutraceutical Res. 2017;15:63–6.

52. Prasad C, Cicero AFG, Petrini O. Planning meaningful clinical trials with botanicals and nutraceuticals: need for a cross-talk between science, business and the regulatory demand. Curr Top Nutraceutical Res. 2017;15:49–56.
53. HMPC. Guideline on the assessment of clinical safety and efficacy in the preparation of community herbal monographs for well-established and of community herbal monographs/entries to the community list for traditional herbal medicinal products/substances/preparations. EMEA/HMPC/104613/2005. 7 September 2006.
54. Borghi C, Cicero AF. Nutraceuticals with a clinically detectable blood pressure-lowering effect: a review of available randomized clinical trials and their meta-analyses. Br J Clin Pharmacol. 2017 Jan;83:163–71.
55. Cicero AF, Ferroni A, Ertek S. Tolerability and safety of commonly used dietary supplements and nutraceuticals with lipid-lowering effects. Expert Opin Drug Saf. 2012;11:753–66.
56. Chiesa G, Busnelli M, Manzini S, Parolini C. Nutraceuticals and bioactive components from fish for dyslipidemia and cardiovascular risk reduction. Mar Drugs. 2016 Jun; 08:14.
57. Cicero AF, Colletti A. Nutraceuticals and blood pressure control: results from clinical trials and meta-analyses. High Blood Press Cardiovasc Prev. 2015 Sep;22:203–13.
58. Cicero AF, Colletti A. Combinations of phytomedicines with different lipid lowering activity for dyslipidemia management: the available clinical data. Phytomedicine. 2016 Oct 15;23:1113–8.
59. Micucci M, Malaguti M, Toschi TG, et al. Cardiac and vascular synergic protective effect of Olea europea L. leaves and *Hibiscus sabdariffa* L. flower extracts. Oxidative Med Cell Longev. 2015;2015:318125.
60. Sanidas E, Grassos C. The role of nutraceuticals in the treatment of primary dyslipidemia. [letter]. Hell J Cardiol. 2018 Aug 07;

Chapter 4
Dietary Patterns and Cardiovascular Disease Risk: From Epidemiology to Intervention Study

Laura García Molina

Cardiovascular diseases are the leading cause of death in industrialized countries. For this reason, primary prevention of cardiovascular disease is one of the main objectives of public health worldwide. Nowadays, there is scientific evidence to ensure that by modifying five factors, the risk of cardiovascular disease can be reduced by more than 80% [62]. The five factors include:

- No Smoking
- BMI <25 kg/m^2
- Frequent physical activity
- Moderate alcohol consumption
- Healthy diet

Three of the five risk factors can be controlled by dietary changes and all the factors involve a lifestyle modification. A healthy and balanced diet with low-alcohol consumption will most likely result in a BMI below 25 kg/m^2. In addition, the prevention of chronic noncommunicable diseases, such as diabetes, can be achieved by 91% with lifestyle intervention, where diet plays an important and fundamental role [21].

Throughout history, nutrition has been interpreted by various approaches to improve health. Recently, the aim of nutritional epidemiology focused on the effect of a specific nutrient from food and its direct relationship with public health. However, nutrition is a multidimensional discipline, where individual nutrients are not consumed, but rather immersed in typical meals like a lunch, dinner or breakfast that includes a multitude of nutrients consumed in a short period of time [5, 32, 49, 60]. In fact, it is quite complicated to analyse the individual effect of a nutrient without considering the other components. Generally, we consume a combination

L. G. Molina (✉)
Department of Preventive Medicine and Public Health, University of Granada, Granada, Spain
e-mail: lgarmol@ugr.es

© Springer Nature Switzerland AG 2021
A. F.G. Cicero, M. Rizzo (eds.), *Nutraceuticals and Cardiovascular Disease*,
Contemporary Cardiology, https://doi.org/10.1007/978-3-030-62632-7_4

of vegetables with either meat, rice, or fish. As a result, the dietary pattern under-stood as a set of nutrients and its effect on health has gained relevance in recent years, which involves evaluating multiple dietary components in a single discipline [22, 28, 45].

Accordingly, this chapter will address different dietary patterns to date in relation to the scientific evidence that supports them. In addition, each dietary pattern will include a summary table found at the end of each chapter, as well as an example of a menu for each.

Mediterranean Diet

History of the Mediterranean Diet

Since 2013, the Mediterranean Diet (MD) has been part of UNESCO Intangible Cultural Heritage [57] and, it represents a lifestyle, beyond a simple food pattern. The Mediterranean dimension uses a combination of local agriculture, homemade recipes, traditions, physical exercise and leisure time. The benefits attributed to the MD were unknown until the twentieth century. The origin of the alimentary pattern was first proposed in 1948 when the epidemiologist Leland Allbaugh carried out his main investigation in the island of Crete. His research followed a request of the Greek government and subsidized by the Rockefeller Foundation. The objective was to evaluate the possibility and feasibility of increasing the living standard of the island, in terms of economy, society and health. After the Second World War, the island experienced a serious situation of poverty and a scarcity of assets. In addition, the study could verify if the resources and management tools of industrialized coun-tries with a better socioeconomic position could help the growth and development of Crete. The results were published in 1953 in a report entitled: "Crete: A Case Study of an Underdeveloped Area". One of the main findings was in relation to the feeding of the island. Their diet was based on frequent consumption of olives, cere-als, fresh fruits, vegetables, wild plants, and bread. On the contrary, the consump-tion of meat and dairy products was relatively low. The core meals always contained bread, olive oil, and, olives. The conclusions highlighted by this study stated that the level of food consumption in the diet was quite favorable and the eating habits were well adapted to the natural resources found on the island [1].

Another contemporary study by the physiologist Ancel Keys began to show interest in the same subject and focused his research on the relationship of food and lifestyle with cardiovascular risk. Thus, he planned a large study on 13,000 men between 40 and 59 years of age from seven different countries: the Seven Country Study. The purpose was to see the effect of the typical diet of each country on the frequency of coronary heart disease. This was the first study that systematically examined the relationship between diet, these region's lifestyle, risk factors and coronary heart disease and stroke rates. The countries were chosen for their diversity in eating patterns: Italy, Greece, Finland, Netherlands, Yugoslavia, Japan, and the United States. The follow-up lasted over 25 years after the original study. The main conclusions showed a direct relationship between the consumption of saturated fats and mortality rates from cardiovascular disease. Additionally, a protective effect was found when there was a positive ratio between the consumption of polyunsaturated and monounsaturated fatty acids regarding to saturated fatty acids [9, 39]. Therefore, the conclusions were an indicative of the differences between Mediterranean countries typical diet, Japan, United States, and the rest of Europe. The study showed a correlation between high intake of saturated fats (typical diet of United States) and high presence of blood cholesterol with a greater number of deaths due to cardiovascular disease. However, a high consumption of carbohydrates, polyphenols, and polyunsaturated and monounsaturated fatty acids found in the typical diet of Mediterranean countries had a cardioprotective effect. As a result, the concept of the MD began to emerge and over the years has undergone various modifications.

Currently, the MD is considered a healthy and balanced lifestyle that combines recipes, ways of cooking, celebrations, customs, fresh and typical products, and diverse human activities. It is not a simple nutritional guideline [18].

Mediterranean Diet Pyramid and Its Components

The Mediterranean Diet is presented as a lifestyle typical of the countries within the Mediterranean area, often characterized by a temperate climate. This denotation directly favors agriculture, the development of native crops of the area that is known as the Mediterranean triad: olive, vine, and wheat. It also favors social and cultural aspects that allow the interaction of citizens among themselves and with the environment [56]. However, it is logical to assume that every region has variants and there is great diversity, depending on the resources and the climate of each. Nevertheless, this model fulfils a series of common characteristics [30]. It is characterized for being a dietary pattern relatively high in fats. However, these are not saturated fats since they come mainly from extra virgin olive oil. It is a diet high in antioxidants and anti-inflammatory components. The MD highlights a high ingestion of fruits, vegetables, legumes, nuts and whole grains; the ingestion of olive oil as the main source of dietary fat; a frequent but moderate intake of red wine at meals; moderate ingestion of fresh fish and dairy products (especially low-fat cheese and yogurt), poultry and eggs; and a low ingestion in frequency and quantity of red meats and sausages [14, 19, 31, 51]. Fresh, unprocessed and typical foods of each season are prevalent. Figure 4.1 is resuming the MD model in the famous MD pyramid.

It can be observed that at the base of the pyramid of healthy eating is the realization of daily physical activity. It is also essential the social dimension in which the experiences of each day during the main meals are shared with friends and family. The homemade recipes and the development of the healthy culinary techniques of

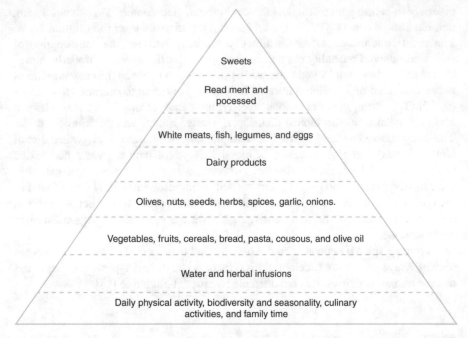

Fig. 4.1 Mediterranean Diet Pyramid

each region, always with seasonal foods, are also part of the pyramid's base. Hydration is a fundamental pillar with water as the main source. Occasionally, fermented alcoholic beverages that are not distilled, such as wine and beer, can be consumed. However, it always accompanied by meals and in moderation, avoiding the ingestion in fasting.

The intake of more than one glass of wine per day in women and more than two drinks in men is discouraged. Extra virgin olive oil is used as the fat par excellence, high in antioxidants, monounsaturated fatty acids, vitamin E and specific aromas that make it unique. Consumption should be moderate, due to its high caloric load but a daily intake of 4–5 tablespoons is considered, preferably crude for all types of culinary procedures. Perhaps, this aspect is one of the most important, since the MD, in addition to the beneficial properties attributed to it, has a high palatability and produces great satiety: a fact that facilitates its long-term follow-up. The diet should be colorful, rich in fresh fruit and vegetables. Fruit consumption is two to three servings per day (approximately 100–150 grams of fruits). Smaller fruits such as tangerines, figs or grapes will represent more than one unit in the same serving, and vegetables ration is two servings per day as well, preferably one of them raw, in the form of salad, cream or cold soup. The reason to eat raw vegetables is to ensure the daily vitamin intake, since the heat treatment of the vegetables allows increased digestibility, the thermolabile vitamins disappear during the cooking process. This point is also important for frozen vegetables, which sometimes lack nutritional benefits. Fruits and vegetables also provide a large amount of water, dietary fiber, vitamins, minerals and simple sugars necessary for the proper development of the organism in their daily activity. In the MD, approximately 50–60% of the total daily calories are represented by high quality carbohydrates. It consists of pasta, legumes, rice, breads and cereals, but better consumed with the integral or semi-integral version [6, 13, 47].

It is interesting to note how younger generations are unaware of what specific fruits and vegetables are produced at each time of the year. International trade allows for many fruits and vegetables like tomatoes, strawberries, eggplants, cucumbers and peppers to be available throughout the year. They are readily available at any supermarket year-round. In this sense, the pattern of Mediterranean life promotes a reasonable consumption of seasonal foods. The nutritional dimension, since the contribution of vitamins and minerals will be much greater in its epoch, and the hedonic dimension, since the aroma and flavor of the food will make the consumer fully enjoy it. The cooked preserves with fresh products make that they can be consumed out of season, conserving still the flavor from they were collected.

Another important point is dairy, mainly yogurt and cheese, preferably in its semi-skimmed or skimmed version. Two servings of dairy are consumed daily. Dairy consumption is frequently consumed with these food groups: poultry meats, eggs, legumes and fish. It is a food group that allows a protein contribution of high biological value, representing 2–3 times of the weekly intake each one of them. The consumption of fatty fish should be included at least once a week. Despite the recent controversy with eggs intake, the MD includes this food up to 5 times per week. On the contrary, the intake of red meat, such as veal, lamb and pork, is low. It is at the top of the healthy food pyramid and should not be consumed more than once a week. Processed meat products like sausages, burgers, etc., will have a very occasional ingestion and reserved for specific days. Fresh fruit is presented as the only dessert after the main meals. Sweets, cakes and pastries (even homemade), represent a very casual consumption, always less than two times a week, and preferably made at home.

In short, a pattern of Mediterranean life includes a frugal and varied diet with a strong social component that, unfortunately embodies more of a utopian ideology than a real situation. Over the last few years, this lifestyle has sparked great scientific interest and there have been many clinical trials that have been carried out to verify its effect on health. More specifically, one of the effects with the greatest scientific evidence is its cardioprotective action.

Scientific Evidence

One of the clinical trials with highest impact worldwide is the PREvención con DIeta MEDiterránea (PREDIMED) study. This is a multicenter randomized trial with parallel groups that was developed in Spain as of 2003, with a mean follow-up of 4.8 years. 7447 participants with high cardiovascular risk and aged between 55 and 80 years were randomized to three possible 1:1:1 groups, a first group with intervention based on a MD supplemented with extra virgin olive oil, a second group with a MD supplemented with walnuts and, a third group with a low fat diet as a control group. The recommendations and intervention were based on improving adherence to the diet based on a 14-point questionnaire that included food groups that scored positively or negatively. For example, the daily intake of extra virgin olive oil, consumption of fruits, nuts, vegetables were positive, and, contrary to, the intake of sweets, sugary drinks and red meats. The main end points were myocardial infarction, stroke, or death from cardiovascular causes; however, numerous variables have been measured in different investigations. One of the main findings of this study for the previous end points were the results that showed a Hazard Ratio of 0.69 (0.53–0.91) for the intervention group with MD and extra virgin olive oil and 0.72 (0.54–0.95) for the group with MD and nuts compared to the control group with low fat diet [16].

The same study demonstrates a positive effect regarding weight gain; prevents overweight and obesity and avoids the excessive increase of waist circumference, coming from the visceral adipose tissue [15]. However, results were not so clear in the first year of follow-up, when it was possible to see, according to the inflammatory index of the diet, how the parameters related to cardiovascular risk and inflammation fluctuated between them, and it was highlighted an absence of change in the levels of total cholesterol and triglycerides. The levels of LDL-cholesterol dropped significantly, and the HDL-cholesterol also rose significantly. However, this situation occurred in all three groups, without differentiating by intervention, as demonstrated in a subpopulation within the PREDIMED study. In the same way, 284 participants of the same study were subjected to a control of blood pressure of 24 h. In this study it was found that after 1 year of intervention, the group with MD supplemented in olive oil showed a change of the systolic blood pressure values of −3.14 mm Hg (−5.30 to −0.98) and diastolic of −1.68 mm Hg (−3.11 to −0.24) regarding baseline values. This same study showed the effect of the MD compared to the control group on blood glucose, which significantly decreased in the MD group supplemented with olive oil, −6.13 mg/dL (−11.62 to −0.64) and, a significantly effect on total blood cholesterol −13.6 mg/dL (−18.3 to −9.0) in the MD group supplemented in walnuts. On the contrary, LDL-cholesterol levels decreased in all groups equally, nor was change in HDL-cholesterol significantly observed [38].

The effect is favorable when the prevention of type 2 diabetes mellitus is assessed. In this study published in 2017, an inverse relationship was observed between the consumption of legumes in the PREDIMED population, and the risk of developing type 2 diabetes mellitus [8]. Among the many benefits that are attributed to the MD from the PREDIMED study, is the protective effect of the MD supplemented in extra virgin olive oil on breast cancer, which manages to reduce the risk by more than 60% respect to the control group [55]. It also has a positive effect on cognitive function, depression and prevents the risk of dementia [37, 50, 58].

Also, in Spain, the "Seguimiento Universidad de Navarra – SUN" study was carried out with a dynamic cohort of university students over 20 years old, since December 1999 and with a total of 22,786 participants (February 2018). The follow-up consists of a several questionnaires biannually about lifestyle, diet and health. In the study by Álvarez-Alvarez et al. the results of most of the participants were analyzed and found a significant association between a better adherence to the MD with a lower risk of mortality from all causes [2]. Various studies have also shown positive effects in the same cohort in relation to adherence to the MD and the reduction of cardiovascular disease. In 2011, a study was published by Martínez-González [35], where the questionnaire of adherence to the MD was assessed using a 136-item food consumption frequency questionnaire and associated a higher score significantly with a lower risk of cardiovascular diseases, in particular, those with higher score had a 59% lower risk than those with a lower score. In addition, in a recent review published in 2018, it is also concluded that the greater adherence to the MD contributes to the reduction of risk factors for type 2 diabetes in the SUN cohort. It is also associated with a lower rate of overweight and obesity, decreased risk of depression and higher quality of life, however, no evidence was found in the prevention and improvement of arterial hypertension [10].

On the other hand, in Athens, Greece, in the year 2001–2002, the distribution of cardiovascular risk factors was examined in a total population of 3042 participants with ages between 18 and 89 years, in order to relate them to sociodemographic variables, lifestyles and psychological characteristics. As well as assessing the prognosis at 5–10 years from baseline levels. After 10 years from the first evaluation, a greater adherence to a MD (estimated by the MedDietScore) was associated with a 90% lower risk of cardiovascular event compared to the lowest tertile [44].

The MD also shows its effect on secondary cardiovascular prevention, in the randomized Lyon Diet Heart Study, the recurrence rate after a first myocardial infarction was evaluated at 46 months of follow-up, with a MD in the experimental group compared with a control group. The ratio of cardiac deaths and non-fatal infarction in the experimental group was 1.24 per 100 patients per year with a value for the risk ratio 0.28 (0.15–0.53, $p = 0.001$) vs. 4.97 for every 100 patients and year [12].

Mediterranean Foods and Example of a Mediterranean Daily Menu

Foods included in the Mediterranean Diet
Extra Virgin Olive Oil (EVOO)
Seasonal fruits and vegetables
Poultry meat and fresh fish
Eggs
Dairy products (mostly fermented)
Nuts
Whole grains
Red wine with meals

Foods not included in the Mediterranean Diet
High-sugar drinks
Ultra-processed foods and fast food
Red meat
Processed meat (hamburgers, sausages…)
Butter and animal fats
Distilled alcoholic beverages
Pre-packaged foods and refined grains
Snacks and chips

Mediterranean Menu

- **1°) Greek salad.** Ingredients: Fresh tomatoes, cucumber, red pepper, green pepper, red onion, olives and feta cheese. For lemon vinaigrette, extra virgin olive oil, lemon, pepper and salt.
- **2°) Grilled mackerel with potatoes**. Ingredients: Fresh mackerel, lemon, extra virgin olive oil and salt. Potatoes, rosemary, oregano, bay leaf, pepper and salt.
- **3°) Fruit Macedonia**. Ingredients: Seasonal fruits, cinnamon and the juice of an orange.
- **Drink:** natural water or a glass of red wine.

Dietary Approaches to Stop Hypertension (DASH)

History of the DASH Diet

The Dietary Approaches to Stop Hypertension (DASH) diet is the result from one of the most relevant studies that has assessed the relationship between dietary patterns and blood pressure: The DASH trial. In this study, a total of 459 22-years-old individuals were randomized in one of the three possible diets for 8 weeks: a diet control, a diet of fruits and vegetables, and a diet called "combination" (DASH diet).

DASH and Its Components

The DASH diet consists of a high intake of vegetables, fruits, whole grains, fish and meat, nuts, vegetable oils and low-fat dairy products. This dietary pattern avoids the consumption of foods saturated fats-rich, such as copious fat meals or the fatty cuts of red meat. The consumption of high-fat milk products, trans fats and palm and coconut oils is also avoided. Also, the recommendation should be avoiding sugary drinks and sweets.

As far as micronutrients are concerned, it is a diet with a high content of potassium, calcium, magnesium, proteins and fiber, however, it is about reducing the consumption of sodium, mainly from processed foods, fast food, canned food and table salt, among others.

Regarding the daily serving, it is the following distribution:

- 6–8 serving/day of grains
- 6 or less serving/day of meats, poultry, fish and eggs
- 5 or less serving/week of sweets
- 4–5 serving/day of vegetables
- 4–5 serving/day of fruits
- 4–5 serving/week of dry fruits
- 2–3 serving/day of low-fat dairy products
- 2–3 serving/day fats and oils

Each serving corresponds to a certain amount, for whole grains it means a slice of bread, half a cup of rice, pasta or cooked cereals. It represents a source of fiber and complex carbohydrates. For vegetables it is estimated a consumption of one cup for raw vegetables and half a cup if vegetables are cooked. It also counts half a cup for vegetable or fruit juice. For natural fruits an average piece is estimated, for nuts a quarter of a cup approximately. A cup of milk or yogurt are considered as low-fat dairy products. For meat and fish each portion correspond to 30 grams, and the eggs would be a unit.

Regarding the amount of added fats and oils, an amount of one teaspoon of margarine, vegetable oil or mayonnaise is estimated. Finally, the consumption of sweets, although sporadic, contemplates a spoonful of sugar or jam as daily serving.

It is a dietary pattern with a high content of dietary fiber, antioxidants and minerals indispensable in the management of hypertension, such as magnesium, potassium and calcium, as well as less sodium. The daily caloric distribution of the DASH diet is similar to the Mediterranean Diet, between 50% and 55% of the total daily caloric intake is represented by carbohydrates. A lower percentage, 30% fats and finally, between 15% and 20% of calories, are represented by proteins. Diet composition is show in Table 4.1 [3].

One of the main differences between DASH and the Mediterranean Diet is that the Dietary Approaches to Stop Hypertension aims to reduce blood pressure, through certain nutritional recommendations similar to MD, although it advises the consumption of low-fat dairy products, and the reduction of total sodium intake. In addition, it advises to increase the intake of potassium, magnesium, calcium, total proteins and fiber.

Scientific Evidence

The DASH diet is the result of the clinical trial "Dietary approaches to stop hypertension". This is a multicentre, randomized study whose aim was to evaluate the effect of a specific dietary pattern on blood pressure values. The study included 459

Table 4.1 Diet components in the dietary approaches to stop hypertension [3]

	Control diet		Fruits and vegetables diet		Combination diet	
	Nutrient target	Menu analysis	Nutrient target	Menu analysis	Nutrient target	Menu analysis
Nutrients						
Fat (% of total kcal)	37	35.7	37	35.7	27	25.6
Saturated	16	14.1	16	12.7	6	7.0
Monounsatured	13	12.4	13	13.9	13	9.9
Polynsaturated	8	6.2	8	7.3	8	6.8
Carbohydrates (% of total kcal)	48	50.5	48	49.2	55	56.5
Protein (% of total kcal)	15	13.8	15	15.1	18	17.9
Cholesterol (mg/day)	300	233	300	184	150	151
Fiber (g/day)	9	NA	31	NA	31	NA
Potassium (mg/day)	1700	1752	4700	4101	4700	4415
Magnesium (mg/day)	165	176	500	423	500	480
Calcium (mg/day)	450	443	450	534	1240	1265
Sodium (mg/day)	3000	3028	3000	2816	3000	2859
Food groups (no. of servings/day)						
Fruits and juices	1.6		5.2		5.2	
Vegetables	2.0		3.3		4.4	
Grains	8.2		6.9		7.5	
Low-fat dairy	0.1		0.0		2.0	
Regular-fat dairy	0.4		0.3		0.7	
Nuts, seeds, and legumes	0.0		0.6		0.7	
Beef, pork, and ham	1.5		1.8		0.5	
Poultry	0.8		0.4		0.6	
Fish	0.2		0.3		0.5	
Fat, oils, and salad dressing	5.8		5.3		2.5	
Snacks and sweets	4.1		1.4		0.7	

22-years-old adult subjects and figures of systolic blood pressure less than 160 mm Hg and diastolic 80–95 mm Hg, without antihypertensive medication taken. The exclusion criteria were: poorly controlled diabetes mellitus, BMI greater than 35, pregnancy or lactation and hyperlipidaemia among others. The subjects were randomized to receive a control diet, typical of the United States, a diet with fruits and vegetables or a combined diet. This combined diet was high in fruits and vegetables, whole grains, low-fat dairy products, with a cholesterol, saturated and total fat reduction. Subjects were recommended not to consume more than three drinks with caffeine per day or more than two alcoholic drinks per day. The main outcome was the change in diastolic blood pressure and changes in systolic blood pressure. After the intervention in the different groups, the study of Appel et al. [3] showed an over-all reduction in systolic blood pressure of 5.5 mm Hg (−7.4 to −3.7) in favor of the combined diet compared to the control diet. This reduction was higher in women −6.2 mm Hg (−9.2 to −3.3) with significant results (p < 0.001).

Similar values were found for diastolic blood pressure, −3.0 mm Hg (−4.3 to −1.6), however, the reduction was greater in men, −3.3 mm Hg (−5.1 to −1.5), both had significant results (p < 0.001). When the effect of the high vegetables and fruits diet was compared with the control diet, the results were also positive, however, the effect of the reduction on blood pressure was lower, with the reduction in systolic blood pressure −2.8 mm Hg (−4.7 to −0.9) in total, with the greatest effect in men. And the total reduction in diastolic blood pressure of −1.1 mm Hg (−2.4 to 0.3), with the reduction also being higher in men. In addition, when comparing the con-trol diet with a DASH diet low in sodium intake, the results show a reduction in systolic and diastolic blood pressure levels [25, 48].

Despite being the main outcome changes in blood pressure, different studies have evaluated the effect of the DASH diet on several parameters. Thus, in the study by Chen et al. [11] the objective was to estimate 10-year coronary heart disease risk (CHD) as the primary outcome. Compared with control group, the relative risk ratio comparing 8-week with baseline 10-year coronary heart disease risk was 0.93 (0.85–1.02) for vegetables and fruits diet, and 0.82 (0.75–0.90) for combinate diet. On the other hand, comparing this diet with vegetables and fruits diet, the relative risk ratio was 0.89 (0.81–0.97). The conclusion of the study showed a reduction of 18% and 11% of the CHD risk by combinate diet and vegetables diet respectively. Similar results have been demonstrated in diabetic patients with the same interven-tion and cardiovascular risk [4]. However, in another more recent study, 80 partici-pants with type 2 diabetes and prehypertension underwent an intervention and follow-up with the DASH diet and the control diet. Participants were aged between 18 and 65 years and were followed for 12 weeks.

After the intervention, a systolic blood pressure reducing effect was shown, how-ever, there was no change in the diastolic blood pressure values [20]. As far as cholesterol levels are concerned, this diet helped reduce total cholesterol levels by −0.35 mmol/L, LDL-C by −0.28 mmol/L and finally HDL-C by −0.09 mmol/L to the intervention group compared to the control group (p < 0.001). However, there were no effects on triglyceride levels [43].

In other recent study recruited 131 participants with obesity or overweight and hypertension, divided into two groups, one who followed the DASH diet and one comparison control group. A follow-up was carried out for 3 months to see the effect of this dietary pattern on blood pressure, cholesterol levels, weight, BMI among others.

After this time of intervention, a reduction was observed for the intervention group of body weight, waist and hip volume, an improvement in body composition, decrease in glucose, insulin and leptin values, compared to the control group. However, the main differences and the decrease in values were observed in body weight −4.09 kg for the intervention group and +0.65 kg in the control group. And, the values of systolic blood pressure −4.63 mm Hg for the group with DASH diet and a reduction of −0.84 mm Hg for the control group. And the values of diastolic blood pressure −2.64 mm Hg intervention group and +1.74 mm Hg control group [33]. These results are similar to the study by Kawamura et al. [29], in which a Japanese population is selected and a clinical trial is conducted to assess the effect of the modified DASH diet (DASH-JUMP), for local tastes, introducing soups on a daily basis, more Fish and local dishes, compared to a control group. It was a clinical trial with 60 participants, aged between 35 and 70 years and with high blood pressure levels.

After 2 months of intervention, a reduction in biochemical parameters was observed, as well as an improvement in the body mass index, fasting glucose levels, insulin levels and systolic and diastolic blood pressure.

DASH Foods and Example of a DASH Daily Menu

Foods included in the DASH Diet
Seasonal fruits and vegetables
Poultry meat and fresh fish
Eggs
Low-fat dairy products
Nuts
Whole grains
Vegetable oil

Foods not included in the DASH Diet
High-sugar drinks
Ultra-processed foods and fast food
Trans fat
Fat meals, high-fat dairy
Pre-packaged foods and refined grains
Palm and coconut oil

DASH Menu
- **1°) Spinach salad.** Ingredients: Spinach, chickpeas, natural and raw almonds onion, tomato, extra virgin olive oil, lemon, pepper and salt.
- **2°) Chicken and veggie brochette.** Ingredients: Chicken breast, green and red pepper, sweet onion, mushrooms, cherry tomatoes.
- **3°) Yogurt**. Ingredients: Yogurt with strawberry jam.
- **Drink:** natural water.

Vegetarian Diet

Vegetarian Diet and Its Components

The vegetarian diet is a dietary pattern based on the consumption of vegetable foods and the decrease of total or partial animal food. The International Vegetarian Union defines vegetarianism as "a diet of foods derived from plants, with or without dairy products, eggs and/or honey" [23]. Currently, there are several variants depending on which food is consumed:

- Ovo-Lacto Vegetarian: diet where people include plant food plus eggs and milk products. Common in the West.
- Lacto-Vegetarian: diet where people include plant foods and milk products. Common in India.
- Vegan: excludes any use of animal products for any purpose, including animal flesh (meat, poultry, fish and seafood), animal products (eggs, dairy, honey); the wearing and use of animal products (leather, silk, wool, lanolin, gelatin); also excludes animal use in entertainment, sport, research etc.

The vegetarian diet includes seasonal fruits and vegetables, cereals and legumes, nuts, seeds, eggs, dairy products and honey. On the other hand, it excludes products such as meat, fish, shellfish and their derivatives from food. Nor would insects, gelatins or animal rennet or animal fats be included [59]. The term vegan could include more of a lifestyle, while the term vegetarian only refers to a dietary pattern.

It is important to mention that the fact of eating a vegetarian or vegan diet does not imply that it is healthy. In this section, an analysis of healthy vegetarian diet will be elaborated, the one that has shown a beneficial effect for health in general and for the protection of cardiovascular diseases.

Healthy vegetarian food includes five different servings of fresh fruits and vegetables a day are recommended, such as oranges, bananas, apples, pears, courgettes, aubergines, leeks, etc. On the other hand, whole grains and high fiber versions with less fat, salt and added sugar, such as potatoes, whole meal bread, pasta and brown rice, are chosen as the main source of carbohydrates. Protein foods are mainly beans, peas, chickpeas, lentils, eggs and tofu. Dairy products can also be part of the vegetarian diet, always trying to eat the low-fat and low-sugar version. Vegetable drinks, such as soy drinks, rice, almonds ... are also consumed.

Special attention should be paid to these products, as it is not uncommon to find them with a high content of sugar and low content of nutrients. The fats in this diet are mainly oils and margarines in small quantities. As a drink, a daily intake of 6–8 glasses of water is recommended. If water is not consumed, low-sugar drinks, low-fat dairy products, and unsweetened tea and coffee are preferred. As for sauces, artificial condiments, snacks, industrial sweets, ice cream and cookies, their consumption is left for special occasions and occasional consumption.

In recent years, there has been a high interest about this dietary pattern and its possible risks, since by radically eliminating some food groups could also be eliminating essential nutrients from the diet. This can lead to an appearance of vitamin deficiencies and minerals, with its corresponding impact on health. However, in a vegetarian diet, with dairy and egg consumption, the only nutrient at risk of deficit, and therefore necessary to supplement, would be vitamin B12. According to the EFSA [17] the recommended daily intake of cobalamin is 4 micrograms/day for people over 15 years of age, being higher in pregnant women and lactating mothers.

To be able to reach these recommendations through vegetarian food, it is needed to consume more than 6 eggs a day or more than 4 glasses of milk in the same day. Therefore, the supplementation of this vitamin would be justified.

Another recommendation is related to the quality of fats and omega-3 fatty acids, present in high fat fish. The omega-3 fatty acids or their precursors, can be found easily in the plant world, a correct consumption of nuts, seaweed, or flax seed would ensure the contribution of this nutrient. It is important to mention that the seeds must be crushed or consumed in their crushed form so that the nutrients inside them can be absorbed, otherwise, they would be excreted from the organism in the same way they were consumed.

According to the Vegetarian Society to ensure a complete and safe diet based on foods of plant origin is necessary to pay special attention to the following nutrients: vitamin B12, omega-3 fatty acids, calcium, iron, vitamin D, iodine, zinc and the total protein intake. In the vitamin D case, it is of great importance to sun exposure, and control vitamin D levels.

Scientific Evidence

One of the first experimental studies conducted to test the utility of the vegetarian diet in order to prevent cardiovascular risk factors, was the study published in 1983 by Rouse et al. [46]. In it, 59 healthy subjects, aged between 25 and 63 years and with an omnivorous diet, were randomized to receive a control diet, or an experimental diet. The experimental diet consisted mainly of an ovolactovegetarian diet. After 14 weeks of intervention, the study showed evidence in the results that saw an improvement in the systolic and diastolic blood pressure figures in normotensive subjects who took an ovolactovegetarian diet regarding to the control diet.

In a more recent study [40], a vegetable-based diet was evaluated in order to reduce body weight and cardiovascular risk factors. 291 adult subjects with a BMI of ≥ 25 kg/m^2 were randomized and assigned a low-fat vegan diet or a control diet for 18 weeks. After the follow-up there was a significant difference between groups in total cholesterol levels -8.5 mg/dL (-13.1 to -3.8), LDL-Cholesterol -7.2 mg/dL (-11.4 to -3.2) y peso corporal -2.8 kg (-3.8 to -1.8). However, no favourable results were found for the vegan diet group for diastolic, systolic and triglyceride blood pressure values. These results are similar to the findings of Najjar et al. [42], where for 4 weeks, 31 adults followed a diet rich in vegetables, seeds, raw fruits and avocado. All foods of animal origin were excluded. A reduction of all biochemical parameters mentioned above was observed in addition to blood pressure and triglyceride values.

When the diet is based on whole foods of vegetable origin, similar results are obtained for values of body weight and total cholesterol [63]. Several cohort studies have also showed a lower prevalence of cardiovascular disease and the presence of risk factors with a vegetarian diet [24, 34, 52]. A curious fact is that the follow-up of an alimentary diet pattern based on a Mediterranean diet, taking preference for foods derived from vegetables and fruits, has beneficial effects for health, among others reduces mortality from all causes in high risk individuals cardiovascular [36].

Finally, the effectiveness of the vegetative or pro-vegetarian diet is also reflected when it comes to a vegan food pattern. Some studies show the effectiveness of this diet based on 100% plant-based foods for diseases such as type 2 diabetes or even to lose weight.

In a study by Barnard et al. [7], 99 adult individuals with type 2 diabetes mellitus were randomized to receive a low-fat vegan diet or a diet based on the Standards of Medical Care in Diabetes recommendations [53]. After 22 weeks of intervention, both groups showed significant improvements, however, the differences were greater in the group that followed the vegan diet, for the values of fasting plasma glucose, body weight and HbA1c. The metabolic improvement of type 2 diabetes is due to a stimulation of incretin secretion and insulin thanks to the vegan diet [27]. Similar findings were found for the values of insulin resistance markers and fat mass with the vegan diet in overweight patients [26].

Vegetarian Diet Foods and Example of a Vegetarian Daily Menu

Foods included in the Vegetarian Diet
Dry fruits and seeds
Seasonal fruits and vegetables
Whole grains and cereals
Eggs, dairy products and honey (optional)
Seed oil

Foods not included in the Vegetarian Diet
Fish and fish products
Meat and meat products
Insects and seafood
Animal gelatine
Fat from animals

Vegetarian Menu
- **1°) Hummus with carrot.** Ingredients: Chickpeas, tahini, sesame, carrots, lemon, garlic and salt.
- **2°) Tomato salad**. Ingredients: fresh red tomatoes, avocado, red onion, cucumber, green olives, asparagus, extra virgin olive oil and salt.
- **3°) Roasted apple with walnuts**. Ingredients: Yellow apple, walnuts and cinnamon.
- **Drink:** natural water.

Okinawa Diet

History of the Okinawa Diet

The Okinawa archipelago is located at the southern tip of Japan. It is a series of islands located between the East China Sea and the Pacific Ocean. These islands have become famous throughout history for being the region that includes the world record number of people with more than 100 years per capita.

The Okinawa diet began to gain more interest when the Japanese Ministry designed and subsidized a study called the Okinawa Centenarian Study in 1975, which followed more than 600 centenarians of the island. Into the main results, a life expectancy far superior to the rest of the countries of the world was observed. This study was carried out for more than 25 years and brought to light that the incidence of cancer, cardiovascular disease and cerebrovascular disease was lower in this region. In addition, not only quantitative data but the quality of life in these population was higher. However, despite this dietary pattern, the new generations no longer have the same life expectancy, due to the new incorporation of fast food establishments and foods rich in low quality fats that have invaded the island.

Okinawa Diet and Its Components

As any nutritional pattern, it includes some variables more than diet. The Okinawa archipelago has a more relaxed lifestyle, devoid of stress, a peaceful climate, special care for the members of society, especially the elderly, a social community life and even great weight to emphasis the physical activity and meditation. The care of the quality of mental, physical and social life make this lifestyle pattern different from others, and very similar to the priorities of the Mediterranean lifestyle.

In Japanese culture, and more specifically in the islands of Okinawa, there is a term on which life revolves around: *"ikigai"*, that term is defined by them as "the reason to get up every morning". Although it seems to get out of the eating pattern, it could be important to emphasize that they have a constant search for the meaning of life, and the culture of the place favours this search. In fact, some authors have suggested that the success of this society in terms of longevity is concerned, not only in food, but in the search for *"ikigai"*, in introspection and self-knowledge of everyone to be able to self-fulfil in life.

Therefore, key points in this pattern:

- Varied and balanced diet
- Minimum quantities of food
- Physical activity, including meditation
- High quality of social life
- Search of the *"ikigai"*

The Okinawa diet is mainly characterized by being a pro-vegetarian dietary pattern, where fruits and vegetables predominate and a little of each group of food is consumed, and in small quantities. It is a follow-up of guidelines where 80% of the foods are of vegetable origin, seasonal vegetables and fruits, whole grains, algae, soybeans in various forms, low consumption of meat (mostly pork), eggs, high-fat fish and a low consumption of dairy products. In this important dietary pattern are the characteristics of the products consumed as the hours and the caloric distribution throughout the day. The main caloric intake is done in the morning, that is, breakfast and lunch, leaving lighter meals for the snack and dinner. The adepts to this diet try to end the lunch with a sensation of fullness of 80%, leaving them the 20 min relevant to reach the point of satiety. Predominantly a high consumption of natural and little processed foods, seasonality and little addition of salt and sugar to the dishes. In addition, the consumption of alcohol is minimal, the main drink is water and green tea.

It treats of a feeding where the low caloric density and the high density of nutrients are prioritized. It is a diet high in antioxidants, present in foods such as green tea, turmeric, ginger, fruits and varied vegetables. In high quality fatty acids, omega-3 from fish and algae and minerals, also present in seaweed, shellfish and seeds.

The distribution of the food pyramid is very similar to that of the Mediterranean Diet. Vegetables and fruits followed by whole grains and legumes. On the next step foods such as seaweed, oils, sauces and condiments. Next, high-fat fish rich in omega-3. Finally, meats and eggs would be located, followed by the top, where the sweets and processed cakes are.

Scientific Evidence

Unlike the dietary patterns cited above, most of the scientific studies that have been conducted around the Okinawa diet have been related to providing a plausible explanation for the high longevity of its population. Some studies have focused on analysing the genetic component of part of the population [61]. After the first findings of the Okinawa Centenarian Study, some of the principal investigators of the study carried out several analyses where they found a cumulative survival advantage for centennial siblings of the study of 5.43 times compared to the female sisters, with a probability of 2.58 times. Within this same study, genetic research was carried out, showing a higher prevalence of anti-inflammatory alleles, as well as a lower prevalence of proinflammatory alleles in centenarians of the cohort [54].

However, these values are not found in Japanese from the island of Okinawa who have migrated to Brazil. In this population, mortality from cardiovascular disease was higher and they had a shorter life expectancy compared to their counterparts living in Japan. Therefore, the results suggest that the cardiovascular risk factors related to the state of health of the inhabitants of the island of Okinawa are related to lifestyle, mainly with diet, than with the genetic component of individuals [41].

Okinawa Diet Foods and Example of an Okinawa Daily Menu

Foods included in the Okinawa Diet
Fresh fish
Seasonal fruits and vegetables
Legumes (mostly soybean) and algae
Eggs
Green tea
Herbs and ginger
Sweet potato

Foods not included in the Okinawa Diet
High-sugar food
Ultra-processed foods and fast food
Red meat
Dairy products
Moderate alcohol consumption
Pre-packaged foods and refined grains
Snacks and chips

Okinawa Menu
- **1°) Whole rise salad with mushrooms.** Ingredients: Whole rise, mushrooms, green pepper, onion and garlic.
- **2°) Salmon with eggs**. Ingredients: Fresh salmon, eggs, mix of vegetables, rapeseed oil and salt.
- **3°) Fruit**. Ingredients: Seasonal fruit.
- **Drink:** natural water or green tea.

Other Dietary Patterns

Alternatively, there are other minority dietary patterns. The Ketogenic diet is based on the high reduction of carbohydrates, with the intention of induce the body into a ketosis state. Almost 90% of the total energy is represented by lipids and proteins and, this diet is a very restrictive, where long-term follow-up is not advised. Nevertheless, it has demonstrated a positive impact for type 2 diabetes management, since blood glucose and haemoglobin levels were reduced and regulated. This diet has been experimented on refractory epileptic patients with positive results. However, there is no conclusive, long-term evidence that considers this dietary pattern as a reducer of cardiovascular risk factors.

Other alternative diets like the Dukan and Atkins diet focuses on weight loss within a short period of time. The treatment contains different phases in which carbohydrates are eliminated immediately, and low-carbohydrates vegetables are consumed, nuts and high proteins food (egg, meat, fish). The last phase consists of a weight maintenance through a balance diet. This diet should not be practiced over a long period of time, since evidence has shown that it could negatively affect kidney and liver function.

High caloric restriction diets (VLCD) are implemented for patients who have a high BMI (> 30 m²/kg) and is usually practiced as a last resort. Caloric consumption in this diet is usually no higher than 800–1000 kcal/day. Food intake is generally in the form of shakes, energy bars and soups. It is usually recommended for patients under constant medical supervision. The duration should not be longer than 12 weeks. It is a diet whose benefit is immediate and closely related to weight loss. For example, this diet is used before or after a surgical intervention that requires significant weight loss. Therefore, it has no preventive effect at the cardiovascular level beyond that reported by weight loss and the short-term effects they present.

Conclusions

After an intensive analysis of the main nutritional patterns and their relationship with cardiovascular risk factors, one of the conclusions that the reader could interpret is that a varied diet with a pro-vegetarian tendency, low processed and seasonal food intake, and moderate food quantity might significantly improve cardiovascular diseases, as well as the quality of life.

Nowadays, society is saturated in information, influenced by everyday television advertisement and trends in social networks. These stimuli play a factor in the food choices we make. Despite breakthrough moments for nutrition-related scientific evidence, this information does not reach the general population. The rates of overweight and obesity demonstrate this problem. In conclusion to this chapter, it would be worthwhile to delve deeper into how to put this theory into practice and how to move from scientific evidence to clinical and social practice, without intermediaries that dissipate the message.

References

1. Allbaugh LG. Crete, a case study of an underdeveloped area. Am J Public Health Nations Health. 1953;43(7):928–9.
2. Alvarez-Alvarez I, Zazpe I, Pérez de Rojas J, Bes-Rastrollo M, Ruiz-Canela M, Fernandez-Montero A, et al. Mediterranean diet, physical activity and their combined effect on all-cause mortality: the Seguimiento Universidad de Navarra (SUN) cohort. Prev Med (Baltim). 2018;106:45–52.
3. Appel LJ, Thomas JM, Obarzanek E, Vollmer WM, Svetkey LP, Sacks FM, et al. A clinical trial of the effects of dietary patterns on blood pressure. N Engl J Med. 1997;336(16):1117–24.
4. Azadbakht L, Fard NRP, Karimi M, Baghael MH, Surkan PJ, Rahimi M, et al. Effects of the Dietary Approaches to Stop Hypertension (DASH) eating plan on cardiovascular risks among type 2 diabetic patients: a randomized crossover clinical trial. Diabetes Care. 2011;34(1):55–7.
5. Bach A, Serra-Majem L, Carrasco JL, Roman B, Ngo J, Bertomeu I, et al. The use of indexes evaluating the adherence to the Mediterranean diet in epidemiological studies: a review. Public Health Nutr. 2006;9(1A):132–46.
6. Bach-Faig A, Berry EM, Lairon D, Reguant J, Trichopoulou A, Dernini S, et al. Mediterranean diet pyramid today. Science and cultural updates. Public Health Nutr. 2011;14(12A):2274–84.
7. Barnard ND, Cohen J, Jenkins DJA, Turner-McGrievy G, Gloede L, Jaster B, et al. A low-fat vegan diet improves glycemic control and cardiovascular risk factors in a randomized clinical trial in individuals with type 2 diabetes. Diabetes Care. 2006;29(8):1777–83.
8. Becerra-Tomás N, Díaz-López A, Rosique-Esteban N, Ros E, Buil-Cosiales P, Corella D, et al. Legume consumption is inversely associated with type 2 diabetes incidence in adults: a prospective assessment from the PREDIMED study. Clin Nutr. 2018;37(3):906–13.
9. Buckland G, Bach-Faig A, Serra Majem L. Eficacia de la dieta mediterránea en la prevención de la obesidad. Una revisión de la bibliografía. Rev Esp Obe. 2008;6(6):329–39.
10. Carlos S, De La Fuente-Arrillaga C, Bes-Rastrollo M, Razquin C, Rico-Campà A, Martínez-González MA, et al. Mediterranean diet and health outcomes in the SUN cohort. Nutrients. 2018;10(4):1–24.
11. Chen ST, Maruthur NM, Appel LJ. The effect of dietary patterns on estimated coronary heart disease risk: results from the Dietary Approaches to Stop Hypertension (DASH) trial. Circ Cardiovasc Qual Outcomes. 2010;3(5):484–9.
12. De Lorgeril M, Salen P, Martin J-L, Monjaud I, Delaye J, Mamelle N. Mediterranean diet, traditional risk factors, and the rate of cardiovascular complications after myocardial infarction. Circulation. 1999;99(6):779–85.
13. Dinu M, Pagliai G, Casini A, Sofi F. Mediterranean diet and multiple health outcomes: an umbrella review of meta-analyses of observational studies and randomised trials. Eur J Clin Nutr. 2018;72(1):30–43.
14. Dontas AS, Zerefos NS, Panagiotakos DB, Vlachou C, Valis DA. Mediterranean diet and prevention of coronary heart disease in the elderly. Clin Interv Aging. 2007;2(1):109–15.
15. Estruch R, Martínez-González MA, Corella D, Salas-Salvadó J, Fitó M, Chiva-Blanch G, et al. Effect of a high-fat Mediterranean diet on bodyweight and waist circumference: a prespecified secondary outcomes analysis of the PREDIMED randomised controlled trial. Lancet Diabetes Endocrinol. 2016;4:666–76.
16. Estruch R, Ros E, Salas-Salvadó J, Covas M-I, Corella D, Arós F, et al. Primary prevention of cardiovascular disease with a Mediterranean diet supplemented with extra-virgin olive oil or nuts. N Engl J Med. 2018;378(25):e34.
17. European Food Safety Authority. Scientific opinion on dietary reference values for cobalamin (vitamin B12). EFSA J. 2015;13(7):1–64.
18. Fundación Dieta Mediterránea. ¿Qué es la Dieta Mediterránea?, 2019.
19. González CA, Argilaga S, Agudo A, Amiano P, Barricarte A, Beguiristain JM, et al. Sociodemographic differences in adherence to the Mediterranean dietary pattern in Spanish populations. Gac Sanit. 2002;16(3):214–21.

20. Hashemi R, Rahimlou M, Baghdadian S, Manafi M.Investigating the effect of DASH diet on blood pressure of patients with type 2 diabetes and prehypertension: Randomized clinical trial. Diabetes & Metabolic Syndrome: Clinical Research & Reviews. 2019;13(1):1–4.
21. Hu FB, Manson JE, Stampfer MJ, Colditz G, Simin L, Solomon CG, et al. Diet, lifestyle, and the risk of type 2 diabetes mellitus in women. N Engl J Med. 2001;345(11):790–7.
22. Hu FB. Dietary pattern analysis: a new direction in nutritional epidemiology. Curr Opin Lipidol. 2002;13(1):3–9.
23. International Vegetarian Union [Internet]. Definitions. 2019. Available from: https://ivu.org/definitions.html
24. Jin Y, Kanaya AM, Kandula NR, Rodriguez LA, Talegawkar SA. Vegetarian diets are associated with selected cardiometabolic risk factors among middle-older aged South Asians in the United States. J Nutr. 2018;148(12):1954–60.
25. Juraschek SP, Miller ER, Weaver CM, Appel LJ. Effects of sodium reduction and the DASH diet in relation to baseline blood pressure. J Am Coll Cardiol. 2017;70(23):2841–8.
26. Kahleova H, Fleeman R, Hlozkova A, Holubkov R, Barnard ND. A plant-based diet in overweight individuals in a 16-week randomized clinical trial: metabolic benefits of plant protein. Nutr Diabetes. 2018;8(1):58.
27. Kahleova H, Tura A, Klementova M, Thieme L, Haluzik M, Pavlovicova R, et al. A plant-based meal stimulates incretin and insulin secretion more than an energy- and macronutrient-matched standard meal in type 2 diabetes: a randomized crossover study. Nutrients. 2019;11(3):486.
28. Kant AK. Dietary patterns and health outcomes. J Am Diet Assoc. 2004;104(4):615–35.
29. Kawamura A, Kajiya K, Kishi H, Inagaki J, Mitarai M, Oda H, et al. Effects of the DASH-JUMP dietary intervention in Japanese participants with high-normal blood pressure and stage 1 hypertension: an open-label single-arm trial. Hypertens Res. 2016;39(11):777–85.
30. Keys A, Menotti A, Aravanis C, Blackburn H, Djordevic BS, Buzina R, et al. The seven countries study: 2289 deaths in 15 years. Prev Med. 1984;13:141–54.
31. Keys A, Menotti A, Karvonen MJ, Aravanis C, Blackburn H, Buzina R, et al. The diet and 15-year death rate in the seven countries study. Am J Epidemiol. 1986;124(6):903–15.
32. Kourlaba G, Panagiotakos DB. Dietary quality indices and human health: a review. Maturitas. 2009 Jan 20;62(1):1–8.
33. Kucharska A, Gajewska D, Kiedrowski M, Sińska B, Juszczyk G, Czerw A, et al. The impact of individualised nutritional therapy according to DASH diet on blood pressure, body mass, and selected biochemical parameters in overweight/obese patients with primary arterial hypertension: a prospective randomised study. Kardiol Pol. 2017;76(1):158–65.
34. Matsumoto S, Beeson WL, Shavlik DJ, Siapco G, Jaceldo-Siegl K, Fraser G, et al. Association between vegetarian diets and cardiovascular risk factors in non-Hispanic white participants of the Adventist Health Study-2. J Nutr Sci. 2019;8:e6.
35. Martínez-González MA, García-López M, Bes-Rastrollo M, Toledo E, Martínez-Lapiscina EH, Delgado-Rodriguez M, et al. Mediterranean diet and the incidence of cardiovascular disease: a Spanish cohort. Nutr Metab Cardiovasc Dis. 2011;21(4):237–44.
36. Martínez-González MA, Sánchez-Tainta A, Corella D, Salas-Salvadó J, Ros E, Arós F, et al. A provegetarian food pattern and reduction in total mortality in the Prevención con Dieta Mediterránea (PREDIMED) study. Am J Clin Nutr. 2014;100(Suppl 1):320–8.
37. Martínez-Lapiscina EH, Clavero P, Toledo E, Estruch R, Salas-Salvadó J, San Julián B, et al. Mediterranean diet improves cognition: the predimed-navarra randomised trial. J Neurol Neurosurg Psychiatry. 2013;84:1318–25.
38. Medina-Remón A, Casas R, Tressserra-Rimbau A, Ros E, Martínez-González MA, Fitó M, et al. Polyphenol intake from a Mediterranean diet decreases inflammatory biomarkers related to atherosclerosis: a substudy of the predimed trial. Br J Clin Pharmacol. 2017;83(1):114–28.
39. Menotti A, Puddu PE. How the seven countries contributed to the definition and development of the Mediterranean diet concept: a 50-year journey. Nutr Metab Cardiovasc Dis. 2015;25(3):245–52.

40. Mishra S, Xu J, Agarwal U, Gonzales J, Levin S, Barnard ND. A multicenter randomized controlled trial of a plant-based nutrition program to reduce body weight and cardiovascular risk in the corporate setting: the GEICO study. Eur J Clin Nutr. 2013;67(7):718–24.
41. Moriguchi EH, Moriguchi Y, Yamori Y. Impact of diet on the cardiovascular risk profile of Japanese immigrants living in Brazil: contributions of World Health Organization CARDIAC and MONALISA studies. Clin Exp Pharmacol Physiol. 2004;31(Suppl 2):S5–7.
42. Najjar RS, Moore CE, Montgomery BD. A defined, plant-based diet utilized in an outpatient cardiovascular clinic effectively treats hypercholesterolemia and hypertension and reduces medications. Clin Cardiol. 2018;41(3):307–13.
43. Obarzanek E, Sacks FM, Vollmer WM, Bray GA, Miller ER, Lin PH, et al. Effects on blood lipids of a blood pressure–lowering diet: the Dietary Approaches to Stop Hypertension (DASH) Trial. Am J Clin Nutr. 2018;74(1):80–9.
44. Panagiotakos DB, Georgousopoulou EN, Pitsavos C, Chrysohoou C, Metaxa V, Georgiopoulos GA, et al. Ten-year (2002-2012) cardiovascular disease incidence and all-cause mortality, in urban Greek population: the ATTICA study. Int J Cardiol. 2015;180:178–84.
45. Román-Viñas B, Barba LR, Ngo J, Martínez-González MA, Wijnhoven TMA, Serra-Majem L. Validity of dietary patterns to assess nutrient intake adequacy. Br J Nutr. 2009;101(Suppl 2):S12–20.
46. Rouse IANL, Armstrong BK, Beilin LJ, Vandongen R. Vegetarian diet: controlled trial in normotensive subjects. Lancet. 1983;321(8314):5–10.
47. Rumawas ME, Dwyer JT, McKeown NM, Meigs JB, Rogers G, Jacques PF. The development of the Mediterranean-style dietary pattern score and its application to the American diet in the Framingham Offspring Cohort. J Nutr. 2009;139(6):1150–6.
48. Sacks FM, Svetkey LP, Vollmer WM, Appel LJ, Bray GA, Harsha D, et al. Effects on blood pressure of reduced dietary sodium and the Dietary Approaches to Stop Hypertension (Dash) diet. J Cardpulm Rehabil. 2001;21(3):176.
49. Sánchez-Villegas A, Martínez JA, De Irala J, Martínez-González MA. Determinants of the adherence to an "a priori" defined Mediterranean dietary pattern. Eur J Nutr. 2002 Dec;41(6):249–57.
50. Sanchez-Villegas A, Martinez-Gonzalez MA, Estruch R, Salas-Salvado J, Corella D, Covas MI, et al. Mediterranean dietary pattern and depression: the PREDIMED randomized trial. BMC Med. 2013;11:208.
51. Schroder H, Marrugat J, Vila J, Covas MI, Elosua R. Adherence to the traditional Mediterranean diet is inversely associated with body mass index and obesity in a Spanish population. J Nutr. 2004 Dec;134(12):3355–61.
52. Shridhar K, Dhillon PK, Bowen L, Kinra S, Bharathi AV, Prabhakaran D, et al. The association between a vegetarian diet and cardiovascular disease (cvd) risk factors in India: the Indian migration study. PLoS One. 2014;9(10):1–8.
53. Standards of Medical Care in Diabetes—2019. Diabetes care. 2019;42:S1–S2. Available from: https://doi.org/10.2337/dc19-Sint01.
54. Takata H, Suzuki M, Ishii T, Sekiguchi S, Iri H. Influence of major histocompatibility complex region genes on human longevity among Okinawan-Japanese centenarians and nonagenarians. Lancet. 1987;10:824–6.
55. Toledo E, Salas-Salvado J, Donat-Vargas C, Buil-Cosiales P, Estruch R, Ros E, et al. Mediterranean diet and invasive breast cancer risk among women at high cardiovascular risk in the predimed trial a randomized clinical trial. JAMA Intern Med. 2015;175(11):1752–60.
56. Trichopoulou A, Lagiou P. Healthy traditional Mediterranean diet: an expression of culture, history, and lifestyle. Nutr Rev. 1997;55(11):383–9.
57. United Nations Educational, Scientific and Cultural Organization. Annual report 2014. 2014. Available from: https://unesdoc.unesco.org/ark:/48223/pf0000232794_eng
58. Valls-Pedret C, Sala-Vila A, Serra-Mir M, Corella D, De La Torre R, Martínez-González MÁ, et al. Mediterranean diet and age-related cognitive decline: a randomized clinical trial. JAMA Intern Med. 2015;175(7):1094–103.

59. Vegetarian Society. 2019. Available from: https://www.vegsoc.org/info-hub/definition/
60. Waijers PMCM, Feskens EJM, Ocké MC. A critical review of predefined diet quality scores. Br J Nutr. 2007;97(2):219–31.
61. Willcox DC, Willcox BJ, Hsueh WC, Suzuki M. Genetic determinants of exceptional human longevity: insights from the Okinawa centenarian study. Age (Omaha). 2006;28(4):313–32.
62. World Health Organization (WHO). World Health statistics 2018: monitoring health for the SDGs. 2018. Available from: https://www.who.int/gho/publications/world_health_statistics/2018/en/
63. Wright N, Wilson L, Smith M, Duncan B, McHugh P. The BROAD study: a randomised controlled trial using a whole food plant-based diet in the community for obesity, ischaemic heart disease or diabetes. Nutr Diabetes. 2017;7(3)

Chapter 5
Nutraceuticals and Cardiovascular Disease

Roberta Chianetta, Alexandros Sachinidis, Dragana Nikolic,
Luca Marco Luzzu, Anca Pantea Stoian, Peter P. Toth, and Manfredi Rizzo

Introduction

Cardiovascular disease (CVD) remains the primary cause of mortality in the world, in particular, coronary heart disease (CHD) [1, 2]. Unhealthy dietary habits are closely linked to obesity and dyslipidemia [3]. Dyslipidemia management, one of the key modifiable cardiometabolic risk factors, and especially high low-density cholesterol (LDL-C), can be achieved by certain changes in the macronutrient composition of the diet [4]. Dietary habits significantly differ between regions and countries, and reducing the unhealthfulness of diets may, consequently, reduce the increased incidence and prevalence of CVD [5]. In addition, physical activity,

R. Chianetta · D. Nikolic · L. M. Luzzu
PROMISE Department, School of Medicine, University of Palermo, Palermo, Italy
e-mail: roberta.chianetta@you.unipa.it; dragana.nikolic@unipa.it; lucamarco.luzzu@unipa.it

A. Sachinidis
PROMISE Department, School of Medicine, University of Palermo, Palermo, Italy

2nd Propaedeutics Department of Internal Medicine, Hippocration Hospital, Medical School of Aristotle University Thessaloniki, Thessaloniki, Greece

A. P. Stoian
Department of Diabetes, Nutrition and Metabolic Diseases, Carol Davila University of Medicine and Pharmacy, Bucharest, Romania

P. P. Toth
Department of Preventive Cardiology, CGH Medical Center, Sterling, IL, USA

Cicarrone Center for the Prevention of Cardiovascular Disease, Johns Hopkins University School of Medicine, Baltimore, MD, USA
e-mail: Peter.Toth@cghmc.com

M. Rizzo (✉)
PROMISE Department, School of Medicine, University of Palermo, Palermo, Italy

Italian Nutraceutical Society (SINut), Bologna, Italy
e-mail: manfredi.rizzo@unipa.it

© Springer Nature Switzerland AG 2021
A. F.G. Cicero, M. Rizzo (eds.), *Nutraceuticals and Cardiovascular Disease*,
Contemporary Cardiology, https://doi.org/10.1007/978-3-030-62632-7_5

avoidance of alcohol abuse and smoking cessation may also improve dyslipidemia and decrease CVD risk [4].

Nutraceuticals are specific nutrients that can be used for the prevention and/or treatment of certain diseases and can be consumed as part of a conventional food or as a dietary supplement. Overall, they represent an alternative option to treat dyslipidemia in combination with statins or as a monotherapy in case of statin-intolerance [6, 7]. The commonly used nutraceuticals for the management of dyslipidemia and CVD risk are red yeast rice, phytosterols and fish oil, while other nutraceuticals include bergamot and chitosan [8]. Very recently a number of certain dietary patterns (DPs) which promote adherence and implementation of healthy habits, such as the Mediterranean Diet (MedDiet) [9], the dietary approaches to stop hypertension (DASH) [10], the Portfolio diet [11], the Vegetarian [12], the Nordic diet [13] and low-carbohydrate diets [14] have been evaluated including their usefulness in managing dyslipidemia, different cardiometabolic risk factors and CVD risk [15].

In this chapter we discuss recent data on the effects of nutraceuticals on different cardiometabolic risk factors and CVD risk. In addition, we briefly summarize available data about application of the Mediterranean Diet (MedDiet) in improving cardiovascular (CV) health, including the international guideline which support this dietary intervention.

Nutraceuticals That Improve Lipids and Other Cardiometabolic Parameters

Red Yeast Rice

Monascus purpureus is a mold that ferments rice to produce Red Yeast Rice (RYR), which contains molecules that inhibit hepatic cholesterol synthesis and 70–83% of these molecules actually are monacolin K, identical to the statin lovastatin and inhibits 3-hydroxy-3-methylglutaryl-coenzyme A (HMG-CoA) reductase, the rate-limiting enzyme in cholesterol biosynthesis and even more bioavailable than pure lovastatin [16]. Monacolin K, at doses of 3–10 mg/day, reduces LDL-C up to 20–25% [17].

The results from a randomized controlled trial (RCT) performed on 5000 subjects with previous coronary events, including myocardial infarction (China Coronary Secondary Prevention Study), showed an average reduction in LDL-C levels of about 20% after use of RYR extracts (xuezhikang) with 2.5–3.2 mg of monacolin. This reduction in LDL-C was associated with significant reductions in fatal and nonfatal coronary events, stroke, and all-cause mortality (−31%, −44%, and −32%, respectively) [18]. The dose of 10 mg/day has been suggested with medical supervision [19]. The combination of monacolin K with statins should be avoided [19], while its co-administration with medicines containing clarithromycin, erythromycin, itraconazole, ketoconazole, telithromycin, HIV protease inhibitors, cyclosporine, nefazodone, in addition to grapefruit juice (≥ 0.2 L/day) is contraindicated.

One meta-analysis confirmed the safety and efficacy of RYR to treat dyslipidemia and CVD risk in statin intolerant subjects [20], while some clinical data showed a reduction in the estimated CVD (eCVD) risk after a short-term supplementation with a combined nutraceutical containing RYR (10 mg), phytosterols (800 mg), and L-tyrosol (5 mg) [21]. It is highlighted that there was also a decrease in systolic blood pressure (SBP) (-5.6%, $p < 0.05$ vs baseline and placebo), improvement in endothelial reactivity (-13.2%, $p < 0.001$ vs baseline), favorable changes in total cholesterol (TC) and LDL-C (-16.3% vs 9.9%, and -23.4% vs -13.2%, respectively, $p < 0.001$ for both), and hepatic steatosis index (-2.8%, $p < 0.01$ vs -1.8%, $p < 0.05$). Moreover, ALT (alanine aminotransferase -27.7%, $p < 0.001$), AST (aspartate aminotransferase -13.8%, $p = 0.004$), and serum uric acid (-12.3%, $p = 0.005$) were reduced by this nutraceutical compound [21].

Phytosterols and Stanols

Phytosterols in a dose-dependent way inhibit intestinal absorption of both dietary and biliary sources of cholesterol. A significant cholesterol-lowering effect was seen after intakes of more than 1.5 g of phytosterols per day, reducing LDL-C by about 9–10% [22], while in subjects with type 2 diabetes mellitus (T2DM) both LDL-C and trglyceride (TG) levels decreased significantly [23]. In addition, phytosterols exert anti-inflammatory actions and may improve endothelial function [24, 25]. However, subjects treated with phytosterols should consume higher amounts of vegetables and fruits containing such nutrients [24]. Their use is recommended in subjects with dyslipidemia at low and high CVD risk (in combination with statins), but also in subjects with familial hypercholesterolemia [26]. However, further trials are needed to show if the reductions in lipids (LDL-C and TG) induced by phytosterols may lead to an improvement in CVD risk [27, 28]. Two meta-analyses by Genser et al. [27] involving 11182 participants and Silbernagel et al. [28] were performed based on the results from observational studies, however, data from RCTs are scarce and predominantly assess the reduction in the eCVD risk after supplementation with phytosterols [29, 30].

Marine-Derived Omega-3 Fatty Acids

Fish oil is rich in the omega-3 polyunsaturated fatty acids eicosapentaenoic acid (EPA) and docosahexaenoic acid (DHA) with a recommended daily dose 2–4 g. The TG-lowering effect of fish oil supplements, especially in patients with hypertriglyceridemia, has been shown by several meta-analyses [31–34], accompanied by small, reductions in LDL-C levels, with the exception krill oil [35]. Interestingly, DHA has been shown to be more efficient in lowering TG levels than EPA; DHA and EPA also increase HDL-C and apolipoprotein (apo) AI concentrations, increase the number of large LDL and HDL particles, and decrease very low-density lipoprotein cholesterol (VLDL-C) [32, 36]. DHA may also have a more favorable effect on endothelial function than EPA [37], inflammation [38], as well as blood pressure (BP) [39], though this is controversial. EPA has been shown to improve pulse wave velocity (PWV) [40].

It has been shown that the combination of DHA/EPA reduces TG but does not reduce risk for CV events [41, 42]. The Reduction of Cardiovascular Events with Icosapent Ethyl–Intervention Trial (REDUCE-IT) trial [43] using 4.0 g of purified EPA (Icosapent ethyl) in addition to statin therapy demonstrated significant incremental reductions in myocardial infarction, ischemic stroke, need for revascularization, sudden death, as well as CV mortality compared to statin monotherapy among patients with established atherosclerotic cardiovascular disease (ASCVD) or diabetic patients with multiple major CVD risk factors. Two recent meta-analyses failed to demonstrate CV benefit [44, 45] when using DHA/EPA combination therapies.

Fish oil supplements improve other CV risk factors such as body weight (by 5.6 +/− 0.8 kg [46]) and BP (DHA reduced SBP −5.8 ± 2.1 mm Hg, p = 0.022 and diastolic BP (DBP) −3.3 ± 1.3 mm Hg, p = 0.029 [39]), but also reduce adipose tissue mass [47], especially when combined with lifestyle modification interventions [48]. However, a large meta-analysis [34] did not demonstrate a reduction in total mortality, cardiac mortality or cardiac events. However, in terms of mortality and admission to hospital for CV reasons a significant protective effect on heart failure was observed [49], and some analyses found a significantly reduced risk of cardiac death and all-cause mortality in high-risk groups consuming fish oil supplements (recommended daily dose 2–4 g) [50].

A beneficial role of n-3 PUFA in CVD prevention has been suggested [51] and also the other nutrients included in this food (proteins, vitamins, minerals, etc.) may play a role [52]. A previous meta-analysis [53] indicates an inverse association between fish intake and coronary heart disease (CHD) risk [relative risk (RR) 0.79; 95% confidence interval (CI): 0.70–0.89]. Similar findings were found by Del Gobbo et al. [54]. Fish consumption may be associated with a reduction in ischemic stroke (IS) risk [55]. In addition, in 2018 the American Heart Association (AHA) has included new recommendations to consume fish with n-3 PUFA twice weekly, with benefits in the secondary prevention of heart failure (HF), IS and cardiac death risk, in addition to the secondary prevention of CHD [56]. By contrary, they do not include specific advice in relation to fish and n-3 PUFA intake for the primary prevention of CVD and atrial fibrillation due to the lack of beneficial effects in these endpoints. Thus, future, long-term RCTs are needed to confirm these possible benefits of fish consumption.

Soluble Fiber: The Case for Beta-Glucan

Beta-glucan can be found in larger quantities in barley and oats as well as in some supplements and functional foods, and in small amounts in grains, cereals, and certain mushrooms [19]. One meta-analysis reported that beta-glucan (at a daily dose of 3.5 g) reduces LDL-C, non-HDL-C and apo B [57]. Moreover, glucomannan, plantago/psyllium, and chitosan are also effective in lipid management [58]. At doses ranging between 1.24 and 15.1 g/d glucomannan significantly reduces LDL-C and TG (by −0.41 mmol/L and −0.13 mmol/L, respectively, $p < 0.05$ for both) as shown by one meta-analysis [59] including 14 RCTs (n = 531 subjects). These findings have been confirmed by another meta-analysis [60] where intake of 3 g glucomannan/day resulted in reductions in LDL- and non-HDL-C cholesterol of 10% and 7%, respectively. An average intake of psyllium of 10 g/day resulted in an average reduction of LDL-C of 7% as observed in a meta-analysis [61], while LDL-C reduced by 0.278 mmol/L (95% CI: 0.213–0.312 mmol/L) compared to placebo. Regarding chitosan, a non-fiber lipid-lowering agent isolated from shellfish and sea crustaceans, a recent meta-analysis including 14 RCTs [62] demonstrated that chitosan supplementation (mean dosage 2 g/day) leads to significant weight loss (−1.01 kg, 95% CI: −1.67 to −0.34), improves the plasma lipid profile (LDL-C −0.83 mmol/L, 95% CI: −1.64 to −0.01; TG −1.06 mmol/L (95% CI: −1.67 to −0.45)) and decreases SBP and DBP: −2.68 mm Hg (95% CI: −4.19 to −1.18) and −2.14 mm Hg (95% CI: −4.14 to −0.14), respectively) compared to placebo.

Berberine

Berberine, an alkaloid found in and extracted from the root of *Berberis aristata* and other congeners, exerts LDL-C lowering effects (in the range 10–20%), decreases plasma TG (the standardized mean difference (SMD) = −0.50 mmol/L; 95% CI: −0.69 to −0.31), and increases HDL-C concentrations (SMD = 0.05 mmol/L; 95% CI: 0.02–0.09) [63]. A safe limit for daily intake for berberine is about 500–1500 mg [64], however, it has mainly been studied in Asian populations and in the Western world is under investigation (often found in products containing also RYR) [24]. In addition, its possible anti-atherosclerotic effects were observed in animal models [19, 65] and are associated with an increased growth of specific bacterial taxa *Akkermansia* in the gut and consequently modulation of gut microbiota. A recent randomized, double-blind, placebo-controlled, single-center pilot study [66], showed that supplementation with *A. muciniphila* bacteria improves several metabolic parameters, including TC (−8.68 ± 2.38%, p = 0.02). Currently there is a high scientific interest in the possible development of effective dietary interventions able to reduce cardiometabolic risk markers by modulating the gut microbiome [67].

Soy Protein and Dietary Oils

Soy, lupin and its products contain isoflavones, lecithin, and proteins that promote the expression of LDL receptors. A consumption of high amounts of soy protein (25 g/day) was not associated with very high reduction (4–6%) in plasma TC and LDL-C and is mostly seen in persons with high basal cholesterol concentrations [19]. Interestingly, when animal proteins were replaced with soybeans, reductions in LDL-C, non-HDL-C and apo B levels were observed [68]. Although one meta-analysis including 10 RCTs did not report significant effects of soy isoflavones on plasma lipoprotein(a) (Lp(a)) concentrations [69], another meta-analysis including 5 prospective cohort and 6 case-control studies with a total of 4954 participants, has shown an inverse relationship between soy protein intake and CHD and IS risk only in case control studies [70]. Similarly, Nagata et al. [71] found in a cohort of 29079 subjects that total soy protein and soy isoflavone intake was significantly associated with IS mortality but not with total CVD mortality. Also, epidemiological studies explored the association between soy protein intake and CVD risk [72].

Polyphenols, namely flavonoids such as quercetin and those contained in berga-mot extracts (that might competitively inhibit 3-hydroxy-3-methyl-glutaryl-CoA (HMG-CoA) reductase), have been studied in subjects with dyslipidemia and metabolic syndrome (MetS) [73], showing not only beneficial effects on the lipid profile (TC decreased form 6.6 +/− 0.4 to 5.8 +/− 1.1 mmol/l, $p < 0.0001$; LDL-C from 4.6 +/− 0.2 to 3.7 +/− 1.0 mmol/l, $p < 0.0001$ and TG from 1.8 +/− 0.6 to 1.5 +/− 0.9 mmol/l, $p = 0.002$, while HDL-C increased from 1.3 +/− 0.2 to 1.4 +/− 0.4 mmol/l, $p < 0.0007$), but also favorable changes in LDL-C quality, a shift toward larger and more buoyant LDL particles (LDL-1 particles increased from 41.2 +/− 0.2 to 49.6 +/− 0.2%, $p < 0.0001$, while small, dense LDL-3, -4, and 5 particles decreased from 14.5 +/− 0.1 to 9.0 +/− 0.1% $p < 0.0001$; 3.2 +/− 0.1 to 1.5 +/− 0.1% $p = 0.0053$; 0.3 +/− 0.0% to 0.1 +/− 0.0% $p = 0.0133$, respectively) [74], that further may be associated with decreased CV risk.

Dietary oils rich in MUFA (e.g. olive and canola oils) and PUFA (e.g. sunflower and soy oils) may beneficially affect dyslipidemia and CVD risk. Olive oil has a high nutritional quality due to its components such as polyphenols, and only extra virgin olive oil (EVOO) is known by its health benefits [75]: reduces LDL-C [76], but also lipoprotein oxidation and inflammation [77]. One meta-analysis has shown that a high intake of MUFA from EVOO was associated with a decrease in CVD events (by 9%), IS (by 17%), and CVD mortality (by 12%) and all-cause death (by 11%), when compared with a low MUFA intake [78].

Vitamin D

A large meta-analysis of 41 RCTs including 3434 participants evaluated the effect of vitamin D supplementation on lipids [79], showing a beneficial effect on serum TC (SMD = −0.17 (−0.28 to −0.06)), LDL-C (SMD = −0.12 (−0.23 to −0.01)); and TG (SMD = −0.12 (−0.25 to 0.01)), but not on HDL-C. In addition, there is growing evidence that vitamin D deficiency significantly increases the risk of a CV event, while a sufficient or optimum vitamin D status is protective [80]. Furthermore, it should be mentioned that changes in vitamin D status may confound some statin studies finding CV risk reduction [81]. Dinca et al. wanted to clarify the role of vitamin D supplementation on adipokines through a systematic review and meta-analysis of 9 RCTs [82]. There was no significant change in plasma concentrations of adiponectin and leptin after vitamin D supplementation. In meta-regression, changes in plasma leptin and adiponectin concentrations following vitamin D supplementation were found to be independent of the duration of treatment. Nimitphong et al. investigated the effects of vitamin D supplementation for 3 months on anthropometric measurements [83]. Forty-seven subjects with impaired fasting glucose (IFG) and/or impaired glucose tolerance (IGT) were randomized into three groups: control (n = 18), vitamin D2 (20,000 IU weekly, n = 19) or vitamin D3 (15,000 IU weekly, n = 10). After 3 months, waist circumference had significantly decreased in subjects in the vitamin D supplementation group. Body weight (BW), body mass index (BMI), SBP, and the homeostasis model assessment index insulin resistance (HOMA-IR) also decreased, but not significantly. However, subjects with an increase of total 25(OH)D levels > 10 ng/ml (23 of 29 subjects) had significant reductions in HOMA-IR and an increase in disposition index [83].

Coenzyme Q10

CoQ10 is the only lipid-soluble antioxidant that slows lipid peroxidation in the circulation, plays a crucial role in oxidative phosphorylation (i.e. ATP biosynthesis), and stabilises Ca-dependent channels, cell signalling and cell growth by regulating levels of cytosolic redox intermediates (e.g., nicotinamide adenine dinucleotide phosphate (NADPH)) [84]. Its deficiency may play an etiologic role in the development and progression of HF [85].

It has been shown that supplementation with CoQ10 beneficialy impacts hypercholesterolemia and hypertriglyceridemia. A combination of CoQ10 with astaxanthin, RYR, berberina, policosanol, and folic acid decreased TC (−26.15 mg/dL, p < 0.001), LDL-C (−23.85 mg/dL, p < 0.001), TG (−13.83 mg/dL, p < 0.001), increased HDL-C (2.53 mg/dL, p < 0.001) levels [86] and also an inverse association was observed between administered CoQ10 dose and Lp(a) lowering (slope: 0.04; 95% CI: 0.01, 0.07; p = 0.004) [87]. In addition, its health benefits against CVD are provided by lowering lipid peroxidation of LDL particles [84, 88]. In subjects with HF who used coenzyme Q10, a lower mortality and a higher exercise capacity improvement were found compared with the placebo-treated subjects with HF [89]. However, no significant differences in the left heart ejection fraction and NYHA classification were observed. Yet, the combination of aged garlic extract and CoQ10 was independently associated with significant beneficial changes in vascular elasticity and endothelial function, highlighting the important role of this combination in atherosclerosis prevention [90]. Furthermore, the data from one meta-analysis indicate that CoQ10 should be considered as a prophylactic treatment for preventing complications in subjects undergoing cardiac surgery with cardiopulmonary bypass [91]. However, future RCTs are needed to clarify the roles of CoQ10 in the prevention and management of CVD.

Turmeric and Curcumin

Turmeric (*Curcuma longa*), a yellow pigment, is a traditional Indian spice, used frequently as a food additive in Southeast Asia, improving color and flavor of food preparations, but also is used worldwide in cosmetics, dyes, and medicines [92]. Curcumin (diferuloylmethane) is an active component of turmeric. A large meta-analysis has shown a cardioprotective effect associated with reduced LDL-C (SMD = −0.340, 95% CI: −0.530 to −0.150, p < 0.0001) and TG (SMD = −0.214, 95% CI: −0.369 to −0.059, p = 0.007) levels in subjects who received turmeric and curcumin compared to those who did not receive this supplement [93]. Also in subjects with the MetS and higher CVD risk, the efficacy of turmeric and curcumin on serum TC levels (−0.934, 95% CI: −1.289 to −0.579, p < 0.0001) has been reported [93] and such effect in TC lowering may be greater by turmeric extract (SMD = −0.584, 95% CI: −0.980 to −0.188, p = 0.004). However, these findings need to be confirmed by future studies and it remains premature to recommend the use of these compounds in clinical practice. The supplementation with curcuminoids (1000 mg/day) plus piperine as an absorption enhancer (10 mg/day) or placebo, showed a reduction in atherogenic lipid indices including non-HDL-C (−23.42 +/− 25.13 versus −16.84 +/− 41.42, respectively; p = 0.014) and Lp(a) (−1.50 +/− 1.61 versus −0.34 +/− 1.73, respectively; p = 0.001) in T2DM subjects [94]. Furthermore, the curcumin effects in CVD through its anti-hypercholesterolemic and anti-atherosclerotic effects as well as its protective properties against cardiac ischemia and reperfusion have been suggested [95]. Di Pierro et al. in a randomized, controlled study evaluated the tolerability and the efficacy of curcumin in overweight subjects with the MetS, with a focus on impaired glucose intolerance and android-type fat accumulation [96]. Forty-four subjects, selected among those who after 30 days of diet and intervention lifestyle had a weight loss <2%, were treated for 30 days with either daily treatment of a curcumin-based product or pure phosphatidylserine. Curcumin administration increased weight loss from 1.88% to 4.91%, enhanced percentage reduction of body fat (from 0.70% to 8.43%), increased waistline reduction (from 2.36% to 4.14%), improved hip circumference reduction from 0.74% to 2.51%, and enhanced reduction of BMI (from 2.10% to 6.43%) (p < 0.01 for all comparisons) [96]. In addition, a natural supplement (Kepar) containing curcuma longa, silymarin, guggul, chlorogenic acid, and inulin, at a dose of 2 pills/day for 4 months, significantly reduced TC (from 4.8 ± 1.4 to 4.5 ± 1.0 mmol/l, p = 0.03) as well as evaluated anthropometric parameters in subjects with the MetS [97]: significant reductions in BW (from 81.1 ± 13.5 to 79.4 ± 12.5 kg, p < 0.0001), BMI (from 29.6 (23.7) to 29.3 (21.9) kg/m^2, p = 0.001), and waist circumference (from 105 ± 11 to 102 ± 10 cm, p = 0.0004), as well as in fasting glucose (from 6.5 (11.7) to 6.4 (7.6) mmol/l, p = 0.014), while no significant changes were found in investigated markers of oxidative stress.

Green Tea

The major components of green tea, one of the most popular beverages worldwide, are polyphenols, including catechins (about 30% of its dry weight), alkaloids, and polysaccharide [98, 99]. Supplementation with green tea extract is associated with an improved lipid profile: reduced TC (from 5.4 ± 1.0 mmol to 5.0 ± 0.9 mmol; p = 0.009), LDL-C (from 3.5 ± 1.0 mmol to 3.1 ± 0.9 mmol; p = 0.011) and TG (from 1.4 ± 0.6 mmol to 1.1 ± 0.5 mmol; p = 0.004), while HDL-C increased (from 1.2 ± 0.2 mmol to 1.4 ± 0.3 mmol; p < 0.001) [100]. A recent animal study [101] showed that a basal diet plus 10 g/kg green tea powder increased lipoprotein lipase expression in the liver after 8–12 weeks feeding (a basal diet plus 10 g/kg green tea powder) when compared to the control group (p < 0.05) [101]; apo B, TG, TC (p < 0.01, respectively), and LDL (p < 0.05) decreased after 8 weeks feeding, while after 12 weeks HDL, apo A, and very high-density lipoprotein (VHDL) increased (p < 0.01, respectively). Increased HDL and apo A was observed also in Portuguese adults to whom 1 liter of green tea per day was given for 4 weeks [102].

Green tea is a natural source of antioxidants in the form of catechins, particularly epigallocatechin gallate (EGCG) [103]. Flavonoids of this group inhibit the expression of inducible NO synthase that potentiates inflammation, platelet aggregation, and oxidative stress [104]. Experimentally drinking or eating green tea significantly reduces both body fat and body weight (BW) [100]. Obese hypertensive patients were treated for 3 months with extracts of green tea. The study group experienced a decrease in anthropometric parameters (BW from 73.2 to 71.9 kg, $p < 0.001$; BMI from 27.4 to 26.9 kg/m^2, $p < 0.001$, and waist circumference from 95.8 to 91.5 cm, $p < 0.001$) [105].

Resveratrol

Resveratrol (3,5,4′-trihydroxy-trans-stilbene) is a natural polyphenolic compound in grapes, nuts, fruits, and vegetables [106], that has been approved as a dietary supplement by the Food and Drug Administration (FDA) because of its multiple functions and low cytotoxicity. Resveratrol has health promoting functions such as anti-inflammatory, antioxidant, and anti-tumor activity, as well as cardioprotective effects [107].

One recent meta-analysis [108] showed that resveratrol supplementation (up to 3000 mg/day) in subjects with the MetS significantly reduced TC, while in subjects with dyslipidemia resveratrol supplementation (100 mg/day) also significantly reduces TC (201.4 +/− 34.4 versus 220.6 +/− 37.4, p = 0.04) and TG triglycerides (133.4 +/− 55.3 versus 166.7 +/− 68.5, p = 0.04) compared with placebo [109]. A systematic review has shown that resveratrol does not consistently improve BMI or BW, fat mass, fat volume, or abdominal fat distribution. Instead this polyphenol has been shown to have a significant positive effect ($p < 0.05$) on inflammatory markers [110]. However, dietary supplementation with an extract from black chokeberry (*Aronia melanocarpa*) fruit, that is a condensed source of polyphenols (714 mg/g) represents a promising supplementary therapeutic option in both prevention and treatment of the MetS, as well as its complications [111, 112].

*Artichoke (*Cynara scolymus, Cynara cardunculus*)*

Artichoke leaf extract (ALE) has potential hypolipidemic as well as hepatoprotective effects that can be attributed to its antioxidant action and the main compounds include: mono- and dicaffeoylquinic acid (chlorogenic acid and cynarin), caffeic acid (1%), volatile sesquiterpene, and flavonoids (1% which include the glycosides luteolin-7-beta-rutinoside (scolymoside), luteolin-7- beta-D-glucoside, and luteolin-4-beta-D-glucoside) [58]. A recent randomized, double-blind, placebo-controlled study [113], using a natural supplement containing chlorogenic acid and luteolin for 6-months, demonstrated a significant improvement in lipid profiles (TC −19.59 mg/dl (95% CI: −23.71, −15.47), TG −35.14 mg/dl (95% CI: −44.83, −25.45) and LDL-C −24.79 mg/dl (−95% CI: 31.43, −18,16), p < 0.001 for all) as well as other investigated cardio-metabolic parameters including BW (−2.40% (95% CI: −3.79, −1.01); p < 0.001), waist circumference (−2.76% (95% CI: −4.55, −0.96); p = 0.003), HbA1c (−0.95% (95% CI: −1.22, −0.67); p < 0.001), hepatic transaminases, flow-mediated dilation (10.56% (95% CI: 5.00, 16.12); p < 0.001), and carotid intima-media thickness (−39.48% (95% CI: −47.98, −30.97); p < 0.001). Importantly, the improvements in these cardiometabolic variables were independent of the degree of hepatic steatosis [113]. These findings are in accordance with the most recent meta-analysis of 9 RCTs including 702 participants [114]. A hepatoprotective effect observed after ALE supplementation suggests possible benefit in statin-intolerant patients with elevated alanine transaminase levels. However, long-term safety studies are needed to confirm such findings.

Legumes

Legumes are mainly composed of complex carbohydrates, as well as proteins, fiber, and some micronutrients that may affect lipids and CVD risk. The consumption of a large amount of legumes is associated with a significant decrease in TC (by 7.2%), LDL-C (by 6.2%) and TG (by 16.6%) as it has been shown by some studies [115] and confirmed in a meta-analysis performed by Bazzano et al. [116]. Moreover, legume consumption (4 weekly 100 g servings) has been associated with a 14% CHD risk reduction [117]. Furthermore, it has been reported that a high daily intake of whole grains is associated with the decreased risk of CHD (by 12%), IS (by 19%)

and total CVD (by 22%), as well as reduced all-cause death (by 15%), and T2DM (by 26%) risk [118]. Chen et al. [119] have obtained similar findings with a risk reduction of total mortality (by 12%), CVD mortality (by 30%) and CHD mortality (by 32%).

Nutraceuticals and Blood Pressure

Pomegranate has been widely used as a folk medicine in many cultures [120]. The content of soluble polyphenols in pomegranate juice (PJ) varies within the limits of 0.2–1.0%, and they include tannins, ellagic tannins, anthocyanins, catechins, as well as gallic and ellagic acids [121]. The consumption of PJ reduces BP, and in hypertensive patients affects the activity of angiotensin-converting enzyme (ACE) [122]. Aviram et al. [123] noted a 36% decrease in serum ACE activity and a 5% reduction in SBP. PJ has also been shown to beneficially impact oxidative stress [123].

When measured over 8 weeks of treatment, as mentioned above, green tea also lowers SBP (from 126.2 mm Hg to 118.6 mm Hg; $p < 0.05$) [100]. In another study in obese persons, green tea reduced BP (SBP from 145 ± 10 mm Hg to 141 ± 8 mm Hg, $p = 0.004$; DBP from 88 ± 4 mm Hg to 84 ± 3 mm Hg, $p < 0.01$), serum insulin levels, and improved the lipid profile ($p < 0.05$) [124].

The pro-health properties of garlic (*Allium sativum*), including the prevention of atherosclerosis, are due to its chemical composition [125, 126]. High levels of allicin and sulfur reduced blood pressure [127]. Data from clinical studies indicate that garlic powder is an antihypertensive agent in patients with hypertension and reduces both SBP (aged garlic extract Δ: -2.59 ± 1.91 vs. placebo, Δ: -1.72 ± 1.60) and DBP (aged garlic extract Δ: -1.07 ± 1.32 vs. placebo, Δ: -0.31 ± 1.17) [128]. The above results demonstrate that garlic as a food supplement may be useful in the treatment of the MetS [129]. EPA and DHA also impact SBP and DBP in hypertensive patients. It has been suggested that the hypotensive properties of omega-3 fatty acids are associated with angiotensin II antagonism and increased production of NO [130, 131].

Nutraceuticals, Cardiovascular Risk and Prevention: Current Knowledge and Future Prospective

Nutraceuticals may be used to improve health, support the structure or function of the body, delay the aging process, prevent chronic diseases and increase life expectancy and consequently have received considerable scientific interest due to potential nutritional, safety and therapeutic effects [132]. Numerous preclinical and clinical studies indicate that cardioprotection and lifespan extension is possible through a nutritional, dietary and exercise approach or their combination. However, both randomized trials and observational studies with concrete CVD endpoints are needed.

In addition, the lack of pharmacokinetic and pharmacodynamic studies represents one of the biggest limitations to nutraceutical use in cardiometabolic prevention.

The MedDiet is the most recommended DP to reduce CVD risk in different populations by some scientific societies. It is well-known that the MedDiet can improve glycemic control, dyslipidemia, chronic inflammation, oxidative stress and endothelial dysfunction [133], resulting in reduced CVD risk, especially in "high risk" subjects [134], with favorable effects also on obesity and high BP [135], and even may prevent CVD [136]. Liyanage et al. [137] showed that the MedDiet was associated with a significant decrease in CVD (by 31%) and IS risk (by 34%). Similar results were found in two meta-analyses [138, 139], reporting an inverse association between MedDiet and CHD or IS risk. Finally, the Primary Prevention of Cardiovascular Disease with a Mediterranean Diet (PREDIMED) trial [140] provided additional important evidence on the role of the MedDiet in CVD prevention, further supporting the existing positive data. This multicenter clinical trial included 7447 subjects at high CVD risk but without established CVD at baseline. Such links between the MedDiet and CVD risk should be further investigated and there are currently 2 ongoing clinical trials, PREDIMED-PLUS (ISRCTN89898870) and the CORonary Diet Intervention With Olive Oil and Cardiovascular PREVention trial (CORDIOPREV; NCT00924937). It should be emphasized that the European Society of cardiology/European Atherosclerosis Society (ESC/EAS) guidelines acknowledge that the MedDiet may reduce CVD risk and contribute to CVD prevention [141]. Similarly, the Canadian Cardiovascular Society (CCS) recommends the implementation of the MedDiet to lower CVD risk [142], while the American Diabetes Association guidelines suggest adherence to the MedDiet to prevent the development of T2DM [143].

The benefits of DPs may differ between individuals and age, gender, genetics, BMI and health status have been suggested to be crucial predictors in the response to lifestyle changes, and specifically to diet. In this context, the research in nutrigenetics has shown that nutritional advice could be tailored to the individual's genetic background [144, 145]. Future research from long-term dietary interventions and nutrigenetics could provide new data and an effective health tool to improve cardiometabolic risk factors, and consequently not only treat, but also prevent CVD. Thus, further research in the field of nutraceuticals is very important and may allow us to prevent the development of chronic diseases, such as CVD, with an adequate risk-benefit balance in comparison to pharmacological therapies [15]. Clinicians should adapt their advice regarding the most appropriate DP for each individual.

Overall, a healthy lifestyle is critical to prevent and/or delay the onset of MetS as well as to prevent CVD and T2DM in those with MetS. In this context, the recommendations that should help both subjects and clinicians in understanding and implement of the most effective lifestyle approaches in order to improve cardiometabolic health have recently been presented in detail [146].

Conclusions

Through the consumption of nutraceuticals, functional foods as soluble fiber and soy protein could be included in the diet. These foods may exert beneficial effects not only on lipid metabolism, but also overall CVD risk. Consequently, nutraceuticals and functional foods might be indeed used for the prevention or delaying, but also management, as adjunct therapy, of CVD along with modified lifestyle patterns and drugs of standard care. However, further research in this field is required to provide unequivocal evidence.

References

1. Hartley A, Marshall DC, Salciccioli JD, Sikkel MB, Maruthappu M, Shalhoub J. Trends in mortality from ischemic heart disease and cerebrovascular disease in Europe: 1980 to 2009. Circulation. 2016;133:1916–26.
2. Cardiovascular disease in Europe 2016: an epidemiological update. Eur Heart J. 2016;37:3182–3.
3. Siri-Tarino PW, Krauss RM. Diet, lipids, and cardiovascular disease. Curr Opin Lipidol. 2016;27:323–8.
4. Authors/Task Force M, Catapano AL, Graham I, De Backer G, Wiklund O, Chapman MJ, et al. 2016 ESC/EAS guidelines for the management of dyslipidaemias: the task force for the management of dyslipidaemias of the European Society of Cardiology (ESC) and European Atherosclerosis Society (EAS) developed with the special contribution of the European Association for Cardiovascular Prevention & Rehabilitation (EACPR). Atherosclerosis. 2016;253:281–344.
5. Imamura F, Micha R, Khatibzadeh S, Fahimi S, Shi P, Powles J, et al. Dietary quality among men and women in 187 countries in 1990 and 2010: a systematic assessment. Lancet Glob Health. 2015;3:e132–42.
6. Cicero AFG, Colletti A, Bajraktari G, Descamps O, Djuric DM, Ezhov M, et al. Lipid lowering nutraceuticals in clinical practice: position paper from an International Lipid Expert Panel. Arch Med Sci. 2017;13:965–1005.
7. Banach M, Patti AM, Giglio RV, Cicero AFG, Atanasov AG, Bajraktari G, et al. The role of nutraceuticals in statin intolerant patients. J Am Coll Cardiol. 2018;72:96–118.
8. Toth PP, Patti AM, Giglio RV, Nikolic D, Castellino G, Rizzo M, et al. Management of statin intolerance in 2018: still more questions than answers. Am J Cardiovasc Drugs. 2018;18:157–73.
9. Willett WC, Sacks F, Trichopoulou A, Drescher G, Ferro-Luzzi A, Helsing E, et al. Mediterranean diet pyramid: a cultural model for healthy eating. Am J Clin Nutr. 1995;61:1402S–6S.
10. Appel LJ, Champagne CM, Harsha DW, Cooper LS, Obarzanek E, Elmer PJ, et al. Effects of comprehensive lifestyle modification on blood pressure control: main results of the PREMIER clinical trial. JAMA. 2003;289:2083–93.
11. Jenkins DJ, Jones PJ, Lamarche B, Kendall CW, Faulkner D, Cermakova L, et al. Effect of a dietary portfolio of cholesterol-lowering foods given at 2 levels of intensity of dietary advice on serum lipids in hyperlipidemia: a randomized controlled trial. JAMA. 2011;306:831–9.

12. Expert Panel on Detection E, Treatment of High Blood Cholesterol in A. Executive summary of the third report of the National Cholesterol Education Program (NCEP) expert panel on detection, evaluation, and treatment of high blood cholesterol in adults (adult treatment panel III). JAMA. 2001;285:2486–97.

13. Nordisk Råd and Nordisk Ministerråd, 2005. Nordic Nutrition Recommendations NNR 2004: integrating nutrition and physical activity. Nordic Council of Ministers.

14. Oh R, Gilani B, Uppaluri KR. Low carbohydrate diet. StatPearls, Treasure Island; 2020.

15. Gomez-Delgado F, Katsiki N, Lopez-Miranda J, Perez-Martinez P. Dietary habits, lipoprotein metabolism and cardiovascular disease: from individual foods to dietary patterns. Crit Rev Food Sci Nutr. 2020;2020:1–19.

16. Chen CH, Yang JC, Uang YS, Lin CJ. Improved dissolution rate and oral bioavailability of lovastatin in red yeast rice products. Int J Pharm. 2013;444:18–24.

17. Li Y, Jiang L, Jia Z, Xin W, Yang S, Yang Q, et al. A meta-analysis of red yeast rice: an effective and relatively safe alternative approach for dyslipidemia. PLoS One. 2014;9:e98611.

18. Ye P, Lu ZL, Du BM, Chen Z, Wu YF, Yu XH, et al. Effect of xuezhikang on cardiovascular events and mortality in elderly patients with a history of myocardial infarction: a subgroup analysis of elderly subjects from the China Coronary Secondary Prevention Study. J Am Geriatr Soc. 2007;55:1015–22.

19. Poli A, Visioli F. Pharmacology of nutraceuticals with lipid lowering properties. High Blood Press Cardiovasc Prev. 2019;26:113–8.

20. Gerards MC, Terlou RJ, Yu H, Koks CH, Gerdes VE. Traditional Chinese lipid-lowering agent red yeast rice results in significant LDL reduction but safety is uncertain – a systematic review and meta-analysis. Atherosclerosis. 2015;240:415–23.

21. Cicero AFG, Fogacci F, Bove M, Veronesi M, Rizzo M, Giovannini M, et al. Short-term effects of a combined nutraceutical on lipid level, fatty liver biomarkers, hemodynamic parameters, and estimated cardiovascular disease risk: a double-blind, placebo-controlled randomized clinical trial. Adv Ther. 2017;34:1966–75.

22. Ras RT, Geleijnse JM, Trautwein EA. LDL-cholesterol-lowering effect of plant sterols and stanols across different dose ranges: a meta-analysis of randomised controlled studies. Br J Nutr. 2014;112:214–9.

23. Trautwein EA, Koppenol WP, de Jong A, Hiemstra H, Vermeer MA, Noakes M, et al. Plant sterols lower LDL-cholesterol and triglycerides in dyslipidemic individuals with or at risk of developing type 2 diabetes; a randomized, double-blind, placebo-controlled study. Nutr Diabetes. 2018;8:30.

24. Poli A, Barbagallo CM, Cicero AFG, Corsini A, Manzato E, Trimarco B, et al. Nutraceuticals and functional foods for the control of plasma cholesterol levels. An intersociety position paper. Pharmacol Res. 2018;134:51–60.

25. Rocha VZ, Ras RT, Gagliardi AC, Mangili LC, Trautwein EA, Santos RD. Effects of phytosterols on markers of inflammation: a systematic review and meta-analysis. Atherosclerosis. 2016;248:76–83.

26. Gylling H, Plat J, Turley S, Ginsberg HN, Ellegard L, Jessup W, et al. Plant sterols and plant stanols in the management of dyslipidaemia and prevention of cardiovascular disease. Atherosclerosis. 2014;232:346–60.

27. Genser B, Silbernagel G, De Backer G, Bruckert E, Carmena R, Chapman MJ, et al. Plant sterols and cardiovascular disease: a systematic review and meta-analysis. Eur Heart J. 2012;33:444–51.

28. Silbernagel G, Genser B, Nestel P, Marz W. Plant sterols and atherosclerosis. Curr Opin Lipidol. 2013;24:12–7.

29. Banuls C, Martinez-Triguero ML, Lopez-Ruiz A, Morillas C, Lacomba R, Victor VM, et al. Evaluation of cardiovascular risk and oxidative stress parameters in hypercholesterolemic subjects on a standard healthy diet including low-fat milk enriched with plant sterols. J Nutr Biochem. 2010;21:881–6.

30. Granado-Lorencio F, Lagarda MJ, Garcia-Lopez FJ, Sanchez-Siles LM, Blanco-Navarro I, Alegria A, et al. Effect of beta-cryptoxanthin plus phytosterols on cardiovascular risk and bone turnover markers in post-menopausal women: a randomized crossover trial. Nutr Metab Cardiovasc Dis. 2014;24:1090–6.
31. Eslick GD, Howe PR, Smith C, Priest R, Bensoussan A. Benefits of fish oil supplementation in hyperlipidemia: a systematic review and meta-analysis. Int J Cardiol. 2009;136:4–16.
32. Hartweg J, Farmer AJ, Perera R, Holman RR, Neil HA. Meta-analysis of the effects of n-3 polyunsaturated fatty acids on lipoproteins and other emerging lipid cardiovascular risk markers in patients with type 2 diabetes. Diabetologia. 2007;50:1593–602.
33. Wei MY, Jacobson TA. Effects of eicosapentaenoic acid versus docosahexaenoic acid on serum lipids: a systematic review and meta-analysis. Curr Atheroscler Rep. 2011;13:474–83.
34. Hooper L, Thompson RL, Harrison RA, Summerbell CD, Moore H, Worthington HV, et al. Omega 3 fatty acids for prevention and treatment of cardiovascular disease. Cochrane Database Syst Rev. 2004;4:CD003177.
35. Berge K, Musa-Veloso K, Harwood M, Hoem N, Burri L. Krill oil supplementation lowers serum triglycerides without increasing low-density lipoprotein cholesterol in adults with borderline high or high triglyceride levels. Nutr Res. 2014;34:126–33.
36. Nikolic D, Katsiki N, Montalto G, Isenovic ER, Mikhailidis DP, Rizzo M. Lipoprotein subfractions in metabolic syndrome and obesity: clinical significance and therapeutic approaches. Nutrients. 2013;5:928–48.
37. Mori TA, Watts GF, Burke V, Hilme E, Puddey IB, Beilin LJ. Differential effects of eicosapentaenoic acid and docosahexaenoic acid on vascular reactivity of the forearm microcirculation in hyperlipidemic, overweight men. Circulation. 2000;102:1264–9.
38. Kelley DS, Siegel D, Fedor DM, Adkins Y, Mackey BE. DHA supplementation decreases serum C-reactive protein and other markers of inflammation in hypertriglyceridemic men. J Nutr. 2009;139:495–501.
39. Mori TA, Bao DQ, Burke V, Puddey IB, Beilin LJ. Docosahexaenoic acid but not eicosapentaenoic acid lowers ambulatory blood pressure and heart rate in humans. Hypertension. 1999;34:253–60.
40. Satoh N, Shimatsu A, Kotani K, Himeno A, Majima T, Yamada K, et al. Highly purified eicosapentaenoic acid reduces cardio-ankle vascular index in association with decreased serum amyloid A-LDL in metabolic syndrome. Hypertens Res. 2009;32:1004–8.
41. Alexander DD, Miller PE, Van Elswyk ME, Kuratko CN, Bylsma LC. A meta-analysis of randomized controlled trials and prospective cohort studies of eicosapentaenoic and docosahexaenoic long-chain omega-3 fatty acids and coronary heart disease risk. Mayo Clin Proc. 2017;92:15–29.
42. Kromhout D, Giltay EJ, Geleijnse JM. Alpha omega trial G. n-3 fatty acids and cardiovascular events after myocardial infarction. N Engl J Med. 2010;363:2015–26.
43. Bhatt DL, Steg PG, Miller M. Cardiovascular risk reduction with icosapent ethyl. reply. N Engl J Med. 2019;380:1678.
44. Manson JE, Cook NR, Lee IM, Christen W, Bassuk SS, Mora S, et al. Marine n-3 fatty acids and prevention of cardiovascular disease and cancer. N Engl J Med. 2019;380:23–32.
45. Abdelhamid AS, Brown TJ, Brainard JS, Biswas P, Thorpe GC, Moore HJ, et al. Omega-3 fatty acids for the primary and secondary prevention of cardiovascular disease. Cochrane Database Syst Rev. 2018;11:CD003177.
46. Mori TA, Bao DQ, Burke V, Puddey IB, Watts GF, Beilin LJ. Dietary fish as a major component of a weight-loss diet: effect on serum lipids, glucose, and insulin metabolism in overweight hypertensive subjects. Am J Clin Nutr. 1999;70:817–25.
47. Poudyal H, Panchal SK, Diwan V, Brown L. Omega-3 fatty acids and metabolic syndrome: effects and emerging mechanisms of action. Prog Lipid Res. 2011;50:372–87.
48. Du S, Jin J, Fang W, Su Q. Does fish oil have an anti-obesity effect in overweight/obese adults? A meta-analysis of randomized controlled trials. PLoS One. 2015;10:e0142652.

49. Tavazzi L, Maggioni AP, Marchioli R, Barlera S, Franzosi MG, Latini R, et al. Effect of n-3 polyunsaturated fatty acids in patients with chronic heart failure (the GISSI-HF trial): a randomised, double-blind, placebo-controlled trial. Lancet. 2008;372:1223–30.
50. Hunter PM, Hegele RA. Functional foods and dietary supplements for the management of dyslipidaemia. Nat Rev Endocrinol. 2017;13:278–88.
51. Abdelhamid AS, Martin N, Bridges C, Brainard JS, Wang X, Brown TJ, et al. Polyunsaturated fatty acids for the primary and secondary prevention of cardiovascular disease. Cochrane Database Syst Rev. 2018;7:CD012345.
52. Torris C, Smastuen MC, Molin M. Nutrients in fish and possible associations with cardiovascular disease risk factors in metabolic syndrome. Nutrients. 2018;10(7):952.
53. Leung Yinko SS, Stark KD, Thanassoulis G, Pilote L. Fish consumption and acute coronary syndrome: a meta-analysis. Am J Med. 2014;127:848–57 e2.
54. Del Gobbo LC, Imamura F, Aslibekyan S, Marklund M, Virtanen JK, Wennberg M, et al. Omega-3 polyunsaturated fatty acid biomarkers and coronary heart disease: pooling project of 19 cohort studies. JAMA Intern Med. 2016;176:1155–66.
55. Xun P, Qin B, Song Y, Nakamura Y, Kurth T, Yaemsiri S, et al. Fish consumption and risk of stroke and its subtypes: accumulative evidence from a meta-analysis of prospective cohort studies. Eur J Clin Nutr. 2012;66:1199–207.
56. Rimm EB, Appel LJ, Chiuve SE, Djousse L, Engler MB, Kris-Etherton PM, et al. Seafood long-chain n-3 polyunsaturated fatty acids and cardiovascular disease: a science advisory from the American Heart Association. Circulation. 2018;138:e35–47.
57. Ho HV, Sievenpiper JL, Zurbau A, Blanco Mejia S, Jovanovski E, Au-Yeung F, et al. The effect of oat beta-glucan on LDL-cholesterol, non-HDL-cholesterol and apoB for CVD risk reduction: a systematic review and meta-analysis of randomised-controlled trials. Br J Nutr. 2016;116:1369–82.
58. Cicero AFG, Colletti A, Bajraktari G, Descamps O, Djuric DM, Ezhov M, et al. Lipid-lowering nutraceuticals in clinical practice: position paper from an International Lipid Expert Panel. Nutr Rev. 2017;75:731–67.
59. Sood N, Baker WL, Coleman CI. Effect of glucomannan on plasma lipid and glucose concentrations, body weight, and blood pressure: systematic review and meta-analysis. Am J Clin Nutr. 2008;88:1167–75.
60. Ho HVT, Jovanovski E, Zurbau A, Blanco Mejia S, Sievenpiper JL, Au-Yeung F, et al. A systematic review and meta-analysis of randomized controlled trials of the effect of konjac glucomannan, a viscous soluble fiber, on LDL cholesterol and the new lipid targets non-HDL cholesterol and apolipoprotein B. Am J Clin Nutr. 2017;105:1239–47.
61. Wei ZH, Wang H, Chen XY, Wang BS, Rong ZX, Wang BS, et al. Time- and dose-dependent effect of psyllium on serum lipids in mild-to-moderate hypercholesterolemia: a meta-analysis of controlled clinical trials. Eur J Clin Nutr. 2009;63:821–7.
62. Moraru C, Mincea MM, Frandes M, Timar B, Ostafe V. A meta-analysis on randomised controlled clinical trials evaluating the effect of the dietary supplement chitosan on weight loss, lipid parameters and blood pressure. Medicina (Kaunas). 2018;54(6):109.
63. Dong H, Zhao Y, Zhao L, Lu F. The effects of berberine on blood lipids: a systemic review and meta-analysis of randomized controlled trials. Planta Med. 2013;79:437–46.
64. Caliceti C, Franco P, Spinozzi S, Roda A, Cicero AF. Berberine: new insights from pharmacological aspects to clinical evidences in the management of metabolic disorders. Curr Med Chem. 2016;23:1460–76.
65. Zhu L, Zhang D, Zhu H, Zhu J, Weng S, Dong L, et al. Berberine treatment increases Akkermansia in the gut and improves high-fat diet-induced atherosclerosis in Apoe(−/−) mice. Atherosclerosis. 2018;268:117–26.
66. Depommier C, Everard A, Druart C, Plovier H, Van Hul M, Vieira-Silva S, et al. Supplementation with Akkermansia muciniphila in overweight and obese human volunteers: a proof-of-concept exploratory study. Nat Med. 2019;25:1096–103.

67. Marungruang N, Tovar J, Bjorck I, Hallenius FF. Improvement in cardiometabolic risk markers following a multifunctional diet is associated with gut microbial taxa in healthy overweight and obese subjects. Eur J Nutr. 2018;57:2927–36.
68. van Nielen M, Feskens EJ, Rietman A, Siebelink E, Mensink M. Partly replacing meat protein with soy protein alters insulin resistance and blood lipids in postmenopausal women with abdominal obesity. J Nutr. 2014;144:1423–9.
69. Simental-Mendia LE, Gotto AM Jr, Atkin SL, Banach M, Pirro M, Sahebkar A. Effect of soy isoflavone supplementation on plasma lipoprotein(a) concentrations: a meta-analysis. J Clin Lipidol. 2018;12:16–24.
70. Lou D, Li Y, Yan G, Bu J, Wang H. Soy consumption with risk of coronary heart disease and stroke: a meta-analysis of observational studies. Neuroepidemiology. 2016;46:242–52.
71. Nagata C, Wada K, Tamura T, Konishi K, Goto Y, Koda S, et al. Dietary soy and natto intake and cardiovascular disease mortality in Japanese adults: the Takayama study. Am J Clin Nutr. 2017;105:426–31.
72. Talaei M, Koh WP, van Dam RM, Yuan JM, Pan A. Dietary soy intake is not associated with risk of cardiovascular disease mortality in Singapore Chinese adults. J Nutr. 2014;144:921–8.
73. Giglio RV, Patti AM, Nikolic D, Li Volti G, Al-Rasadi K, Katsiki N, et al. The effect of bergamot on dyslipidemia. Phytomedicine. 2016;23:1175–81.
74. Toth PP, Patti AM, Nikolic D, Giglio RV, Castellino G, Biancucci T, et al. Bergamot reduces plasma lipids, atherogenic small dense LDL, and subclinical atherosclerosis in subjects with moderate hypercholesterolemia: a 6 months prospective study. Front Pharmacol. 2015;6:299.
75. Flori L, Donnini S, Calderone V, Zinnai A, Taglieri I, Venturi F, et al. The nutraceutical value of olive oil and its bioactive constituents on the cardiovascular system. Focusing on main strategies to slow down its quality decay during production and storage. Nutrients. 2019;11:1962.
76. Lapointe A, Couillard C, Lemieux S. Effects of dietary factors on oxidation of low-density lipoprotein particles. J Nutr Biochem. 2006;17:645–58.
77. Jimenez-Gomez Y, Lopez-Miranda J, Blanco-Colio LM, Marin C, Perez-Martinez P, Ruano J, et al. Olive oil and walnut breakfasts reduce the postprandial inflammatory response in mononuclear cells compared with a butter breakfast in healthy men. Atherosclerosis. 2009;204:e70–6.
78. Schwingshackl L, Hoffmann G. Monounsaturated fatty acids, olive oil and health status: a systematic review and meta-analysis of cohort studies. Lipids Health Dis. 2014;13:154.
79. Dibaba DT. Effect of vitamin D supplementation on serum lipid profiles: a systematic review and meta-analysis. Nutr Rev. 2019;77:890–902.
80. Giustina A, Adler RA, Binkley N, Bollerslev J, Bouillon R, Dawson-Hughes B, et al. Consensus statement from 2(nd) international conference on controversies in vitamin D. Rev Endocr Metab Disord. 2020;21:89–116.
81. Ware WR. The JUPITER lipid lowering trial and vitamin D: is there a connection? Dermatoendocrinoloy. 2010;2:50–4.
82. Dinca M, Serban MC, Sahebkar A, Mikhailidis DP, Toth PP, Martin SS, et al. Does vitamin D supplementation alter plasma adipokines concentrations? A systematic review and meta-analysis of randomized controlled trials. Pharmacol Res. 2016;107:360–71.
83. Nimitphong H, Samittarucksa R, Saetung S, Bhirommuang N, Chailurkit LO, Ongphiphadhanakul B. The effect of vitamin D supplementation on metabolic phenotypes in thais with prediabetes. J Med Assoc Thail. 2015;98:1169–78.
84. Hernandez-Camacho JD, Bernier M, Lopez-Lluch G, Navas P. Coenzyme Q10 supplementation in aging and disease. Front Physiol. 2018;9:44.
85. Cicero AFG, Colletti A, von Haehling S, Vinereanu D, Bielecka-Dabrowa A, Sahebkar A, et al. Nutraceutical support in heart failure: a position paper of the International Lipid Expert Panel (ILEP). Nutr Res Rev. 2020;16:1–25.

86. Pirro M, Mannarino MR, Bianconi V, Simental-Mendia LE, Bagaglia F, Mannarino E, et al. The effects of a nutraceutical combination on plasma lipids and glucose: a systematic review and meta-analysis of randomized controlled trials. Pharmacol Res. 2016;110:76–88.

87. Sahebkar A, Simental-Mendia LE, Stefanutti C, Pirro M. Supplementation with coenzyme Q10 reduces plasma lipoprotein(a) concentrations but not other lipid indices: a systematic review and meta-analysis. Pharmacol Res. 2016;105:198–209.

88. Littarru GP, Tiano L. Bioenergetic and antioxidant properties of coenzyme Q10: recent developments. Mol Biotechnol. 2007;37:31–7.

89. Lei L, Liu Y. Efficacy of coenzyme Q10 in patients with cardiac failure: a meta-analysis of clinical trials. BMC Cardiovasc Disord. 2017;17:196.

90. Larijani VN, Ahmadi N, Zeb I, Khan F, Flores F, Budoff M. Beneficial effects of aged garlic extract and coenzyme Q10 on vascular elasticity and endothelial function: the FAITH randomized clinical trial. Nutrition. 2013;29:71–5.

91. de Frutos F, Gea A, Hernandez-Estefania R, Rabago G. Prophylactic treatment with coenzyme Q10 in patients undergoing cardiac surgery: could an antioxidant reduce complications? A systematic review and meta-analysis. Interact Cardiovasc Thorac Surg. 2015;20:254–9.

92. Pulido-Moran M, Moreno-Fernandez J, Ramirez-Tortosa C, Ramirez-Tortosa M. Curcumin and health. Molecules. 2016;21:264.

93. Qin S, Huang L, Gong J, Shen S, Huang J, Ren H, et al. Efficacy and safety of turmeric and curcumin in lowering blood lipid levels in patients with cardiovascular risk factors: a meta-analysis of randomized controlled trials. Nutr J. 2017;16:68.

94. Panahi Y, Khalili N, Sahebi E, Namazi S, Reiner Z, Majeed M, et al. Curcuminoids modify lipid profile in type 2 diabetes mellitus: a randomized controlled trial. Complement Ther Med. 2017;33:1–5.

95. Salehi B, Del Prado-Audelo ML, Cortes H, Leyva-Gomez G, Stojanovic-Radic Z, Singh YD, et al. Therapeutic applications of curcumin nanomedicine formulations in cardiovascular diseases. J Clin Med. 2020;9(3):746.

96. Di Pierro F, Bressan A, Ranaldi D, Rapacioli G, Giacomelli L, Bertuccioli A. Potential role of bioavailable curcumin in weight loss and omental adipose tissue decrease: preliminary data of a randomized, controlled trial in overweight people with metabolic syndrome. Preliminary study. Eur Rev Med Pharmacol Sci. 2015;19:4195–202.

97. Patti AM, Al-Rasadi K, Katsiki N, Banerjee Y, Nikolic D, Vanella L, et al. Effect of a natural supplement containing Curcuma longa, guggul, and chlorogenic acid in patients with metabolic syndrome. Angiology. 2015;66:856–61.

98. Onakpoya I, Spencer E, Heneghan C, Thompson M. The effect of green tea on blood pressure and lipid profile: a systematic review and meta-analysis of randomized clinical trials. Nutr Metab Cardiovasc Dis. 2014;24:823–36.

99. Khalesi S, Sun J, Buys N, Jamshidi A, Nikbakht-Nasrabadi E, Khosravi-Boroujeni H. Green tea catechins and blood pressure: a systematic review and meta-analysis of randomised controlled trials. Eur J Nutr. 2014;53:1299–311.

100. Basu A, Sanchez K, Leyva MJ, Wu M, Betts NM, Aston CE, et al. Green tea supplementation affects body weight, lipids, and lipid peroxidation in obese subjects with metabolic syndrome. J Am Coll Nutr. 2010;29:31–40.

101. Chen X, He K, Wei C, Yang W, Geng Z. Green tea powder decreased egg weight through increased liver lipoprotein lipase and decreased plasma total cholesterol in an indigenous chicken breed. Animals (Basel). 2020;10(3):370.

102. Erba D, Riso P, Bordoni A, Foti P, Biagi PL, Testolin G. Effectiveness of moderate green tea consumption on antioxidative status and plasma lipid profile in humans. J Nutr Biochem. 2005;16:144–9.

103. Serban C, Sahebkar A, Antal D, Ursoniu S, Banach M. Effects of supplementation with green tea catechins on plasma C-reactive protein concentrations: a systematic review and meta-analysis of randomized controlled trials. Nutrition. 2015;31:1061–71.

104. Chacko SM, Thambi PT, Kuttan R, Nishigaki I. Beneficial effects of green tea: a literature review. Chin Med. 2010;5:13.

105. Mousavi A, Vafa M, Neyestani T, Khamseh M, Hoseini F. The effects of green tea consumption on metabolic and anthropometric indices in patients with Type 2 diabetes. J Res Med Sci. 2013;18:1080–6.
106. Giovinazzo G, Ingrosso I, Paradiso A, De Gara L, Santino A. Resveratrol biosynthesis: plant metabolic engineering for nutritional improvement of food. Plant Foods Hum Nutr. 2012;67:191–9.
107. Salehi B, Mishra AP, Nigam M, Sener B, Kilic M, Sharifi-Rad M, et al. Resveratrol: a double-edged sword in health benefits. Biomedicine. 2018;6(3):91.
108. Akbari M, Tamtaji OR, Lankarani KB, Tabrizi R, Dadgostar E, Haghighat N, et al. The effects of resveratrol on lipid profiles and liver enzymes in patients with metabolic syndrome and related disorders: a systematic review and meta-analysis of randomized controlled trials. Lipids Health Dis. 2020;19:25.
109. Simental-Mendia LE, Guerrero-Romero F. Effect of resveratrol supplementation on lipid profile in subjects with dyslipidemia: a randomized double-blind, placebo-controlled trial. Nutrition. 2019;58:7–10.
110. Christenson J, Whitby SJ, Mellor D, Thomas J, McKune A, Roach PD, et al. The effects of resveratrol supplementation in overweight and obese humans: a systematic review of randomized trials. Metab Syndr Relat Disord. 2016;14:323–33.
111. Jurgonski A, Juskiewicz J, Zdunczyk Z. Ingestion of black chokeberry fruit extract leads to intestinal and systemic changes in a rat model of prediabetes and hyperlipidemia. Plant Foods Hum Nutr. 2008;63:176–82.
112. Kowalczyk E, Fijalkowski P, Kura M, Krzesinski P, Blaszczyk J, Kowalski J, et al. The influence of anthocyanins from Aronia melanocarpa on selected parameters of oxidative stress and microelements contents in men with hypercholesterolemia. Pol Merkur Lekarski. 2005;19:651–3.
113. Castellino G, Nikolic D, Magan-Fernandez A, Malfa GA, Chianetta R, Patti AM, et al. Altilix((R)) supplement containing chlorogenic acid and luteolin improved hepatic and cardiometabolic parameters in subjects with metabolic syndrome: a 6 month randomized, double-blind, placebo-controlled study. Nutrients. 2019;11:11.
114. Sahebkar A, Pirro M, Banach M, Mikhailidis DP, Atkin SL, Cicero AFG. Lipid-lowering activity of artichoke extracts: a systematic review and meta-analysis. Crit Rev Food Sci Nutr. 2018;58:2549–56.
115. Anderson JW, Major AW. Pulses and lipaemia, short- and long-term effect: potential in the prevention of cardiovascular disease. Br J Nutr. 2002;88(Suppl 3):S263–71.
116. Bazzano LA, Thompson AM, Tees MT, Nguyen CH, Winham DM. Non-soy legume consumption lowers cholesterol levels: a meta-analysis of randomized controlled trials. Nutr Metab Cardiovasc Dis. 2011;21:94–103.
117. Afshin A, Micha R, Khatibzadeh S, Mozaffarian D. Consumption of nuts and legumes and risk of incident ischemic heart disease, stroke, and diabetes: a systematic review and meta-analysis. Am J Clin Nutr. 2014;100:278–88.
118. Aune D, Keum N, Giovannucci E, Fadnes LT, Boffetta P, Greenwood DC, et al. Whole grain consumption and risk of cardiovascular disease, cancer, and all cause and cause specific mortality: systematic review and dose-response meta-analysis of prospective studies. BMJ. 2016;353:i2716.
119. Chen GC, Tong X, Xu JY, Han SF, Wan ZX, Qin JB, et al. Whole-grain intake and total, cardiovascular, and cancer mortality: a systematic review and meta-analysis of prospective studies. Am J Clin Nutr. 2016;104:164–72.
120. Langley P. Why a pomegranate? BMJ. 2000;321:1153–4.
121. Gil MI, Tomas-Barberan FA, Hess-Pierce B, Holcroft DM, Kader AA. Antioxidant activity of pomegranate juice and its relationship with phenolic composition and processing. J Agric Food Chem. 2000;48:4581–9.
122. Stowe CB. The effects of pomegranate juice consumption on blood pressure and cardiovascular health. Complement Ther Clin Pract. 2011;17:113–5.

123. Aviram M, Dornfeld L. Pomegranate juice consumption inhibits serum angiotensin converting enzyme activity and reduces systolic blood pressure. Atherosclerosis. 2001;158:195–8.
124. Bogdanski P, Suliburska J, Szulinska M, Stepien M, Pupek-Musialik D, Jablecka A. Green tea extract reduces blood pressure, inflammatory biomarkers, and oxidative stress and improves parameters associated with insulin resistance in obese, hypertensive patients. Nutr Res. 2012;32:421–7.
125. Mikaili P, Maadirad S, Moloudizargari M, Aghajanshakeri S, Sarahroodi S. Therapeutic uses and pharmacological properties of garlic, shallot, and their biologically active compounds. Iran J Basic Med Sci. 2013;16:1031–48.
126. Sahebkar A, Serban C, Ursoniu S, Banach M. Effect of garlic on plasma lipoprotein(a) concentrations: a systematic review and meta-analysis of randomized controlled clinical trials. Nutrition. 2016;32:33–40.
127. Ried K, Fakler P. Potential of garlic (Allium sativum) in lowering high blood pressure: mechanisms of action and clinical relevance. Integr Blood Press Control. 2014;7:71–82.
128. Gomez-Arbelaez D, Lahera V, Oubina P, Valero-Munoz M, de Las Heras N, Rodriguez Y, et al. Aged garlic extract improves adiponectin levels in subjects with metabolic syndrome: a double-blind, placebo-controlled, randomized, crossover study. Mediat Inflamm. 2013;2013:285795.
129. Bayan L, Koulivand PH, Gorji A. Garlic: a review of potential therapeutic effects. Avicenna J Phytomed. 2014;4:1–14.
130. Houston M. The role of nutrition and nutraceutical supplements in the treatment of hypertension. World J Cardiol. 2014;6:38–66.
131. Zanetti M, Grillo A, Losurdo P, Panizon E, Mearelli F, Cattin L, et al. Omega-3 polyunsaturated fatty acids: structural and functional effects on the vascular wall. Biomed Res Int. 2015;2015:791978.
132. Corina A, Abrudan MB, Nikolic D, Ctoi AF, Chianetta R, Castellino G, et al. Effects of aging and diet on cardioprotection and cardiometabolic risk markers. Curr Pharm Des. 2019;25:3704–14.
133. Delgado-Lista J, Perez-Martinez P, Garcia-Rios A, Perez-Caballero AI, Perez-Jimenez F, Lopez-Miranda J. Mediterranean diet and cardiovascular risk: beyond traditional risk factors. Crit Rev Food Sci Nutr. 2016;56:788–801.
134. Chiva-Blanch G, Badimon L, Estruch R. Latest evidence of the effects of the Mediterranean diet in prevention of cardiovascular disease. Curr Atheroscler Rep. 2014;16:446.
135. Gotsis E, Anagnostis P, Mariolis A, Vlachou A, Katsiki N, Karagiannis A. Health benefits of the Mediterranean diet: an update of research over the last 5 years. Angiology. 2015;66:304–18.
136. Salvia R, D'Amore S, Graziano G, Capobianco C, Sangineto M, Paparella D, et al. Short-term benefits of an unrestricted-calorie traditional Mediterranean diet, modified with a reduced consumption of carbohydrates at evening, in overweight-obese patients. Int J Food Sci Nutr. 2017;68:234–48.
137. Liyanage T, Ninomiya T, Wang A, Neal B, Jun M, Wong MG, et al. Effects of the Mediterranean diet on cardiovascular outcomes – a systematic review and meta-analysis. PLoS One. 2016;11:e0159252.
138. Rosato V, Temple NJ, La Vecchia C, Castellan G, Tavani A, Guercio V. Mediterranean diet and cardiovascular disease: a systematic review and meta-analysis of observational studies. Eur J Nutr. 2019;58:173–91.
139. Grosso G, Marventano S, Yang J, Micek A, Pajak A, Scalfi L, et al. A comprehensive meta-analysis on evidence of Mediterranean diet and cardiovascular disease: are individual components equal? Crit Rev Food Sci Nutr. 2017;57:3218–32.
140. Estruch R, Ros E, Salas-Salvado J, Covas MI, Corella D, Aros F, et al. Retraction and republication: primary prevention of cardiovascular disease with a Mediterranean diet. N Engl J Med 2013;368:1279–90. N Engl J Med 2018; 378:2441–2.

141. Catapano AL, Reiner Z, De Backer G, Graham I, Taskinen MR, Wiklund O, et al. ESC/EAS guidelines for the management of dyslipidaemias The Task Force for the management of dyslipidaemias of the European Society of Cardiology (ESC) and the European Atherosclerosis Society (EAS). Atherosclerosis. 2011;217:3–46.
142. Anderson TJ, Gregoire J, Pearson GJ, Barry AR, Couture P, Dawes M, et al. Canadian Cardiovascular Society guidelines for the management of dyslipidemia for the prevention of cardiovascular disease in the adult. Can J Cardiol. 2016;32:1263–82.
143. Chamberlain JJ, Johnson EL, Leal S, Rhinehart AS, Shubrook JH, Peterson L. Cardiovascular disease and risk management: review of the American Diabetes Association Standards of Medical Care in Diabetes 2018. Ann Intern Med. 2018;168:640–50.
144. Garcia-Rios A, Perez-Martinez P, Delgado-Lista J, Lopez-Miranda J, Perez-Jimenez F. Nutrigenetics of the lipoprotein metabolism. Mol Nutr Food Res. 2012;56:171–83.
145. Gomez-Delgado F, Alcala-Diaz JF, Garcia-Rios A, Delgado-Lista J, Ortiz-Morales A, Rangel-Zuniga O, et al. Polymorphism at the TNF-alpha gene interacts with Mediterranean diet to influence triglyceride metabolism and inflammation status in metabolic syndrome patients: from the CORDIOPREV clinical trial. Mol Nutr Food Res. 2014;58:1519–27.
146. Perez-Martinez P, Mikhailidis DP, Athyros VG, Bullo M, Couture P, Covas MI, et al. Lifestyle recommendations for the prevention and management of metabolic syndrome: an international panel recommendation. Nutr Rev. 2017;75:307–26.

Chapter 6
Antihypertensive Nutraceuticals

José René Romano and Nicolas F. Renna

Introduction

Hypertension is the leading cause of preventable death in the world. The World Health Organization estimates that about 40% of people around the world have hypertension. These statistics are important because hypertension depends on health. The management of the disease and its complications involves the direct costs of health systems and substantial losses in productivity as a result of disability and premature mortality.

Hypertension is also an important risk factor for stroke, heart failure, coronary heart disease, diabetes and kidney disease. Not surprisingly, 55% of the 17 million deaths related to cardiovascular disease (CVD) are related to complications derived from hypertension.

However, there is hope. Hypertension is one of the most cost-effective and powerful conditions to treat. For example, reducing blood pressure has been linked to a 35–40% reduction in the risk of stroke and a 20–25% reduction in the risk of myocardial infarction and heart failure.

The costs of pharmacological treatment, are very high, are estimated for example in 2011, which in the United States were 156,000 million dollars, a global level of ECV is estimated at 906 million dollars in 2015 and is expected to increase in 22% by the year 2030.

J. R. Romano (✉)
Clínica Vrsalovic, Formosa, Argentina

Hospital Centraol de Formosa, Formosa, Argentina

N. F. Renna
Department of Cardiology, Spanish Hospital of Mendoza, Mendoza, Argentina

Laboratory of Cardiovascular Physiopathology, Department of Pathology, School of Medicine, National University of Cuyo, IMBECU-CONICET, Mendoza, Argentina

© Springer Nature Switzerland AG 2021
A. F.G. Cicero, M. Rizzo (eds.), *Nutraceuticals and Cardiovascular Disease*,
Contemporary Cardiology, https://doi.org/10.1007/978-3-030-62632-7_6

The adherence to pharmacological treatment is around 40% then 1 year of treatment. Not less fact is that it also takes into account the economic issue of each patient for the cost of medication. In addition, there is the issue of adverse effects that adherence to pharmacological treatment is reduced in a not lesser percentage, with some adverse effects being more important than others.

In this context, the non-pharmacological treatment, they are very important. The non-pharmacological measures are recommended indicated in all hypertensive patients, and there are including in all the guidelines of management of hypertension, including the new guide of European Society of Hypertension [1].

Clinical and Experimental Evidence in Hypertension

There is a lot medical literature about of the effect of nutraceuticals on cardiovascular disease. Nutraceutical was first defined by DeFelice in 1989 as "a food or part of a food that provides medical or health benefits, including the prevention and/or treatment of diseases." To be considered as such they must comply the following points: be products of natural origin, isolated and purified by nondenaturing methods, which provide beneficial effects for health: a) Improvement of one or more physiological functions; b) Preventive and/or curative action; c) Improvement of the quality of life. In addition, they must provide temporary stability and have reproducible studies of their bioactive properties in experimental animals and in humans, which provide reproducibility, quality, safety and efficacy.

The latter property is what we will try in this section. Beyond the known effects on blood pressure (BP) of dietary approaches to stop hypertension (DASH) and Mediterranean diets, a large number of studies have investigated the possible effect of BP reduction of different dietary and nutraceutical supplements. These are antioxidants with high safety and tolerability profile. In particular, the large body of evidence supports the use of potassium, L-arginine, vitamin C, flavonoids cocoa, beet juice, coenzyme Q10, controlled-release melatonin, different extracts of garlic and onion [2].

Oxidative stress, inflammation and autoimmunity vascular system are the main pathophysiological mechanisms and functional inducing disease [3–17]. The three are closely related. Process begins with endothelial dysfunction, contractile phenotype changes in vascular smooth muscle, hypertension and atherosclerosis with subsequent thrombosis.

The imbalance between radical oxygen species (ROS) and antioxidant defense mechanisms, such as nitric oxide, contributes to the etiology of hypertension in animals [5] and in humans [4, 6]. ROS are generated by multiple cellular sources, including NADPH oxidase, mitochondria, xanthine oxidase, NO synthase derived from the endothelium, cyclooxygenase and lipoxygenase [6]. In addition, several unique nucleotide polymorphisms (SNPs) are found in genes that encode antioxidant enzymes that are directly related to hypertension [17]. These include NADPH oxidase, xanthine oxidase, SOD 3 (superoxide dismutase), catalase, GPx 1 (glutathione peroxidase) and thioredoxin. Numerous epidemiological, observational and interventional studies have shown an increase in ROS production and a reduction in oxidative defense in hypertension in humans [7–9]. ROS directly damage endothelial cells, reduce the bioavailability of NO, modify the metabolism of eicosanoids, oxidize chol-LDL, proteins, carbohydrates, DNA and organic molecules, increase catecholamines, modify gene expression and transcription factors.

The link between inflammation and hypertension has been suggested in cross-sectional and longitudinal studies [12]. Increases in ultrasensitive CRP (hs-CRP), as well as other inflammatory cytokines, occur in hypertension and damage to the target organ related to hypertension, such as increased carotid intima and media thickness (IMT) [13]. Some authors have also suggested different mechanisms that can explain this link, for example, the IL-6 pathway [18] or inflammasomes.

Nutraceuticals

Coconut Oil, Olive Oil or Butter

A recent publication shows that from a 1-year, randomized clinical study, none of these three components of the diet had significant differences among themselves, on blood pressure, weight, central obesity or other cardiovascular risk factors. 50 g daily of one of these three natural fat sources, showed significant changes in LDL-cholesterol, HDL-coly ratio TC/HDL-chol, for coconut oil. Another relevant study is the PREDIMED, a prospective study that managed to reduce cardiovascular events by rabbling extra virgin olive oil against an aggregate of nuts. It also had no effect on blood pressure. [19, 20].

Garlic

Garlic reduces BP by approximately 8.4/7.3 mmHg in meta-analysis reviews [21, 22]. Different compounds derived from raw garlic were investigated in different experimental models: aqueous extract, oily extract, aged garlic and cooked garlic enriched. Together, these derivatives have variables effects [21–26] Garlic showed efficacy even in resistant hypertensive patients [27]. Given the high variability of studies and results, for this compound the authors agree that better-developed studies are needed before reaching any conclusion.

Among the effects found, which could have an anti-hypertensive effect, were ACEI activity, blocking activity of calcium channels, reduction in sensitivity to catecholamines, improved arterial compliance, increases bradykinin and NO, and adenosine, magnesium, flavonoids, sulfur, allicin and phosphorus that reduce BP [23–25].

Ω-3 Polyunsaturated Fatty Acids (FA)

The omega-3 polyunsaturated fatty acids significantly decrease BP in human trials [28–32]. Not all compounds have been shown to be equally effective, for example, docosahexaenoic acid (DHA) is more effective in reducing BP and HR than eicosapentaenoic acid (EPA) [33]. In patients with chronic kidney disease, 4 g of Ω-3 FA reduced BP measured in the 24-h outpatient setting for 8 weeks compared to placebo ($p < 0.0001$) [30, 34].

The authors proposed different mechanism for this effect is that fatty acids Ω-3 FA improve endothelial dysfunction, reduce plasma norepinephrine and increase the tone of the parasympathetic nervous system, suppress ACE activity and improve insulin resistance [35]. The daily dose it is found between 3000–5000 mg per day of DHA and EPA combined in a ratio of 2: 3 [36].

Ω-9 FA

Olive oil, a monounsaturated fatty acid (MUFA), reduces BP [37, 38]. Olive oil and monounsaturated fats have shown consistent reductions in BP in most clinical trials in humans [37–41]. Extra virgin olive oil was more effective than sunflower oil in reducing SBP in a group of 31 elderly hypertensive patients in a double-blind randomized trial, even in diabetic subjects [39, 40].

Vitamin C

The concentration of vitamin C or plasma ascorbate in humans correlates inversely with blood pressure and heart rate [42–51] and a reduced risk of CVD and stroke [45].

An evaluation of published clinical trials suggests that doses of vitamin C 250 mg twice daily reduces the PA at 7.4 mmHg [42–51]. The proposed mechanism was an increase in diuresis of water and sodium, improves endothelial function, increases NO and PGI2, superoxide dismutase will increase, aortic elasticity will improve. Some studies report that vitamin C improves the efficacy of amlodipine, decreases the binding affinity of AT1R for A-II by interrupting the disulfide bridges of AT1R and lowers BP in the elderly with refractory hypertension [23, 24, 46–51].

Vitamin E

The relationship between vitamin E and BP has been very inconsistent, but most studies have shown no reductions in BP with most forms of tocopherols or tocotrienols [23–25].

Vitamin D

Plasma levels of vitamin D3 are associated with BP [52–63]. Vitamin D3 regulates the renin-angiotensin-aldosterone system [53]. If the level of vitamin D is below 30 ng/ml, the levels of circulating PRA are higher, which increases the A-II, increases the BP and attenuates the plasma renal blood flow (74 h). The lower the level of vitamin D3, the higher the risk of incident hypertension, with the lowest serum quartile. Vitamin D3 has a 52% incidence of hypertension versus the highest quartile with an incidence of 20%. [62]. It also reduces ADMA, suppresses proinflammatory cytokines such as TNF-α, increases NO, improves endothelial function and arterial elasticity, reduces hypertrophy of vascular smooth muscle, regulates electrolytes and blood volume, increases insulin sensitivity, reduces the concentration of free FA, regulates the expression of the natriuretic peptide receptor and reduces hs-CRP [55–62].

Vitamin B6

Low levels of vitamin B6 (pyridoxine) in serum are associated with hypertension in humans [64]. Vitamin B6 is a cofactor in the synthesis of neurotransmitters and hormones in the CNS, increases the synthesis of cysteine to neutralize aldehydes, increases the production of glutathione, blocks calcium channels, improves insulin resistance, reduces sympathetic tone central and reduces the response capacity of the final organ to glucocorticoids and mineralocorticoids [23]. Vitamin B6 has an action similar to that of central agonists, diuretics and CCBs. The therapeutical dose is 200 mg per day orally by supplementation.

Tea: Green and Black

The effects of chronic consumption of green or black tea in PA are inconsistent in humans [65].

Seaweed

The wakame seaweed (a natural food, not a supplement) at 3.3 g of dry wakame for 1 month reduced BP [66]. In one study, men with mild hypertension who received a seaweed preparation, mean arterial blood pressure decreased by 11.2 mmHg (p < 0.001) [67].

Seaweed and sea vegetables contain 77 minerals, fiber and alginate in colloidal form [68–70]. Wakame contains ACEIs of several amino acid peptides [71–73].

Healthy Effects of Moderate Red Wine Consumption

Epidemiological studies have shown a protective effect of moderate consumption of red wine (RW) on cardiovascular disease, attributed to the antioxidant properties of polyphenols that this beverage contains.

Since the publication of Drs. Renaud and De Lorgeril on the moderate consumption of red wine have been published more than 1000 articles in medical journals, with a growing interest in recent years. This study published in the prestigious journal *The Lancet* on June 20, 1992, described the MONICA project, a cardiovascular disease monitoring system organized by the World Health Organization, where it shows that cardiovascular diseases are the leading cause of death worldwide, especially in industrialized countries, except in France. This finding was called "French paradox".

This inverse relationship between the moderate consumption of red wine and cardiovascular disease is maintained between 30–50 g of alcohol, that is, approximately 2 glasses of wine per day. In amounts greater than this, these benefits disappear, demonstrating a characteristic pattern of J-shaped curve between dose and risk.

Along with evidence of the harmful effects of excess alcohol, there is a large number of scientific articles that conclude that moderate consumption can be beneficial. A work published in 2012 in the scientific journal *British Medical Journal* (BMJ) estimated that half a glass of wine a day was the optimal amount to protect health. Drinking up to this amount could prevent more than 4500 deaths per year in the United Kingdom, according to the researchers who performed that analysis.

Emanuel Rubin, of the Thomas Jefferson University of Philadelphia (USA), stated in an article recently published in Alcoholism: Clinical and Experimental Research, that "the overwhelming evidence suggests that doctors should advise those who have never drank in their life to enter 40 and 50 relax and have a drink a day, preferably with dinner. ".

Even so, the evidence points to the fact that wine is a perfect product, which maintains the balance between dose effect, of any of these components, which is demonstrated because none of them, administered separately, achieve such favorable effects as drinking as a whole.

Red wine, consumed in moderation, has been considered healthy for the heart. Alcohol and certain substances in red wine, known for their antioxidant effects, can help prevent coronary artery disease, the condition that leads to heart attacks.

Any link between red wine and fewer heart attacks is not fully understood. But part of the benefit could be that antioxidants can increase the levels of cholesterol associated with high density lipoprotein (HDL) (the "good" cholesterol) and protect against the accumulation of cholesterol, as well as protect against damage to cellular structures caused by oxidizing chemical species that are continuously produced in the body.

While news about red wine may sound good if you enjoy a glass of red wine with dinner, doctors are wary of encouraging anyone to start drinking alcohol, especially if they have a family history of alcohol abuse. Too much alcohol can have many harmful effects on your body.

Still, many doctors agree that something in red wine seems to help your heart. Antioxidants, such as flavonoids or a substance called resveratrol, may have heart-healthy benefits. [74–78].

Flavonoids

The more than 4000 flavonoids in fruits, vegetables, red wine, tea, soy and licorice can lower BP [76, 77, 79, 80].

Lycopene

Lycopene (carotenoid) reduces BP [81–85]. The treated hypertensive patients reduced BP when given a standardized tomato extract [83]. Other studies have shown no change in BP with lycopene. The recommended daily intake of lycopene is 10 to 20 mg as a food or supplement.

Coenzyme Q10

Coenzyme Q-10 (Co-Q-10, ubiquinone) is a potent antioxidant in the lipid phase, eliminates free radicals, reduces oxidative stress, regenerates other vitamins and antioxidants, reduces oxidation of LDL and is a cofactor and coenzyme in the mitochondrial oxidant. Phosphorylation that decreases BP [23, 33, 86, 87].

Serum levels of Co-Q-10 are lower in patients with hypertension [24, 25]. Enzymatic assays showed a deficiency of Co-Q-10 in 39% of the 59 patients with essential hypertension versus a deficiency of only 6% in the controls (p < 0.01), oral administration of 100–225 mg a day proved to be effective [88].

However, more data is needed on the long-term safety of a large part of the products mentioned above. In addition, it is advisable to conduct additional clinical investigations.

ALA

ALA is an antioxidant thiol compound that is soluble in both water and lipids, which recirculates other vitamins and antioxidants such as vitamins C and E, glutathione and cysteine [23, 88, 89]. ALA also binds to endogenous aldehydes and provides sulfhydryl groups that help close vascular calcium channels, lower RVS and BPR.

In the QUALITY study, 40 subjects with DM and stage I hypertension were randomized to 40 mg of quinapril per day for 8 weeks or 40 mg of quinapril per day with 600 mg of lipoic acid per day [90]. The excretion of albumin in urine decreased by 30% with quinapril alone and by 53% with the combination of quinapril and lipoic acid (p < 0.005). Fluid-mediated vasodilation increased 58% with quinapril alone and 116% the combination of quinapril and lipoic acid (p < 0.005). BP was significantly reduced in both groups by 10%. However, another study showed no changes in supine BP or pulse wave velocity with 1200 mg of ALA for 8 weeks [91].

The recommended dose is 100–200 mg per day of (R) -lipoic acid with biotin 2–4 mg per day to prevent the depletion of biotin with long-term use of lipoic acid. The (R) -lipoic acid is preferred to the l-isomer due to its preferred use by mitochondria.

L-Arginine

L-arginine and endogenous methylarginines are precursors of NO, mediated by the conversion of L-arginine to NO by eNOS. L-arginine reduces vascular tone, improves coronary artery blood flow, decreases angina, reduces the symptoms of peripheral artery disease, and lowers BP [92–94].

Numerous studies demonstrate an antihypertensive effect of arginine that is similar to that of the DASH I diet [92–98]. BP decreased by 6.2/6.8 mmHg with 10 g per day of l-arginine when it was provided as a supplement or through natural foods to a group of hypertensive subjects. A study of 54 hypertensive subjects who were administered arginine 4 g three times a day for 4 weeks had significant reductions in average blood pressure values of 24 h in one in ambulatory monotherapy [98]. Arginine is recommended for the treatment of hypertension.

Black Chocolate and Cocoa

It has been shown that dark chocolate (100 g) and cocoa with a high polyphenol content (≥30 mg) significantly reduce BP in humans [99–102]. A meta-analysis of 173 hypertensive subjects who were given cocoa for a mean duration of 2 weeks had a significant reduction in BP. Two more recent meta-analyzes of 13 trials and ten trials involving 297 patients found a significant reduction in BP of 3.2/2.0 mmHg and 4.5/3.2 mmHg, respectively [103, 104].

Sesame

Sesame has been shown to reduce BP in several small, randomized, placebo-controlled studies for 30–60 days [105, 106]. It also reduces BP with different anti-hypertensives. Sesame is recommended as a food or as a supplement in the revised forms.

Melatonin

Melatonin demonstrates significant antihypertensive effects in humans in numerous randomized, placebo-controlled, double-blind clinical trials [68–70, 107–111]. Melatonin at 2.5 mg per night for 3 weeks, in a group of 16 hypertensive men, decreased nocturnal BP and reduced the day/night amplitudes of SBP and BPD [107]. Hypertensive patients have altered the function of the circadian pacemaker, have altered the autonomic cardiovascular regulation with a sympathetic and para-sympathetic tone dull from day to night, are the most benefited with this treatment. Beta blockers reduce the secretion of melatonin [111].

Chlorogenic Acids and Green Coffee Bean Extract

Polyphenols, chlorogenic acids (CGA), the ferulic acid metabolite of CGA and di-hydro-caffeine acids decrease BP in a dose-dependent manner, increase eNOS and improve endothelial function in humans [112–117]. The CGAs in the green coffee bean extract at a dose of 140 mg per day significantly reduced SBP and DBP in 28 subjects in a randomized placebo-controlled trial [117]. A study of 122 male subjects demonstrated a dose response in SBP and BPD with a CGA dose of 46–185 mg per day. Another component of coffee beans, hydroxy-hydroquinone, reduces the effectiveness of the CGA in a dose-dependent manner, which partly explains the conflicting results of coffee intake in the BP [116, 117].

Other Various Compounds

Several other nutraceutical compounds have preliminary evidence of modest reductions in BP in humans, including hesperidin, pomegranate juice, grape seed extract and hawthorne [118–124]. Hesperidin significantly reduced BPD and improved microvascular endothelial reactivity in 24 obese male hypertensive subjects in a randomized controlled crossover study for 4 weeks for each of the three treatment groups, consuming 500 ml of orange juice, hesperidin or placebo [118] Pomegranate juice reduces SBP by 5–12%, reduces the activity of ACE in serum by 36% and has anti-atherogenic, antioxidant and anti-inflammatory effects [120–122]. Grape seed extract (GSE) was administered to subjects in nine randomized trials, meta-analysis of 390 subjects and demonstrated a significant reduction in SBP of 1.54 mmHg ($p < 0.02$) [249]. The Hawthorne extract demonstrated limit reductions in BP and significantly reduced DBP ($p < 0.035$) in diabetic patients who took antihypertensive medications at a dose of 1200 mg per day of hawthorn extract [124]. More controlled studies in humans are needed to confirm these initial findings with all compounds.

Conclusions

Where herbals, dietary supplements and functional foods are sold in many different venues outside pharmacies (e.g. in supermarkets, herbalist shops etc.), nutraceuticals are essentially sold in pharmacies and parapharmacies in drug form with a claim to having drug properties. Furthermore one bigger, attractive and sometimes dangerous increasing market is via the Internet. Here, some companies looking to create a wide profit margin may create unregulated products with low-quality or ineffective ingredients.

The medicalisation of today's society and the alleged favourable outcomes with low side effects of such productsi have also lead to the increase in the consumption of these products. Moreover the high cost of prescribing pharmaceuticals and the reluctance of some insurance companies and health national systems to cover the costs of drugs, help nutraceuticals to solidify their presence in the global market of therapies and therapeutic agents. According to CORDIS - the information service of the European Commission for research and development of science – nutraceuticals in 2008 had a European turnover of approximately 1.4 billion Euros in 2008 with an 11% growth compared to the preceding year. Many pharmaceutical and biotechnology companies, detecting good business opportunities, have invested heavily in the nutraceutical sector to create a market that aims to cover 5% of the value of food sales worldwide.

The FDA considers a medical food "to be formulated, consumed or administered internally under the supervision of a physician, and one which is intended for the specific dietary management of a disease or condition for which distinctive nutritional requirements, on the basis of recognised scientific principles, are established by medical evaluation."

In 2000, the European Commission published five horizontal framework directives which identified requirements of public health and safety, consumer information and general food control measurements. The five directives regard: (1) Food labelling and presentation (2) Food additives (3) Materials and articles in contact with food (4) Official control of food stuffs (5) Food for particular nutritional uses (PARNUTS).

In other words, there are a lot of regulations and, there is not, as such, a regulatory framework for 'functional foods' or 'nutraceuticals' in EU food law.

This is why doctors and members of the medical community are asking for the term "nutraceutical" to be clearly defined in order to distinguish the wide varieties of products out there.

However, with all of the aforementioned positive points, nutraceuticals still need support of an extensive scientific study to prove "their effects with reduced side effects." Issues of study quality and bias, true efficacy and toxicity continue to cause uncertainty. The accumulated knowledge regarding nutraceuticals needs to be validated and this need represents a great challenge for many professionals such as nutritionists, physicians, food technologists and food chemists. Only after this process is completed can public health authorities consider prevention and treatment with nutraceuticals as a powerful, natural, and inexpensive tool for the prevention of disease and in maintaining health.

Where herbals, dietary supplements and functional foods are sold in many different venues outside pharmacies (e.g. in supermarkets, herbalist shops etc.), nutraceuticals are essentially sold in pharmacies and parapharmacies in drug form with a claim to having drug properties. Furthermore, one bigger, attractive and sometimes dangerous increasing market is via the Internet. Here, some companies looking to create a wide profit margin may create unregulated products with low-quality or ineffective ingredients. The medicalisation of today's society and the alleged favorable outcomes with low side effects of such products have also lead to the increase in the consumption of these products. Moreover, the high cost of prescribing pharmaceuticals and the reluctance of some insurance companies and health national systems to cover the costs of drugs, help nutraceuticals to solidify their presence in the global market of therapies and therapeutic agents.

In conclusion, we need to pay more attention to nutraceuticals, as well as improved taxonomy, further regulation and the introduction of registers and national surveys to acquire knowledge of today's consumption and indications. More controlled studies will give the scientific evidence essential for the administration of nutraceuticals both in prevention and as therapy for cardiovascular disease. The study and regulation of nutritional genomics might lead to the use of nutraceuticals as an alternative to stem cell transplantation, and would enable the targeting of optimal nutritional advice and the development of food-derived treatments by new nutraceuticals for best treatment, in particular, for uses in groups with cardiovascular risk and individuals with cardiovascular disease.

Bibliography

1. World Health Organization and World Economic Forum. From Burden to "Best Buys": Reducing the economic impact of non-communicable diseases in low- and middle-income countries. Geneva: World Health Organization and World Economic Forum; 2011. http://www.who.int/nmh/publications/best_buys_summary
2. Nayak DU, Karmen C, Frishman WH, Vakili BA. Antioxidant vitamins and enzymatic and synthetic oxygen-derived free radical scavengers in the prevention and treatment of cardiovascular disease. Heart Dis. 2001;3:28–45.
3. Kitiyakara C, Wilcox C. Antioxidants for hypertension. Curr Opin Nephrol Hypertens. 1998;7:531–8.
4. Russo C, Olivieri O, Girelli D, et al. Antioxidant status and lipid peroxidation in patients with essential hypertension. J Hypertens. 1998;16:1267–71.
5. Galley HF, Thornton J, Howdle PD, Walker BE, Webster NR. Combination oral antioxidant supplementation reduces blood pressure. Clin Sci. 1997;92:361–5.
6. Dhalla NS, Temsah RM, Netticadam T. The role of oxidative stress in cardiovascular diseases. J Hypertens. 2000;18:655–73.
7. Saez G, Tormos MC, Giner V, Lorano JV, Chaves FJ. Oxidative stress and enzymatic antioxidant mechanisms in essential hypertension. Am J Hypertens. 2001;14:248A. (Abstract P-653).
8. Ghanem FA, Movahed A. Inflammation in high blood pressure: a clinician perspective. J Am Soc Hypertens. 2007;1(2):113–9.
9. Amer MS, Elawam AE, Khater MS, Omar OH, Mabrouk RA, Taha HM. Association of high-sensitivity C reactive protein with carotid artery intima media thickness in hypertensive older adults. J Am Soc Hypertens. 2011;5(5):395–400.
10. Kvakan H, Luft FC, Muller DN. Role of the immune system in hypertensive target organ damage. Trends Cardiovasc Med. 2009;19(7):242–6.
11. Rodriquez-Iturbe B, Franco M, Tapia E, Quiroz Y, Johnson RJ. Renal inflammation, autoimmunity and salt-sensitive hypertension. Clin Exp Pharmacol Physiol. 2012;39(1):96–103.
12. Mansego ML, Solar Gde M, Alonso MP, et al. Polymorphisms of antioxidant enzymes, blood pressure and risk of hypertension. J Hypertens. 2011;29(3):492–500.
13. Vongpatanasin W, Thomas GD, Schwartz R, et al. C-reactive protein causes downregulation of vascular angiotensin subtype 2 receptors and systolic hypertension in mice. Circulation. 2007;115(8):1020–8.
14. Renna NF, de Las Heras N, Miatello RM. Pathophysiology of vascular remodeling in hypertension. Int J Hypertens. 2013;2013:808353.
15. Renna NF, Lembo C, Diez E, Miatello RM Role of Renin-Angiotensin system and oxidative stress on vascular inflammation in insulin resistence model. Int J Hypertens. 2013;2013:420979
16. Renna NF. Oxidative stress, vascular remodeling, and vascular inflammation in hypertension. Int J Hypertens. 2013;2013:710136.
17. Khaw K, Sharp SJ, Finikarides L, Afzal I, Lentjes M, Luben R, Forouhi NG. Randomised trial of coconut oil, olive oil or butter on blood lipids and other cardiovascular risk factors in healthy men and women. BMJ Open. 2018;8:e020167.
18. Estruch R, Ros E, Salas-Salvadó J, et al. Primary prevention of cardiovascular disease with a Mediterranean diet. N Engl J Med. 2013;368:1279–90.
19. Houston MC. Treatment of hypertension with nutraceuticals. Vitamins, antioxidants and minerals. Expert Rev Cardiovasc Ther. 2007;5(4):681–91.
20. Houston MC. Nutraceuticals, vitamins, antioxidants and mineral in the prevention and treatment of hypertension. Prog Cardiovasc Dis. 2005;47(6):396–449.
21. Reid K, Frank OR, Stocks NP. Aged garlic extract lowers blood pressure in patients with treated but uncontrolled hypertension: a randomized controlled trial. Maturitas. 2010;67(2):144–50.

22. Mori TA, Bao DQ, Burke V, Puddey IB, Beilin LJ. Docosahexaenoic acid but not eicosapentaenoic acid lowers ambulatory blood pressure and heart rate in humans. Hypertension. 1999;34:253–60.
23. Houston MC. Nutrition and nutraceutical supplements in the treatment of hypertension. Expert Rev Cardiovasc Ther. 2010;8(6):821–33.
24. Vazquez-Prieto MA, González RE, Renna NF, Galmarini CR, Miatello RM. Aqueous garlic extracts prevent oxidative stress and vascular remodeling in an experimental model of metabolic syndrome. J Agric Food Chem. 2010;58(11):6630–5. https://doi.org/10.1021/jf1006819.
25. Simons S, Wollersheim H, Thien T. A systematic review on the influence of trial quality on the effects of garlic on blood pressure. Neth J Med. 2009;67(6):212–9.
26. Reinhard KM, Coleman CI, Teevan C, Vacchani P. Effects of garlic on blood pressure in patients with and without systolic hypertension: a meta-analysis. Ann Pharmacother. 2008;42(12):1766–71.
27. Bønaa KH, Bjerve KS, Straume B, Gram IT, Thelle D. Effect of eicosapentaenoic and docosahexanoic acids on blood pressure in hypertension: a population-based intervention trial from the Tromso study. N Engl J Med. 1990;322:795–801.
28. Mori TA, Burke V, Puddey I, Irish A. The effects of omega 3 fatty acids and coenzyme q 10 on blood pressure and heart rate in chronic kidney disease: a randomized controlled trial. J Hypertens. 2009;27(9):1863–72.
29. Ueshima H, Stamler J, Elliot B, Brown CQ. Food omega 3 fatty acid intake of individuals (total, linolenic acid, long chain) and their blood pressure: INTERMAP study. Hypertension. 2007;50(20):313–9.
30. Mon TA. Omega3 fatty acids and hypertension in humans. Clin Exp Pharmacol Physiol. 2006;33(9):842–6.
31. Eaton SB, Eaton SB 3rd, Konner MJ. Paleolithic nutrition revisited: a twelve-year retrospective on its nature and implications. Eur J Clin Nutr. 1997;51:207–16.
32. Chin JP. Marine oils and cardiovascular reactivity. Prostaglandins Leukot Essent Fatty Acids. 1994;50:211–22.
33. Burke BE, Neustenschwander R, Olson RD. Randomized, double-blind, placebo- controlled trial of coenzyme Q10 in isolated systolic hypertension. South Med J. 2001;94:1112–7.
34. Saravanan P, Davidson NC, Schmidt EB, Calder PC. Cardiovascular effects of marine omega-3 fatty acids. Lancet. 2010;376(9740):540–50.
35. Ferrara LA, Raimondi S, d'Episcopa I. Olive oil and reduced need for antihypertensive medications. Arch Intern Med. 2000;160:837–42.
36. Thomsen C, Rasmussen OW, Hansen KW, Vesterlund M, Hermansen K. Comparison of the effects on the diurnal blood pressure, glucose, and lipid levels of a diet rich in monounsaturated fatty acids with a diet rich in polyunsaturated fatty acids in Type 2 diabetic subjects. Diabet Med. 1995;12:600–6.
37. Perona JS, Canizares J, Montero E, Sanchez-Dominquez JM, Catala A, Ruiz-Gutierrez V. Virgin olive oil reduces blood pressure in hypertensive elderly patients. Clin Nutr. 2004;23(5):1113–21.
38. Perona JS, Montero E, Sanchez-Dominquez JM, Canizares J, Garcia M, Ruiz-Gutierrez V. Evaluation of the effect of dietary virgin olive oil on blood pressure and lipid composition of serum and low-density lipoprotein in elderly type 2 subjects. J Agric Food Chem. 2009;57(23):11427–33.
39. Lopez-Miranda J, Perez-Jimenez F, Ros E, et al. Olive oil and health: summary of the II international conference on olive oil and health consensus report, Jaen and Cordoba (Spain) 2008. Nutr Metab Cardiovasc Dis. 2010;20(4):284–94.
40. Sherman DL, Keaney JF, Biegelsen ES, et al. Pharmacological concentrations of ascorbic acid are required for the beneficial effect on endothelial vasomotor function in hypertension. Hypertension. 2000;35:936–41.
41. Ness AR, Khaw KT, Bingham S, Day NE. Vitamin C status and blood pressure. J Hypertens. 1996;14:503–8.

42. Duffy SJ, Bokce N, Holbrook M. Treatment of hypertension with ascorbic acid. Lancet. 1999;354:2048–9.
43. Enstrom JE, Kanim LE, Klein M. Vitamin C intake and mortality among a sample of the United States population. Epidemiology. 1992;3:194–202.
44. Block G, Jensen CD, Norkus EP, Hudes M, Crawford PB. Vitamin C in plasma is inversely related to blood pressure and change in blood pressure during the previous year in young black and white women. Nutr J. 2008;17(7):35–46.
45. Hatzitolios A, Iliadis F, Katsiki N, Baltatzi M. Is the antihypertensive effect of dietary supplements via aldehydes reduction evidence based? A systematic review. Clin Exp Hypertens. 2008;30(7):628–39.
46. Mahajan AS, Babbar R, Kansai N, Agarwai SK, Ray PC. Antihypertensive and antioxidant action of amlodipine and vitamin C in patients of essential hypertension. J Clin Biochem Nutr. 2007;40(2):141–7.
47. Ledlerc PC, Proulx CD, Arquin G, Belanger S. Ascorbic acid decreases the binding affinity of the AT! Receptor for angiotensin II. Am J Hypertens. 2008;21(1):67–71.
48. Plantinga Y, Ghiadone L, Magagna A, Biannarelli C. Supplementation with vitamins C and E improves arterial stiffness and endothelial function in essential hypertensive patients. Am J Hypertens. 2007;20(4):392–7.
49. Sato K, Dohi Y, Kojima M, Miyagawa K. Effects of ascorbic acid on ambulatory blood pressure in elderly patients with refractory hypertension. Arzneimittelforschung. 2006;56(7):535–40.
50. Hanni LL, Huarfner LH, Sorensen OH, Ljunghall S. Vitamin D is related to blood pressure and other cardiovascular risk factors in middle-aged men. Am J Hypertens. 1995;8:894–901.
51. Bednarski R, Donderski R, Manitius L. Role of vitamin D in arterial blood pressure control. Pol Merkur Lekarski. 2007;136:307–10.
52. Li YC, Kong H, Wei M, Chen ZF. 1,25 dihydroxyvitamin D 3 is a negative endocrine regulator of the renin angiotensin system. J Clin Invest. 2002;110(2):229–38.
53. Ngo DT, Sverdlov AL, McNeil JJ, Horowitz JD. Does vitamin D modulate asymmetric dimethylargine and C-reactive protein concentrations? Am. J Med. 2010;123(4):335–41.
54. Rosen CJ. Clinical practice. Vitamin D insufficiency. N Engl J Med. 2011;364(3):248–54.
55. Boldo A, Campbell P, Luthra P, White WB. Should the concentration of vitamin D be measured in all patients with hypertension? J Clin Hypertens. 2010;12(3):149–52.
56. Pittas AG, Chung M, Trikalinos T, et al. Systematic review: vitamin D and cardiometabolic outcomes. Ann Intern Med. 2010;152(5):307–14.
57. Movano Peregrin C, Lopez Rodriguez R, Castilla Castellano MD. Vitamin D and hypertension. Med Clin (Barc). 2011;138(9):397–401.
58. Motiwala SR, Want TJ. Vitamin D and cardiovascular disease. Curr Opin Nephrol Hypertens. 2011;20(4):345–53.
59. Cosenso-Martin LN, Vitela-Martin JF. Is there an association between vitamin D and hypertension? Recent Pat Cardiovasc Drug Discov. 2011;6(2):140–7.
60. Bhandari SK, Pashayan S, Liu IL, et al. 25-hydroxyvitamin D levels and hypertension rates. J Clin Hypertens. 2011;13(3):170–7.
61. Pfeifer M, Begerow B, Minne HW, Nachtigall D, Hansen C. Effects of a short- term vitamin D(3) and calcium supplementation on blood pressure and parathyroid hormone levels in elderly women. J Clin Endocrinol Metab. 2001;86:1633–7.
62. Keniston R, Enriquez JI Sr. Relationship between blood pressure and plasma vitamin B6 levels in healthy middle-aged adults. Ann N Y Acad Sci. 1990;585:499–501.
63. Wahabi HA, Alansary LA, Al-Sabban AH, Glasziuo P. The effectiveness of Hibiscus Sabdariffa in the treatment of hypertension: a systematic review. Phytomedicine. 2010;17(2):83–6.
64. Nakano T, Hidaka H, Uchida J, Nakajima K, Hata Y. Hypotensive effects of wakame. J Jpn Soc Clin Nutr. 1998;20:92.
65. Krotkiewski M, Aurell M, Holm G, Grimby G, Szckepanik J. Effects of a sodium- potassium ion-exchanging seaweed preparation in mild hypertension. Am J Hypertens. 1991;4:483–8.
66. Suetsuna K, Nakano T. Identification of an antihypertensive peptide from peptic digest of wakame (Undaria pinnatifida). J Nutr Biochem. 2000;11:450–4.

67. Sato M, Oba T, Yamaguchi T, et al. Antihypertensive effects of hydrolysates of wakame (Undaria pinnatifida) and their angiotnesin-1-converting inhibitory activity. Ann Nutr Metab. 2002;46(6):259–67.
68. Rechcinski T, Kurpese M, Trzoa E, Krzeminska-Pakula M. The influence of melatonin supplementation on circadian pattern of blood pressure in patients with coronary artery disease-preliminary report. Pol Arch Med Wewn. 2006;115(6):520–8.
69. Merkureva GA, Ryzhak GA. Effect of the pineal gland peptide preparation on the diurnal profile of arterial pressure in middleaged and elderly women with ischemic heart disease and arterial hypertension. Adv Gerontol. 2008;21(1):132–42.
70. Zaslavskaia RM, Scherban EA, Logvinenki SI. Melatonin in combined therapy of patients with stable angina and arterial hypertension. Klin Med (Mosk). 2009;86:64–7.
71. Sato M, Hosokawa T, Yamaguchi T, et al. Angiotensin I converting enzymeinhibitory peptide derived from wakame (Undaria pinnatifida) and their antihypertensive effect in spontaneously hypertensive rats. J Agric Food Chem. 2002;50(21):6245–52.
72. Rodriguez Lanzi C, Perdicaro DJ, Antoniolli A, Fontana AR, Miatello RM, Bottini R, Vazquez Prieto MA. Grape pomace and grape pomace extract improve insulin signaling in high-fat-fructose fed rat-induced metabolic syndrome. Food Funct. 2016;7(3):1544–53.
73. Rodriguez Lanzi C, de Rosas I, Perdicaro DJ, Ponce MT, Martinez L, Miatello RM, Cavagnaro B, Vazquez Prieto MA. Effects of salicylic acid-induced wine rich in anthocyanins on metabolic parameters and adipose insulin signaling in high-fructose fed rats. Int J Food Sci Nutr. 2016;67(8):969–76.
74. Galleano M, Calabro V, Prince PD, Litterio MC, Piotrkowski B, Vazquez-Prieto MA, Miatello RM, Oteiza PI, Fraga CG. Flavonoids and metabolic syndrome. Ann N Y Acad Sci. 2012;1259:87–94.
75. Vazquez-Prieto MA, Renna NF, Diez ER, Cacciamani V, Lembo C, Miatello RM. Effect of red wine on adipocytokine expression and vascular alterations in fructose-fed rats. Am J Hypertens. 2011;24(2):234–40.
76. Vazquez-Prieto MA, Renna NF, Lembo C, Diez ER, Miatello RM. Dealcoholized red wine reverse vascular remodeling in an experimental model of metabolic syndrome: role of NAD(P)H oxidase and eNOS activity. Food Funct. 2010;1(1):124–9.
77. Moline J, Bukharovich IF, Wolff MS, Phillips R. Dietary flavonoids and hypertension: is there a link? Med Hypotheses. 2000;55:306–9.
78. Knekt P, Reunanen A, Järvinen R, Seppänen R, Heliövaara M, Aromaa A. Antioxidant vitamin intake and coronary mortality in a longitudinal population study. Am J Epidemiol. 1994;139:1180–9.
79. Paran E, Engelhard YN. Effect of lycopene, an oral natural antioxidant on blood pressure. J Hypertens. 2001;19:S74.
80. Engelhard YN, Gazer B, Paran E. Natural antioxidants from tomato extract reduce blood pressure in patients with grade-1 hypertension: a double blind placebo controlled pilot study. Am Heart J. 2006;151(1):100.
81. Paran E, Novac C, Engelhard YN, Hazan-Halevy I. The effects of natural antioxidants form tomato extract in treated but uncontrolled hypertensive patients. Cardiovasc Drugs Ther. 2009;23(2):145–51.
82. Reid K, Frank OR, Stocks NP. Dark chocolate or tomato extract for prehypertension: a randomized controlled trial. BMC Complement Altern Med. 2009;9:22.
83. Paran E, Engelhard Y. Effect of tomato's lycopene on blood pressure, serum lipoproteins, plasma homocysteine and oxidative stress markers in grade I hypertensive patients. Am J Hypertens. 2001;14:141A.
84. Langsjoen PH, Langsjoen AM. Overview of the use of Co Q 10 in cardiovascular disease. Biofactors. 1999;9:273–84.
85. Singh RB, Niaz MA, Rastogi SS, Shukla PK, Thakur AS. Effect of hydrosoluble coenzyme Q10 on blood pressure and insulin resistance in hypertensive patients with coronary heart disease. J Hum Hypertens. 1999;12:203–8.
86. Rosenfeldt FL, Haas SJ, Krum H, Hadu A. Coenzyme Q 10 in the treatment of hypertension: a meta-analysis of the clinical trials. J Hum Hypertens. 2007;21(4):297–306.

87. McMackin CJ, Widlansky ME, Hambury NM, Haung AL. Effect of combined treatment with alpha lipoic acid and acetyl carnitine on vascular function and blood pressure in patients with coronary artery disease. J Clin Hypertens. 2007;9:249–55.

88. Salinthone S, Schillace RV, Tsang C, Regan JW, Burdette DN, Carr DW. Lipoic acid stimulates cAMP production via G protein-coupled receptor-dependent and -independent mechanisms. J Nutr Biochem. 2011;22(7):681–90.

89. Rahman ST, Merchant N, Hague T, et al. The impact of lipoic acid on endothelial function and proteinuria in Quinapril-treated diabetic patients with stage I hypertension: results from the Quality Study. J Cardiovasc Pharmacol Ther. 2012;17(2):139–45.

90. Siani A, Pagano E, Iacone R, Iacoviell L, Scopacasa F, Strazzullo P. Blood pressure and metabolic changes during dietary l-arginine supplementation in humans. Am J Hypertens. 2000;13:547–51.

91. Vallance P, Leone A, Calver A, Collier J, Moncada S. Endogenous dimethyl-arginine as an inhibitor of nitric oxide synthesis. J Cardiovasc Pharmacol. 1992;20:S60–2.

92. Ruiz-Hurtado G, Delgado C. Nitric oxide pathway in hypertrophied heart: new therapeutic uses of nitric oxide donors. J Hypertens. 2010;28(Suppl. 1):S56–61.

93. Facchinetti F, Saade GR, Neri I, Pizzi C, Longo M, Volpe A. L-arginine supplementation in patients with gestational hypertension: a pilot study. Hypertens Pregnancy. 2007;26(1):121–30.

94. Neri I, Monari F, Sqarbi L, Berardi A, Masellis G, Facchinetti F. L-arginine supplementation in women with chronic hypertension: impact on blood pressure and maternal and neonatal complications. J Matern Fetal Neonatal Med. 2010;23(12):1456–60.

95. Martina V, Masha A, Gigliardi VR, et al. Long-term N-acetylcysteine and l-arginine administration reduces endothelial activation and systolic blood pressure in hypertensive patients with Type 2 diabetes. Diabetes Care. 2008;31(5):940–4.

96. Ast J, Jablecka A, Bogdanski I, Krauss H, Chmara E. Evaluation of the antihypertensive effect of l-arginine supplementation in patients with mild hypertension assessed with ambulatory blood pressure monitoring. Med Sci Monit. 2010;16(5):CR266–71.

97. Taubert D, Roesen R, Schomig E. Effect of cocoa and tea intake on blood pressure: a meta-analysis. Arch Intern Med. 2007;167(7):626–34.

98. Grassi D, Lippi C, Necozione S, Desideri G, Ferri C. Short-term administration of dark chocolate is followed by a significant increase in insulin sensitivity and a decrease in blood pressure in health persons. Am J Clin Nutr. 2005;81(3):611–4.

99. Taubert D, Roesen R, Lehmann C, Jung N, Schomig E. Effects of low habitual cocoa intake on blood pressure and bioactive nitric oxide: a randomized controlled trial. JAMA. 2007;298(1):49–60.

100. Cohen DL, Townsend RR. Cocoa ingestion and hypertension – another cup please? J Clin Hypertens. 2007;9(8):647–8.

101. Desch S, Kobler D, Schmidt J, et al. Low vs higher-dose dark chocolate and blood pressure in cardiovascular high-risk patients. Am J Hypertens. 2010;23(6):694–700.

102. Desch S, Schmidt J, Sonnabend M, et al. Effect of cocoa products on blood pressure: systematic review and meta-analysis. Am J Hypertens. 2010;23(1):97–103.

103. Sankar D, Rao MR, Sambandam G, Pugalendi KV. Effect of sesame oil on of blood pressure, anthropometry, lipid profile. Am J Med. 2006;119(10):898–902.

104. Maeda H, Kiso Y, Moriyama K. Anti-pattern of blood pressure in patients with hypertensive effects of sesamin in humans. J Nutr Sci Vitaminol (Toyko). 2009;55(1):87–91.

105. Scheer FA, Van Montfrans GA, van Someren EJ, Mairuhu G, Buijs RM. Daily nighttime melatonin reduces blood pressure in male patients with essential hypertension. Hypertension. 2004;43(2):192–7.

106. Cavallo A, Daniels SR, Dolan LM, Khoury JC, Bean JA. Blood pressure response to melatonin in type I diabetes. Pediatr Diabetes. 2004;5(1):26–31.

107. Cavallo A, Daniels SR, Dolan LM, Bean JA, Khoury JC. Blood pressure-lowering effect of melatonin in Type 1 diabetes. J Pineal Res. 2004;36(4):262–6.

108. Cagnacci A, Cannoletta M, Renzi A, Baldassari F, Arangino S, Volpe A. Prolonged melatonin administration decreases nocturnal blood pressure in women. Am J Hypertens. 2005;18(12 Pt 1):1614–8.
109. Grossman E, Laudon M, Yalcin R, et al. Melatonin reduces night blood pressure in patients with nocturnal hypertension. Am J Med. 2006;119(10):898–902.
110. Zamotaev IN, Enikeev AK, Kolomets NM. The use of melaxen in combined therapy of arterial hypertension in subjects occupied in assembly line production. Klin Med (Mosk). 2009;87(6):46–9.
111. Watanabe T, Arai Y, Mitsui Y, et al. The blood pressure-lowering effect and safety of chlorogenic acid from green coffee bean extract in essential hypertension. Clin Exp Hypertens. 2006;28(5):439–49.
112. Ochiai R, Jokura H, Suzuki A, et al. Green coffee bean extract improve human vasoreactivity. Hypertens Res. 2004;27(10):731–7.
113. Yamaquchi T, Chikama A, Mori K, et al. Hydroxyhydroquinone-free coffee: a doubleblind, randomizedcontrolled dose-response study of blood pressure. Nutr Metab Cardiovasc Dis. 2008;18(6):408–14.
114. Chen ZY, Peng C, Jiao R, Wong YM, Yang N, Huang Y. Anti-hypertensive nutraceuticals and functional foods. J Agric Food Chem. 2009;57(11):4485–99.
115. Ochiai R, Chikama A, Kataoka K, et al. Effects of hydroxyhydroquinone-reduce coffee on vasoreactivity and blood pressure. Hypertens Res. 2009;32(11):969–74.
116. Kozuma K, Tsuchiya S, Kohori J, Hase T, Tokimitsu I. Anti-hypertensive effect of green coffee bean extract on mildly hypertensivesubjects. Hypertens Res. 2005;28(9):711–8.
117. Basu A, Penugonda K. Pomegranate juice: a heart-healthy fruit juice. Nutr Rev. 2009;67(1):49–56.
118. Aviram M, Rosenblat M, Gaitine D, et al. Pomegranate juice consumption for 3 years by patients with carotid artery stenosis reduces common carotid intima-media thickness, blood pressure and LDL oxidation. Clin Nutr. 2004;23(3):423–33.
119. Aviram M, Dornfeld L. Pomegranate juice inhibits serum angiotensin converting enzyme activity and reduces systolic blood pressure. Atherosclerosis. 2001;18(1):195–8.
120. Stowe CB. The effects of pomegranate juice consumption on blood pressure and cardiovascular health. Complement Ther Clin Pract. 2011;17(2):113–5.
121. Feringa HH, Laskey DA, Dickson JE, Coleman CI. The effect of grape seed extract on cardiovascular risk markers: a meta-analysis of randomized controlled tirals. J Am Diet Assoc. 2011;111(8):1173–81.
122. Sivaprakasapillai B, Edirsinghe K, Randolph J, Steinberg F, Kappagoda T. Effect of grape seed extract on blood pressure in subjects with the metabolic syndrome. Metabolism. 2009;58(12):1743–6.
123. Edirisinghe I, Burton-Freeman B, Kappagoda CT. Mechanism of the endothelium-dependent relaxation evoked by grape seed extract. Clin Sci (Lond). 2008;114(4):331–7.
124. Walker AF, Marakis G, Morris AP, Robinson PA. Promising hypotensive effect of hawthorn extract: a randomized double-blind pilot study of mile essential hypertension. Phytother Res. 2002;16(1):48–54.

Chapter 7
Nutraceuticals for Insulin Resistance and Type 2 Diabetes Mellitus

Theano Penlioglou and Nikolaos Papanas

Insulin Resistance: Definition and Connection with Type 2 Diabetes Mellitus

The term "insulin resistance" refers to a condition, in which a target cell's response to insulin is decreased, thus leading to impaired glucose homeostasis. Insulin resistance is a powerful risk factor for the development of Type 2 Diabetes Mellitus (T2DM) [1, 2]. Generally, diabetes mellitus (DM) is characterised by hyperglycaemia: this can be caused either by reduced insulin secretion or impaired insulin action, or both [1, 2]. DM has been categorised in two major types [1–4]. Type 1 (T1DM), which is caused mainly by reduced insulin secretion, mostly due to auto-immune causes, is defined by absolute deficiency of insulin secretion; Type 2 (T2DM), the cause of which is a combination of resistance to insulin action and an inadequate insulin secretion [1–4]. Both diabetes types share some common symptoms, mainly polyuria, polydipsia and weight loss [1–4].

Diabetes is now a global pandemic, affecting all people worldwide, [5–9]. Subjects with DM run a high risk of developing diabetes complications, which can cause severe health problems. These include macrovascular (coronary artery disease, stroke, peripheral arterial disease) and microvascular disease (retinopathy, nephropathy, neuropathy) [3–7, 10].

T. Penlioglou · N. Papanas (✉)
Diabetes Centre, Second Department of Internal Medicine, Democritus University of Thrace, University Hospital of Alexandroupolis, Alexandroupolis, Greece

© Springer Nature Switzerland AG 2021
A. F.G. Cicero, M. Rizzo (eds.), *Nutraceuticals and Cardiovascular Disease*,
Contemporary Cardiology, https://doi.org/10.1007/978-3-030-62632-7_7

Pathophysiology of Glucose Metabolism

Glucose is the main source of energy for most cells. Central glucose metabolism is regulated by pancreatic insulin secretion. Normally, there is a complicated inter-relationship between insulin and glucose levels. Glucose homeostasis is also maintained by hepatic glycogenolysis and gluconeogenesis. During fasting, hepatic glycogenolysis and gluconeogenesis become more prominent. Conversely, following meals pancreatic insulin secretion promotes glucose uptake by muscle and adipose cells, at the same time suppressing glycogenolysis and gluconeogenesis [2–4, 11–13]. In the event of insulin resistance, glycogenolysis and gluconeogenesis are not suppressed by insulin, while tissue glucose uptake is also impaired [2–4, 11–13].

Two known transporters involved in this equilibrium are Glut2 and Glut4. Glut4 is involved in glucose transport to muscles and adipose tissue, and so it is a major therapeutic target for T2DM [2–4, 11–13]. In the liver, Glut 2 mediates glucose release. Moreover, the protein kinase "Akt" is activated by the insulin signalling required for normal glucose levels and contributes to glucose homeostasis by various actions, such as .glucose transport to adipocytes and muscle cells, as well as suppression of gluconeogenesis. Normally, insulin is bound to its receptor leading to its tyrosine kinase activation, which in turn phosphorylates the Insulin Receptor Substrate Proteins [2–4, 11–13]. This creates a phospholipid in the membrane which facilitates the interaction between the kinases and Akt, eventually activating the latter. Some of those pathways may lead to systemic insulin resistance and even obesity [2–4, 11–13].

The factors that are involved in developing insulin resistance are complex and are beyond the scope of this brief review. However, excessive visceral adipose tissue as a result of overnutrition is of paramount importance. Interestingly, primary hyperinsulinaemia as the main cause has also been postulated [2–4, 11–13].

Modern Nutraceuticals in the Management of Insulin Resistance and T2DM

Plants have long been widely used for therapeutic purposes, especially in developing countries, for primary care. More than 7000 plants are currently in use as medical treatment for various conditions. Impressively, in some European countries, such as Germany and France, herbal remedies can even be prescribed [14, 15]. Notably, many conventional drugs, like aspirin and digoxin, come from plant sources, while drug companies search out various plants as potential medicaments. In T2DM, metformin, the cornerstone of treatment, was originated from the French lilac *Galega officinalis* [14, 15]. We will briefly discuss nutraceuticals relevant to insulin resistance and T2DM.

Bitter Melon

Bitter gourd (*Momordica charantia L.*), also known as bitter melon, is a tropical and subtropical vine that belongs to the family of Cucurbitaceae [16–22]. For many years, this plant has been often used as a treatment for some medical conditions, such as stomach pain, wounds, malaria and inflammation in the populations of Asia, South America, India and East Africa [16–22]. It is also one of the most common herbs for the treatment of DM and has in fact received the most attention for its antidiabetic properties [16–22]. According to animal studies, bitter melon's fruit extract has a hypoglycaemic effect. This effect is attributed to the stimulation or inhibition of some key enzymes of metabolism and to its active components like charatin, vicine and polypeptide p that are thought to be structurally similar to human insulin [17, 21, 22]. As an example, bitter gourd stimulates enzymes of the hexose monophosphate pathway, increases the utilisation of peripheral glucose, prevents glucose uptake by intestine and increases tissue sensitivity to insulin [17, 21, 22]. In addition, the consumption of bitter melon has been connected with increased β cell function [21, 22]. It has been also implied that it stimulates the secretion of insulin from β cells by depolarisation of β cell membrane, which consequently alters ion flux, a mechanism similar to the one used by some oral hypoglycaemic agents [21, 22]. Finally, it has been shown to also exert hypolipidaemic and antioxidant properties. Importantly, no serious adverse events with use of bitter melon have been reported [16]. Nevertheless, its long-term safety and proper dosage are being discussed [20].

Fenugreek

Fenugreek (*Trigonella foenum-graecum*) is an annual plant, that belongs to the family Fabaceae and is cultivated worldwide. The name Trigonella foenum-graecum is a Latin-Greek name and refers to a typical triangular flower employed as a common fodder for animals in Greece. It is used as a spice all over the world and is also known for its medicinal properties. It has been used for diabetes, cancer and inflammations [23–26]. Fenugreek could be used to delay the onset of diabetes in the stage of prediabetes, through lowering of blood glucose. This is achieved due to insulinotropic effects [23–28]. Soluble fibres in fenugreek, including glucomannan fibre, delay intestinal absorption of ingested sugars. Moreover, some alkaloids such as fenugrecin and trigonelline have demonstrated to possess hypoglycaemic action, and 4 hydroxyisoleucine amino acids act on pancreas to secrete insulin [23–28]. Additionally, Fenugreek has been shown to exert hypolipidaemic effects, reducing low-density lipoprotein cholesterol (LDLc) and total cholesterol [27, 28]. The most studied bioactive compounds of fenugreek with known hypoglycaemic actions are diosgenin, 4-hydroxyisoleucine and the soluble dietary fiber fraction of fenugreek seeds [28]. Their modes of action include: renewal of pancreatic β-cells; stimulation of insulin secretion; antioxidative effects; promotion of adipocyte differentiation; enhancement of insulin-dependent glucose uptake; stimulation of glucose-dependent insulin secretion; reduction of insulin resistance in muscle and/or liver [23, 28–33].

Interestingly, there have been studies evaluating the proper dose of the plant. The best dosage was found to be of 10 g/day [31]. The mode of consumption is also important. Whole fenugreek raw seeds, extracted seed powder, cooked seeds and gum isolate of seeds decreased postprandial glucose levels, whereas degummed seeds showed little effect [31, 34, 35]. With its hypoglycaemic and hypolipidaemic effects, fenugreek emerges as an attractive option for add-on treatment to manage insulin resistance, T2DM and dyslipidaemia.

Cinnamon

Cinnamon belongs to the Lauraceae family, many of whose members are used widely as spices in several cuisines worldwide. It comes from the inner bark of several tree species from the genus Cinnamomum [36, 42, 43]. Today, about 250 species of cinnamon have been identified, but only 4 are as a spice. Cinnamon is currently marketed for the treatment of obesity, glucose intolerance, diabetes mellitus and dyslipidaemia [36–43]. Its basic component, cinnamaldehyde, appears to harbour hypoglycaemic, antioxidant and hypolipidaemic effects [36]. Cinnamon has been reported to reduce postprandial glucose and glycated haemoglobin. Moreover, it reduces insulin resistance [37–39, 41]. The latter action is probably mainly exerted by activating endogenous antioxidant factors and reducing oxidative injury of various tissues [36–39]. Other postulated mechanisms underlying the hypoglycaemic effect include: increased autophosphorylation of the insulin receptor; increased GLUT-4 receptor synthesis and membrane translocation; inhibition of pancreatic and intestinal amylase and glucosidase; increased hepatic glycogen synthesis [37, 38, 41].

More recently, an experimental study in mice has suggested a protective role against hypertension by improved vascular endothelium-dependent diastolic function [36]. Overall, cinnamon has the potential to be a useful add-on therapy in the management of DM. However, more data is needed on its long-term safety and ideal dosage.

Ginseng

Ginseng is the root of plants in the genus *Panax*. To date, there are about 11 available species of ginseng for use [44–48]. Among these, the most famous are the Asian (*Panax ginseng*) and the American (*Panax quinquefolius L*) ginseng. Panax has been used over the years, especially in Chinese traditional medicine, for a wide variety of medical conditions, such as cancer, heart disease and hypertension [44–48]. The pharmacologically active component of ginseng is the triterpene β-glycosides, known as ginsenosides or panaxosides: >150 types of ginsenosides have been identified so far [44–48]. Ginseng is also known and widely used for its hypoglycaemic actions. For these actions, primarily root extracts are used, which contain potent ginsenosides, while other parts are also being investigated for their antidiabetic effects [44, 47]. However, the berries and leaves of ginseng have also been reported to lower blood glucose and decrease body weight. Moreover, according to clinical trials and some animal studies, ginseng could be used to increase insulin sensitivity. It has been suggested that its positive effects on metabolism are achieved through the activation of the peroxisome proliferator-activated receptors (PPARs) by ginsenosides, thus leading to regulation of glucose and lipid metabolism, and the transcription of proteins involved in glucose and fatty-acid uptake [45, 47]. Additionally, according to a meta-analysis of trials in subjects with and without DM, ginseng modestly yet significantly improved fasting blood glucose [44, 48]. However, one study has reported that ginseng failed to improve β cell function in overweight subjects with impaired glucose tolerance or prediabetes [45]. Despite its proven efficacy, again we lack data on its long-term safety and efficacy.

Ginkgo biloba

Ginkgo biloba is a tree growing in East Asia, which has been widely used as traditional herbal medicine in China for many conditions, such as or cough, asthma and skin infections [49]. Ginkgo biloba leaf extracts are made from dried leaves combined with an acetone-water mixture or other solvents through a procedure which results to the enrichment of preferred components and elimination of unwanted substances [49–52]. Ginkgo biloba extracts contain terpenoids and glycosides, that both show antioxidant potency [52–54]. Thus, Ginkgo biloba appears to have potent antioxidant properties, especially via pathways using glutathione peroxidase and superoxide dismutase. Recent experimental evidence in mice has shown shows that ginkgo biloba extracts can improve insulin sensitivity and reduce hyperglycaemia [53, 54]. Similar results have also been obtained in subjects with T2DM [55]. Moreover, Ginkgo biloba plays a protective role against cardiac events in diabetic animals [53, 54].

In addition, Ginkgo biloba has a protective anti antiapoptotic effect on kidneys. Specifically, it has been shown that Ginkgo biloba could rescue renal injury in brain death induced-nephrotoxicity [56, 57]. However, there are still some safety concerns, given that its use may be associated with carcinogenesis [58].

Olive Oil

Olea europaea, also known as olive, is a species of small tree in the family Oleaceae [59–63]. Its oil is commonly used, especially in the Mediterranean cuisine. Olive oil contains polyphenols and iridoids, which explain its anti-atherogenic, antihepatotoxic, anti-inflammatory, antitumor, antiviral and immunomodulator properties [59, 60]. According to some studies, olive oil appears to have a hypogly-caemic effect as well [59–62]. This may be due to the effects of oleuropein on reducing amyloid aggregation and preventing pancreatic β-cell injury from inflammation and cytokine-induced oxidative damage [60]. In practice, reduction of both plasma glucose and glycated haemoglobin has been reported [60, 61]. Finally, there is some data that olive oil may contribute to protection from the development of DM [60, 61].

Red Grapes

Grape is a fruit, botanically a berry, from the vines of the flowering plant genus *Vitis*. Grapes are consumed throughout the world, and are used to produce wine [63–65]. One of the basic components of red wine is quercetin. Quercetin is a flavo-noid naturally present in vegetables, fruit, green tea and red wine. Several beneficial effects have been reported [63–65]. Among them, its antioxidant and anti-inflam-matory actions should be highlighted. In addition, quercetin appears to contribute to body weight reduction, thereby reducing insulin resistance [63]. As regards its hypoglycaemic effects, it is suggested that quercetin may improve insulin-stimulated glucose uptake in mature adipocytes, as well as reduce blood glucose levels by inhibiting GLUT2 [63, 64].

Conclusions

In modern medicine, nutraceuticals are being rediscovered [23–25]. Some of these are gaining importance for the management of insulin resistance and T2DM. Indeed, mostly plant and herb extracts and/or derivatives have been employed and are still being researched. Impressively, scientific enquiries in this area have greatly increased during the last 3 years [23–25].

We now need more data on optimal dosing schemes, treatment duration and long-term safety. Ideally, head-to-head comparisons and more efficacy data to guide us in the selection of appropriate nutraceuticals would be required. It also remains to be ascertained when and how these nutraceuticals may be used instead of and/or on top of mainstream pharmaceutical therapies. Perhaps, patient characteristics and metabolic parameters might prove useful for such therapeutic choices. Obviously, however, there is still a long way to go before these adjunctive therapies can be more widely considered in clinical reality.

Conflicts of Interest None

Funding None

References

1. Czech MP. Insulin action and resistance in obesity and type 2 diabetes. Nat Med. 2017;23:804–14.
2. Kim SH, Reaven GM. Insulin resistance and hyperinsulinemia: you can't have one without the other. Diabetes Care. 2008;31:1433–8.
3. Pippitt K, Li M, Gurgle HE. Diabetes mellitus: screening and diagnosis. Am Fam Physician. 2016;93:103–9.
4. Skyler JS, Bakris GL, Bonifacio E, et al. Differentiation of diabetes by pathophysiology, natural history, and prognosis. Diabetes. 2017;66:241–55.
5. International Diabetes Federation. IDF Diabetes Atlas, 8th Edition, 2017. Available at: http://www.idf.org/diabetesatlas. Last accessed 20th June 2018.
6. Hu FB, Satija A, Manson JE. Curbing the diabetes pandemic: the need of global policy solutions. JAMA. 2015;313:2319–20.
7. Tamayo T, Rosenbauer J, Wild SH, et al. Diabetes in Europe: An update. Diabetes Res Clin Pract. 2014;103:206–17.
8. Papatheodorou K, Banach M, Edmonds M, Papanas N, Papazoglou D. Complications of diabetes. J Diabetes Res. 2015;2015:189525.
9. Seuring T, Archangelidi O, Suhrcke M. The economic costs of type 2 diabetes: a global systematic review. PharmacoEconomics. 2015;33:811–31.
10. Strain WD, Paldánius PM. Diabetes, cardiovascular disease and the microcirculation. Cardiovasc Diabetol. 2018;17:57.
11. Petersen MC, Vatner DF, Shulman GI. Regulation of hepatic glucose metabolism in health and disease. Nat Rev Endocrinol. 2017;13:572–87.
12. Esser N, Legrand-Poels S, Piette J, Scheen AJ, Paquot N. Inflammation as a link between obesity, metabolic syndrome and type 2 diabetes. Diabetes Res Clin Pract. 2014;105:141–50.
13. Ndisang JF, Vannacci A, Rastogi S. Insulin resistance, type 1 and type 2 diabetes, and related complications 2017. J Diabetes Res. 2017;2017:1478294.
14. Karaman E, Erkin O, Senman S, Yildirim Y. The use of herbal supplements by individuals with diabetes mellitus. J Pak Med Assoc. 2018;68:587–94.
15. Ota A, Ulrih NP. An overview of herbal products and secondary metabolites used for management of type two diabetes. Front Pharmacol. 2017;8:436.
16. Mahwish SF, Arshad MS, et al. Hypoglycemic and hypolipidemic effects of different parts and formulations of bitter gourd (Momordica Charantia). Lipids Health Dis. 2017;16:211.
17. Yin RV, Lee NC, Hirpara H, Phung OJ. The effect of bitter melon (Mormordica charantia) in patients with diabetes mellitus: a systematic review and meta-analysis. Nutr Diabetes. 2014;4:e145.
18. Ma C, Yu H, Xiao Y, Wang H. Momordica charantia extracts ameliorate insulin resistance by regulating the expression of SOCS-3 and JNK in type 2 diabetes mellitus rats. Pharm Biol. 2017;55:2170–7.
19. Fachinan R, Fagninou A, Nekoua MP, et al. Evidence of immunosuppressive and th2 immune polarizing effects of antidiabetic Momordica charantia fruit juice. Biomed Res Int. 2017;2017:9478048.
20. Medagama AB, Bandara R. The use of complementary and alternative medicines (CAMs) in the treatment of diabetes mellitus: is continued use safe and effective? Nutr J. 2014;13:102.
21. Rahman IU, Khan RU, Rahman KU, Bashir M. Lower hypoglycemic but higher antiatherogenic effects of bitter melon than glibenclamide in type 2 diabetic patients. Nutr J. 2015;14:13.
22. Mahmoud MF, El Ashry FE, El Maraghy NN, Fahmy A. Studies on the antidiabetic activities of Momordica charantia fruit juice in streptozotocin-induced diabetic rats. Pharm Biol. 2017;55:758–65.
23. Haritha C, Reddy AG, Reddy YR, Anilkumar B. Pharmacodynamic interaction of fenugreek, insulin and glimepiride on biochemical parameters in diabetic Sprague-Dawley rats. Vet World. 2015;8:656–63.

24. Ota A, Ulrih NP. An overview of herbal products and secondary metabolites used for management of type two diabetes. Front Pharmacol. 2017;8:436.
25. Kan J, Velliquette RA, Grann K, Burns CR, Scholten J, Tian F, Zhang Q, Gui M. A novel botanical formula prevents diabetes by improving insulin resistance. BMC Complement Altern Med. 2017;17:352.
26. King K, Lin NP, Cheng YH, Chen GH, Chein RJ. Isolation of positive modulator of glucagon-like Peptide-1 Signaling from Trigonella foenum-graecum (fenugreek) seed. J Biol Chem. 2015;290:26235–48.
27. Sundaram G, Ramakrishnan T, Parthasarathy H, Raja M, Raj S. Fenugreek, diabetes, and periodontal disease: a cross-link of sorts! J Indian Soc Periodontol. 2018;22:122–6.
28. Fuller S, Stephens JM. Diosgenin, 4-hydroxyisoleucine, and fiber from fenugreek: mechanisms of actions and potential effects on metabolic syndrome. Adv Nutr. 2015;6:189–97.
29. Li XY, Lu SS, Wang HL, et al. Effects of the fenugreek extracts on high-fat diet-fed and streptozotocin-induced type 2 diabetic mice. Anim Model Exp Med. 2018;1:68–73.
30. Rampogu S, Parameswaran S, Lemuel MR, Lee KW. Exploring the therapeutic ability of fenugreek against type 2 diabetes and breast cancer employing molecular docking and molecular dynamics simulations. Evid Based Complement Alternat Med. 2018;2018:1943203.
31. Ranade M, Mudgalkar N. A simple dietary addition of fenugreek seed leads to the reduction in blood glucose levels: a parallel group, randomized single-blind trial. Ayu. 2017;38:24–7.
32. Asadi-Samani M, Moradi MT, Mahmoodnia L, Alaei S, Asadi-Samani F, Luther T. Traditional uses of medicinal plants to prevent and treat diabetes; an updated review of ethnobotanical studies in Iran. J Nephropathol. 2017;6:118–25.
33. Gaddam A, Galla C, Thummisetti S, Marikanty RK, Palanisamy UD, Rao PV. Role of Fenugreek in the prevention of type 2 diabetes mellitus in prediabetes. J Diabetes Metab Disord. 2015;14:74.
34. Raghuram TC, Sharma RD, Sivakumar B, Sahay BK. Effect of fenugreek seeds on intravenous glucose disposition in non-insulin dependent diabetic patients. Phytother Res. 1994;8:83–6.
35. Kassaian N, Azadbakht L, Forghani B, Amini M. Effect of fenugreek seeds on blood glucose and lipid profiles in type 2 diabetic patients. Int J Vitam Nutr Res. 2009;79:34–9.
36. Guo X, Sun W, Huang L, Wu L, Hou Y, Qin L, Liu T. Effect of cinnamaldehyde on glucose metabolism and vessel function. Med Sci Monit. 2017;23:3844–53.
37. Medagama AB. The glycaemic outcomes of Cinnamon, a review of the experimental evidence and clinical trials. Nutr J. 2015;14:108.
38. Costello RB, Dwyer JT, Saldanha L, Bailey RL, Merkel J, Wambogo E. Do cinnamon supplements have a role in glycemic control in type 2 diabetes? A narrative review. J Acad Nutr Diet. 2016;116:1794–802.
39. Ranasinghe P, Galappaththy P, Constantine GR, et al. Cinnamomum zeylanicum (Ceylon cinnamon) as a potential pharmaceutical agent for type-2 diabetes mellitus: study protocol for a randomized controlled trial. Trials. 2017;18:446.
40. Van Hul M, Geurts L, Plovier H, et al. Reduced obesity, diabetes, and steatosis upon cinnamon and grape pomace are associated with changes in gut microbiota and markers of gut barrier. Am J Physiol Endocrinol Metab. 2018;314:E334–52.
41. Talaei B, Amouzegar A, Sahranavard S, Hedayati M, Mirmiran P, Azizi F. Effects of cinnamon consumption on glycemic indicators, advanced glycation end products, and antioxidant status in type 2 diabetic patients. Nutrients. 2017;9:pii: E991.
42. Kaur G, Invally M, Khan MK, Jadhav P. A nutraceutical combination of Cinnamomum cassia &Nigella sativa for type 1 diabetes mellitus. J Ayurveda Integr Med. 2018;9:27–37.
43. Kawatra P, Rajagopalan R. Cinnamon: Mystic powers of a minute ingredient. Pharm Res. 2015;7(Suppl 1):S1–6.
44. Gui QF, Xu ZR, Xu KY, Yang YM. The efficacy of ginseng-related therapies in type 2 diabetes mellitus: an updated systematic review and meta-analysis. Medicine (Baltimore). 2016;95:e2584.
45. Reeds DN, Patterson BW, Okunade A, Holloszy JO, Polonsky KS, Klein S. Ginseng and ginsenoside Re do not improve β-cell function or insulin sensitivity in overweight and obese subjects with impaired glucose tolerance or diabetes. Diabetes Care. 2011;34:1071–6.

46. Bai L, Gao J, Wei F, Zhao J, Wang D, Wei J. Therapeutic potential of ginsenosides as an adjuvant treatment for diabetes. Front Pharmacol. 2018;9:423.
47. Ru W, Wang D, Xu Y, et al. Chemical constituents and bioactivities of Panax ginseng (C. A. Mey.). Drug Discov Ther. 2015;9:23–32.
48. Shishtar E, Sievenpiper JL, Djedovic V, et al. The effect of ginseng (the genus panax) on glycemic control: a systematic review and meta-analysis of randomized controlled clinical trials. PLoS One. 2014;9:e107391.
49. Hohmann N, Wolf EM, Rigault P, et al. Ginkgo biloba's footprint of dynamic Pleistocene history dates back only 390,000 years ago. BMC Genomics. 2018;19:299.
50. Rhee KJ, Lee CG, Kim SW, Gim DH, Kim HC, Jung BD. Extract of ginkgo biloba ameliorates streptozotocin-induced type 1 diabetes mellitus and high-fat diet-induced type 2 diabetes mellitus in mice. Int J Med Sci. 2015;12:987–94.
51. Lu Q, Hao M, Wu W, et al. Antidiabetic cataract effects of GbE, rutin and quercetin are mediated by the inhibition of oxidative stress and polyol pathway. Acta Biochim Pol. 2018;65:35–41.
52. Lu Q, Yin XX, Wang JY, Gao YY, Pan YM. Effects of Ginkgo biloba on prevention of development of experimental diabetic nephropathy in rats. Acta Pharmacol Sin. 2007;28:818–28.
53. Banin RM, Hirata BK, Andrade IS, et al. Beneficial effects of Ginkgo biloba extract on insulin signaling cascade, dyslipidemia, and body adiposity of diet-induced obese rats. Braz J Med Biol Res. 2014;47(9):780–8.
54. Vasseur M, Jean T, DeFeudis FV, Drieu K. Effects of repeated treatments with an extract of Ginkgo biloba (EGb 761), bilobalide and ginkgolide B on the electrical activity of pancreatic beta cells of normal or alloxan-diabetic mice: an ex vivo study with intracellular microelectrodes. Gen Pharmacol. 1994;25:31–46.
55. Aziz TA, Hussain SA, Mahwi TO, Ahmed ZA, Rahman HS, Rasedee A. The efficacy and safety of Ginkgo biloba extract as an adjuvant in type 2 diabetes mellitus patients ineffectively managed with metformin: a double-blind, randomized, placebo-controlled trial. Drug Des Devel Ther. 2018;12:735–42.
56. Shi R, Wang Y, An X, et al. Efficacy of co-administration of liuwei dihuang pills and ginkgo biloba tablets on albuminuria in type 2 diabetes: a 24-month, multicenter, double-blind, placebo-controlled, randomized clinical trial. Front Endocrinol (Lausanne). 2019;10:100.
57. Zayed AE, Saleh A, Gomaa AMS, et al. Corrigendum to "protective effect of ginkgo biloba and magnetized water on nephropathy in induced type 2 diabetes in rat". Oxidative Med Cell Longev. 2018;2018:1094650.
58. Mei N, Guo X, Ren Z, Kobayashi D, Wada K, Guo L. Review of Ginkgo biloba-induced toxicity, from experimental studies to human case reports. J Environ Sci Health C Environ Carcinog Ecotoxicol Rev. 2017;35:1–28.
59. Rigacci S, Stefani M. Nutraceutical Properties of olive oil polyphenols. an itinerary from cultured cells through animal models to humans. Int J Mol Sci. 2016;17:pii: E843.
60. Alkhatib A, Tsang C, Tuomilehto J. Olive oil nutraceuticals in the prevention and management of diabetes: from molecules to lifestyle. Int J Mol Sci. 2018;19:pii: E2024.
61. Schwingshackl L, Lampousi AM, Portillo MP, Romaguera D, Hoffmann G, Boeing H. Olive oil in the prevention and management of type 2 diabetes mellitus: a systematic review and meta-analysis of cohort studies and intervention trials. Nutr Diabetes. 2017;7:e262.
62. Guasch-Ferré M, Merino J, Sun Q, Fitó M, Salas-Salvadó J. Dietary polyphenols, mediterranean diet, prediabetes, and type 2 diabetes: a narrative review of the evidence. Oxidative Med Cell Longev. 2017;2017:6723931.
63. de la Iglesia R, Loria-Kohen V, Zulet MA, Martinez JA, Reglero G, Ramirez de Molina A. Dietary strategies implicated in the prevention and treatment of metabolic syndrome. Int J Mol Sci. 2016;17:11.
64. Pandey KB, Rizvi SI. Role of red grape polyphenols as antidiabetic agents. Integr Med Res. 2014;2014(3):119–25.
65. Kim Y, Keogh JB, Clifton PM. Polyphenols and glycemic control. Nutrients. 2016;8:1.

Chapter 8
Nutraceuticals Supporting Body Weight Loss

Andreea Corina, Dragana Nikolic, Adriana Florinela Cătoi, and Pablo Perez-Martinez

Introduction

Obesity and overweightness are major pandemic health problems and, in many cases, appear in close relationship with other cardiovascular disease (CVD) risk factors like glucose intolerance, type 2 diabetes mellitus (T2DM), dyslipidemia, hypertension, and kidney failure [1]. In addition, obesity and overweightness are associated with increased all-cause mortality [2].

According to World Health Organization (WHO) data, obesity has nearly tripled in the last 40 years. In 2016 more than 1.9 billion adults were overweight and, among these, over 650 million were obese, corresponding to 13% of the world's adult population (11% of men and 15% of women) [3].

Overweight and obesity are defined as abnormal or excessive fat accumulation. The calculation of body mass index (BMI) is the most commonly used tool for the classification of overweight and obesity. BMI is calculated as a person's weight in kilograms divided by the square of his height in meters (kg/m^2). For adults, WHO defines overweight as BMI ≥ 25 kg/m^2 and obesity as a BMI ≥ 30 kg/m^2. Furthermore,

A. Corina · P. Perez-Martinez (✉)
Lipid and Atherosclerosis Unit, IMIBIC/Reina Sofia University Hospital/University of Cordoba, Cordoba, Spain

CIBER Fisiopatologia Obesidad y Nutricion (CIBEROBN), Instituto de Salud Carlos III, Madrid, Spain

D. Nikolic
PROMISE Department, School of Medicine, University of Palermo, Palermo, Italy

A. F. Cătoi
Pathophysiology Department, "Iuliu Hațieganu" University of Medicine and Pharmacy, Cluj-Napoca, Romania
e-mail: adriana.catoi@umfcluj.ro

© Springer Nature Switzerland AG 2021
A. F.G. Cicero, M. Rizzo (eds.), *Nutraceuticals and Cardiovascular Disease*, Contemporary Cardiology, https://doi.org/10.1007/978-3-030-62632-7_8

117

obesity is sub-classified into 3 subgroups – class I: BMI between 30–34.9 kg/m^2 (associated with moderate risk); class II: BMI between 35–39.9 kg/m^2 (associated with high risk) and class III: BMI ≥40 kg/m^2 (associated with very high risk). However, in many cases, BMI may not correspond to the same degree of adiposity in different individuals and should be used with caution. Therefore, the use of other indicators such as waist circumference and waist to hip ratio in association with BMI is recommended [4].

Early intervention, even at young ages, should be promoted as obesity prevention is fundamental. The first line treatment in weight management is lifestyle intervention including a hypocaloric diet and increased physical activity. When changing lifestyle fails, pharmacological management should be considered. Bariatric surgery might be recommended for individuals with a BMI ≥40 kg/m^{2}or BMI ≥35 kg/m^2 and other obesity-related comorbidities [5, 6].

Available drugs for weight management in obese patients have a broad mechanism of action including an increase in satiety as well as a decrease in hunger, or a reduction in calorie absorption. Very few drugs are approved for weight loss. At the same time, there are differences between the pharmacological treatments approved by the most important regulatory entities such as the Food and Drug Administration (FDA) and European Medicine Agency (EMA). Considering that the tolerability as well as the efficacy and the safety of anti-obesity drugs for long-term use are still controversial, the consumption of these drugs should be closely supervised [7]. Moreover, the possible interactions between nutraceuticals and other medications are as yet not well enough studied. On the other hand, there are many functional foods and nutraceuticals available for weight loss accessible over the counter and on the internet. The use of dietary supplements for weight loss is quite common and the data from a survey in US adults showed that more than 30% of the subjects who made a serious weight-loss attempt used dietary supplements. At the same time, of those interviewed, more than 60% of users and more than 40% of non-users respond that dietary supplements are effective for weight loss [8]. However, data from the scientific literature is contradictory and the use of these products should be carefully controlled due to increased numbers of documented adverse effects. Moreover, the efficacy of most of the dietary supplements used for weight loss is questionable.

This chapter will provide an overview of the most common nutraceuticals used for body weight management with available scientific data from clinical studies.

Fibers

Fibers are naturally present in the structure of some food plants including vegetables, fruits, grains, and legumes. Fibers are classified as soluble or insoluble, depending on its water-holding capacity or viscous characteristics in solution [9]. Fiber's mechanism of action on body weight is related to fiber proprieties of lowering the absorption of other caloric nutrients, especially carbohydrates and lipids. On the other hand, fibers could have an effect on appetite by increasing satiety while delaying gastric emptying, increasing glucagon-like peptide 1/2 (GLP-1/2) and cholecystokinin (CCK) hormones, as well as lowering ghrelin secretion and serotonin uptake. Generally, both soluble and insoluble fiber intake could increase satiety and hunger, and in obese subjects an intake of an additional 14 g/day of fiber could reduce energy intake by 82% with a further reduction in body weight of 2.4 kg [10]. In addition, the effect of fiber on appetite, acute and long-term energy intake as well as body weight differ depending on the different physicochemical properties of various fibers. For instance, more viscous fibers such as pectins, β-glucans and guar gum reduce appetite around 59%, while less viscous ones showed only a 14% appetite reduction [11].

Due to a low consumption of fiber rich foods like vegetables, fruits, and whole grains, in the USA the average fiber intake of adults does not even rich half of current recommendations. On the other hand, a positive correlation has been established between a low consumption of fiber and obesity. Furthermore, nutraceuticals containing dietary fiber could positively impact obesity [12–15]. Data derived from intervention studies strongly support the use of soluble fiber intake for weight management as well as for metabolic control in overweight and obese subjects. Results from a meta-analysis, including more than 600 patients, conclude a beneficial effect of different soluble fiber consumption (manno-oligosaccharides, galacto-oligosaccharides, fructo-oligosaccharides, β-glucan, flax-seed mucilage, mannans and dextrin) [15]. After 2–17 weeks of follow-up, at a mean dose of 18.5 g/day, overweight and obese subjects experienced reductions of 2.5 kg in weight and 0.4% of body fat.

Psyllium (Psyllium Husk Fiber)

Psyllium husk fiber is a water-soluble, gel-forming mucilage from *Plantago ovata*. As it is less readily fermented it provides less adverse effects than other fibers such as bloating and other gastro-intestinal dysfunction [16, 17]. Its main mechanism of action on body weight includes a delay in gastric emptying as well as increased satiety. Increased satiety at the central level is mediated by the inhibition of ghrelin secretion while up regulating GLP-1/2 and CCK hormones. On the other hand, hepatic cholesterol synthesis is reduced, and fecal excretion of cholesterol and bile salts are increased. Moreover, psyllium has been shown to modulate the gut microbiota by short-chain fatty acids (SCFA) produced by fermentation, lipolysis and lipoprotein lipase (LPL) upregulation [18].

Clinical evidence of psyllium supplementation showed either positive or no effect on weight loss. A very recent systematic review and meta-analysis analyzed the results of 22 randomized controlled trials (RCTs) and included a total 1458 adults [19]. The authors found no effect of psyllium supplementation on body weight, WC, and BMI. However, the results of this publication should be interpreted carefully as not all the participants were obese or overweight. Furthermore, subgroup analysis showed that the effect of psyllium supplementation on body weight and on BMI was significant in studies that used psyllium dosage of more than 10 g/day and with higher duration [19]. Another review concluded that dietary supplementation with psyllium could decrease appetite and has an effect on some components of the metabolic syndrome, such as hyperglycemia, insulin response and the lipid profile [20].

In other clinical studies, in overweight patients with T2DM, an improvement in glycemic control is observed, although there was no effect on BMI, after 8-week consumption of 10.2 g of psyllium daily [21]. In another study, after 7 weeks of high fiber food consumption, the lipid profile improved and there was a minimum reduction in body weight [22], while a 12 month supplementation period with a product containing 5 g of psyllium before meals had beneficial effects on body weight, WC, and body fat percentage [23]. Long-term supplementation with psyllium in addition to a caloric restricted diet showed better effects than short term use of this natural component on weight reduction [24].

Other health effects of soluble fiber, especially psyllium consumption as an adjuvant to a hypocaloric diet, shows that patients experience increased satiety and improvements in CVD related risk factors such as total and low-density lipoprotein (LDL) cholesterol, hypertension as well as an improvement in glycemic response and insulin sensitivity [24–26], findings also corroborated by a recent meta-analysis [27].

In clinical practice, psyllium supplementation could be used in addition to a healthy diet or weight loss plan at a minimum dose of 10 g twice a day for adults for a minimum duration of 10 weeks. Psyllium should be taken with 250 ml water or added to the meal while water consumption should be increased [24]. Psyllium could be a better choice for weight loss than other fibers as it has less adverse effects.

β-Glucans (Oats Bran)

Oats (Avena sativa) is a class of cereal grain belonging to the *Poaceae family*. Oats are rich in protein, lipids, vitamins, minerals, and fibers. Moreover, oats are considered functional food due to its high concentration in a soluble fiber, β-glucan [28]. β-glucan intake might contribute to body weight control and has other health-related beneficial effects such as hypolipidemic, hypoglycaemic, antioxidant and anti-inflammatory [29] efficacy, and could also reduce CVD risk [30]. In overweight subjects oat β-glucan could suppress hunger by increasing gastric emptying time, elevating post-prandial CCK, and decreasing the insulin response [31].

Even if it is largely recommended for obesity treatments, to our knowledge there is not much clinical evidence supporting the use of β-glucan for weight loss. Most of the studies concluded that β-glucan administration has no or has minimal effects on body weight. After 3-months supplementation with 0 g, 5–6 g or 8–9 g of β-glucan, in addition to dietary intervention in overweight women, no significant reduction in body weight was observed among intervention groups [32]. In several other studies investigating health-related benefits of β-glucans, weight loss was also assessed. After an administration of 3–9 g/day of β-glucan for up to 12 weeks, no effect was shown in body weight reduction [33–35]. In conclusion, β-glucan supplementation might not be a good option for treating overweight or obesity, although a recent meta-analysis shows that cereal β-glucan consumption seems to modestly decrease body weight (weighted mean difference (WMD) −0.77 kg, 95% CI: −1.49, −0.04) and BMI (WMD −0.62 kg/m², 95% CI: −1.04, −0.21), respectively, but has no effect on waist circumference and energy intake [36].

Chitosan

Chitosan is the second most abundant naturally occurring polysaccharide next to cellulose. Chitosan results from the deacetylation of chitin [37] and is categorized as an insoluble fiber from animal origin; it reduces cholesterol absorption [38]. The mechanism by which chitosan may exert a weight loss effect is by binding and trapping dietary fat and cholesterol, thus preventing its absorption in the intestinal lumen [39]. Moreover, chitosan might have an effect on the inhibition of adipogenesis in 3T3-L1 cells, as well as on the activation of 5′ adenosine monophosphate-activated protein kinase (AMPK) and by inhibiting lipogenesis-associated genes in the liver and adipose tissue [40]. A recent experimental study demonstrated that chitosan's weight-loss mechanism includes an increase in serum leptin levels, reduced inflammation, and a probiotic effect, leading to a change in gut microbiota by increasing the anti-obesity species such as *Clostridium leptum* and *Coprobacillus cateniformis* and by decreasing *Clostridium lactatifermentans* and *Clostridium cocleatum* [41].

A recent meta-analysis including 15 RCTs with 1130 subjects, studying chitosan consumption in adults, showed a significant reduction in weight (WMD −0.89 kg; 95% confidence interval (CI): −1.41 to −0.38; P = 0.0006) and body fat (WMD −0.69%; 95% CI: −1.02 to −0.35; P = 0.0001) in overweight and obese participants [42]. A meta-analysis by Moraru et al. [43] studying 14 RCT in 1101 individuals with a BMI ≥23.6 kg/m² concluded that the usage of chitosan supplementation might contribute to a slight short- and medium-term effect on weight loss. After an up to 52 week intervention, subjects included in the trials had a reduction of −1.01 kg, (95% CI: −1.67 to −0.34) and an improvement in cardiovascular factors [43]. Another meta-analysis included 13 trials with a total of 1219 participants, investigating the effect of chitosan after 1 to 6 months of supplementation, demonstrated a −1.7 kg (95% CI: −2.1 to −1.3 kg, p < 0.00001) change in weight, compared to placebo [44]. Other beneficial effects of chitosan supplementation includes a decrease in total cholesterol and a decrease in systolic and diastolic blood pressures [44].

The maximum intake recommended by The European Food Safety Authority (EFSA) Panel on Dietetic Products, Nutrition and Allergies (NDA) is 3 g chitosan per day [45].

Glucomannan

Glucomann is a soluble fiber derived from *Amorphophallus konjac*. Glucomaman is specially used for the treatment of constipation, being indicated even in children and during pregnancy [46, 47]. The mechanism of action of glucomanan in body weight loss includes increasing satiety, delaying gastric emptying, and a reduced transit time of food in the small intestine. Therefore, with blunted postprandial insulin excursions, cholesterol absorption is reduced, while there is an increase in fecal fat excretion as well as a reduction in small-bowel transit time [40].

Glucomannan consumption is associated with beneficial effects on body weight in various RCTs and meta-analyses, especially after long-term consumption [48, 49]. After analyzing the results of 14 RCTs on different parameters, Sood et al. [49] revealed that the intake of glucomannan could reduce body weight by −0.79 kg; (95% CI: −1.53, −0.05). On the other hand, a meta-analysis including 8 RCTs showed no difference in weight loss between patients consuming daily dosages ranging from 1000 to 3870 mg glucomannan or placebo (mean difference [MD]: −0.22 kg; 95% CI: −0.62, 0.19; $I(2) = 65\%$) [50]. Some moderate weight loss was observed in obese and overweight subjects in another meta-analysis including results from 6 RCTs by Zalewski et al. [48].

Moreover, supplementation with a soluble viscous fiber complex containing konjac glucomannan, sodium alginate, and xanthan gum reduced the frequency of eating and induced a decrease of body weight and WC [51]. The complex was administered, in the context of a clinical trial, to 83 overweight/obese subjects for a period of 12 weeks. In order to achieve these effects the recommended dose is at least three doses of 1 g each of glucomannan daily with 1–2 glasses of water before meals associated with an energy-restricted diet [49].

African Mango (Irvingia gabonesis)

The soluble fiber of the seed of *Irvingia gabonensis* (IG), similar to other forms of water-soluble dietary fibers, is a "bulk-forming" laxative which delays stomach emptying, leading to a more gradual absorption of dietary sugar, but also can bind to bile acids in the gut and carry them in the feces, which stimulates the liver to convert more cholesterol into bile acids [52].

A double blind randomized study including 40 subjects (28) receiving IG (1.05 g three time a day for 1 month, while 12 were on placebo) was carried out in order to evaluate the efficacy of IG seeds in the management of obesity [53]. The mean body weight of the IG group was decreased by 5.26 +/− 2.37% (p < 0.0001) and that of the placebo group by 1.32 +/− 0.41% (p < 0.02). The difference observed between the 2 groups was significant (p < 0.01). In addition, in the IG group total cholesterol, LDL-cholesterol and triglycerides significantly decreased, while HDL-cholesterol increased [53]. In a 10 week randomized, double-blind, placebo-controlled trial involving 72 obese or overweight participants the Cissus quadrangularis/IF combination resulted in larger reductions in body weight, body fat, waist size; total plasma cholesterol, LDL-cholesterol and fasting glucose level compared to the Cissus quadrangularis-only group [54]. Similarly, in a randomized double-blind placebo controlled study where IG was administered 150 mg twice daily before meals to overweight and/or obese human volunteers, favorable effects on body weight and a variety of parameters of the metabolic syndrome were observed [55]. Finally, the latest meta-analysis including 5 RCTs [56], indicates good overall efficacy of IG seed extract supplementation on weight loss, but due to poor methodological quality and the insufficient clinical reports, further high quality RCTs are necessary.

Fucoxanthin

Among functional ingredients identified from marine algae (such as *Undaria pinnatifida* or *Laminaria japonica*, and microalgae such as *Phaeodactylum tricornutum* or *Cylindrotheca closterium*), fucoxanthin has received particular interest. Anti-obesity effects of fucoxanthin (a xanthophyll) have been reported. Fucoxanthin induces uncoupling protein 1 (an uncoupling protein dissipates protonmotive force without driving ATP biosynthesis) in abdominal white adipose tissue (WAT) mitochondria, leading to the increased oxidation of fatty acids and heat production in WAT; improves insulin resistance and decreases blood glucose levels through the regulation of cytokine secretions from WAT [57]. The carotenoid end of the polyene chromophore, which contains an allenic bond and two hydroxyl groups, has been suggested as the key structure for its anti-obesity effect. Such anti-obesity effects were primarily detected in murine studies, and further studies are needed in order to confirm all these promising scientific results in humans. Xanthigen-600/2.4 mg (300 mg pomegranate seed oil +300 mg brown seaweed extract containing 2.4 mg fucoxanthin) induces weight loss, reduces body and liver fat content, and improves liver function tests in obese non-diabetic women [58]. Finally, recent results suggest that fucoxanthin could be a promising microbiota-targeted functional-food ingredient as the composition of both cecal and fecal microbiota were significantly changed after 4 weeks of fucoxanthin supplementation [59].

Garcinia cambogia

Garcinia is a large genus in the family *Clusiaceae*, and *G. cambogiais,* a tree native to the forests of India, Nepal, and Sri Lanka, and is the most often used for medicinal purposes [60]. Although numerous chemicals have been isolated from G. cambogia fruit, hydroxycitric acid (HCA) is considered the active ingredient for weight loss. It is believed to have multiple sites of action, but primarily in the liver (where inhibits adenosine triphosphate citrate lyase, which cleaves citrate to acetyl coenzyme A (acetyl-CoA) and oxaloacetate), and brain (causes a decrease in serotonin reuptake). Dosages of *G. cambogia* for weight loss have ranged from 1667 to 4668 mg (taken in divided doses) daily [60].

Based on the available evidence from clinical studies published until February 2017, some authors suggest that *G. cambogia* is unlikely to be effective in obese subjects and even may cause harm [60]. On the other hand, the administration of *G. cambogia* and glucomannan for long-term weight loss in people with overweight or obesity led to reduced weight and improved lipid and glucose profiles [61]. Also, these authors suggested that the presence of several polymorphisms, including perilipin 4 (PLIN4), fat mass and obesity-associated (FTO) protein, and β-adrenergic receptor 3 (ADRB3) might hinder to some degree these effects.

Carnitine

In the human body carnitine can be found in almost every cell. Carnitine plays an important role in energy balance, mitochondrial β-oxidation, and in fatty acid metabolism. L-carnitine is the isomer used in weight loss [62]. Some preclinical findings suggest that the expression of microRNAs which play a role in the pathogenesis of obesity might be modulated by dietary agents and supplements including L-carnitine [63]. In human studies, carnitine supplementation as a weight-loss agent leads to increases in its intracellular concentration and triggers increased fat oxidation and a gradual reduction of the body's fat reserves [64].

Data from a systematic review meta-analysis of RCTs investigating the effect of carnitine on body weight loss concluded that carnitine might be an effective adjuvant for weight loss in adults. A daily intake of 1.8–4 g L-carnitine or levocarnitine showed a greater reduction in body weight and BMI. Subjects who received carnitine lost significantly more weight (MD: -1.33 kg; 95% CI: -2.09 to -0.57) and showed a decrease in BMI (MD: -0.47 kg m^{-2}; 95% CI: -0.88 to -0.05) compared with the control group [65]. The effect of carnitine supplementation on body weight decreases over time.

Green Tea

Both green tea and black tea are made from the leaves of the *Camellia sinensis* plant belonging to the *Theaceae family*. Green tea production is characterized by a rapidly steaming process that prevents fermentation, while during black tea production the leaves endure an extra enzymatic oxidation step during the processing [66]. In green tea there are naturally presented a series of components with biological activity, catechins, a class of polyphenols of low molecular weight. Catechins are present mainly as catechin, epicatechin, catechin gallate, gallocatechin, gallocatechin gallate, epicatechin gallate, epigallocatechin and epigallocatechin gallate [67]. The final concentration of these products in green tea drinks is largely variable depending on growing conditions, how the leaves are dried, harvesting and preparation conditions of the formulation that is consumed. Epigallocatechin-3-gallate (EGCG) was identified as the most abundant green-tea catechin and it is responsible for most of the biological properties of green tea [68]. EGCG reduces body weight by decreasing adipocyte differentiation and proliferation during lipogenesis [69]. Moreover, the anti-obesity mechanism of action of EGCG includes inhibition of pancreatic lipase, an increase in glucagon like peptide-1 (GLP-1) levels, and increased satiety (by enhancing serotonin/dopamine uptake) [70, 71]. Furthermore, high-dose green tea extract (EGCG) at a daily dosage of 856.8 mg may influence body weight by decreasing the secretion of ghrelin while increasing adiponectin levels [72]. In addition, green tea polyphenols also modulates the composition of gut microbiota [73].

There is much scientific literature describing the effect of green tea consumption on weight loss. A recent meta-analysis investigated the effect of green tea in 26 RCTs, including 1344 obese adults [74]. Subjects who consumed green tea had a reduction of around -1.78 kg (95% CI: -2.80, -0.75, p = 0.001), as well as a lower BMI WMD: -0.65 kg/m^2 (95% CI: -1.04, -0.25, p = 0.001). Moreover, there was a non-linear dose-response between dose and duration of green tea consumption and the most pronounced reduction in body weight was observed with 500 mg/day green tea for 12 weeks [74]. The effect of green tea extract on weight loss was recently investigated in a meta-analysis of 16 RCTs including 1090 subjects was analyzed [75]. After green tea extract consumption, the study revealed a reduction in BMI of -0.27 kg/m^2 (95% CI: -0.40 to -0.15, p < 0.0001). Moreover, this recent meta-analysis showed a beneficial effect on glycemic profile as well as an increase in high-density lipoprotein (HDL) levels, while all-cause adverse events were minimal [75]. On the other hand, obese women included in another study investigating the high-dose green tea extract intake, experienced significant weight, BMI, as well as WC reduction [72]. Even at a daily dosage of 856.8 mg EGCG for 12 weeks, subjects included in the study reported no side effects or adverse events. Furthermore, significantly lower ghrelin levels and elevated adiponectin levels were found in the active component study group.

For an optimal effect of green tea on weight loss it is essential that the final product contains in the range of 126–300 mg EGCG and 75–150 mg caffeine and

EGCG:caffeine ratio of 1.8:1 to 4:1 per day [76]. Therefore, we conclude that the use of green tea can be useful for the weight management of obese patients.

Hoodia gordonii

Hoodia gordonii (family *Apocynaceae*) is known for its claimed effects of appetite suppression and weight loss [77]. Future studies are needed to elucidate the mechanisms of action (p57 and Hoodigogenin A might not be the active agents responsible for the weight loss associated), as well as side-effects and appropriate doses. Few clinical trials are available, and these show that a 15 days regimen of repeated consumption of H. gordonii purified extract (HgPE) seems to be associated with significant adverse changes in some vital signs and laboratory parameters [78], while 40 days of repeated consumption resulted in statistically significant reductions in body weight, BMI and WC compared with the placebo group [79]. Thus, additional investigations are needed in order to assess safety and efficacy. Interestingly, a very recent randomized blinded controlled trial study, where a 4 weeks long supplementation with *H. Parviflora* at 9 mg + 200 mg of fructo-oligosaccharides was used in 30 overweight and obese patients, favorable effects were reported on weight loss, decreasing satiety, and improving fat mass, in particular visceral adipose tissue [80].

Pyruvate

The efficacy of pyruvate in reducing body weight was assessed in a meta-analysis including 6 RCTs [81] and the results do not convincingly support pyruvate to be efficacious in reducing body weight. However, it should be noted that there is limited evidence and future trials should be more rigorous and better-designed. In addition, pyruvate supplementation seems to be ineffective as a fat loss strategy in young athletes [82].

Caffeine

The daily consumption of coffee and caffeinated beverages between 494 weight loss maintainers and 2129 individuals from the general population controlling for sociodemographic variables, BMI and physical activity level were investigated [83] and the results indicate that weight loss maintainers consume significantly more cups of coffee and caffeinated beverages. Also, a recent meta-analysis demonstrated that caffeine intake might promote weight, BMI and body fat reduction (the overall pooled beta was 0.29 (95%CI: 0.19, 0.40; Q = 124.5, I^2 = 91.2%); 0.23 (95%CI:

0.09, 0.36; Q = 71.0, I^2 = 93.0%) and 0.36 (95% CI: 0.24, 0.48; Q = 167.36, I^2 = 94.0%), respectively) [84]. Thus, consumption of caffeinated beverages might support weight loss maintenance, but further studies are needed to investigate possible mechanisms.

Bitter Orange

Citrus aurantium L. (bitter orange) extracts that contain p-synephrine as the primary protoalkaloid are widely used for weight loss/weight management, appetite control, energy, and mental focus and cognition, although questions have been raised about the safety of p-synephrine as it has some structural similarity to ephedrine [85]. Mechanistic studies suggest that p-synephrine exerts its effects through multiple actions including its binding to β-3 adrenergic receptors that regulate lipid and carbohydrate metabolism, Neuromedin U Receptor 2 (NMUR2s), and AMP-activated protein kinase, cAMP, and Ca(2+)-dependent mechanisms, but also anti-inflammatory effects.

The consumption of bergamot polyphenol extract complex (BPE-C), a novel bergamot juice-derived formulation enriched with flavonoids and pectins, decreased body weight by 14.8% and BMI by 15.9% in obese participants at the dose of 1300 mg daily [86]. This further correlated with a significant, dose-dependent reduction of circulating hormones balancing caloric intake such as leptin and ghrelin, and upregulation of adiponectin. There has been concern that the consumption of orange juice may potentiate weight gain, particularly because of its sugar content. One randomized trial showed that when consumed concomitantly with a reduced-calorie diet, orange juice does not inhibit weight loss (body weight decreased-6.5 kg; p = 0.363 as well as BMI -2.5 kg/m²; p = 0.34), and insulin sensitivity, the lipid profile, and inflammatory status all improved [87].

Chromium

Chromium (III) or trivalent chromium, is a trace element widely present in the human diet (around 1–2% of ingested chromium is absorbed from the diet), and food sources such as meat, nuts, cereal grains, molasses, and brewer's yeast provide an especially abundant source. The exact mechanism is not clear, but it is believed to be associated with carbohydrate and lipid metabolism, and may have roles in the action of insulin and serum glucose regulation, while its effects on weight loss is related to its ability to regulate eating behaviour and food cravings, suppress appetite, stimulate thermo-genesis, enhance resting energy expenditure and improve insulin sensitivity [88–90]. Current dietary recommendations suggest a daily intake range between 25 and 45 µg/d for adults [91].

Although the role of chromium supplementation as a weight loss agent remains questionable, recent meta-analyses have reported reductions in body weight (WMD −0.75 kg, 95% CI: −1.04, −0.45, p < 0.001), BMI (WMD -0.40, 95% CI: −0.66, −0.13, p = 0.003 and body fat percentage (WMD -0.68%, 95% CI: −1.32, −0.03, p = 0.04) in individuals with overweight/obesity [92]. Also, one previous meta-analysis [93] shows that chromium supplementation lead to statistically significant reductions in body weight (MD compared to placebo −0.50 kg; 95% CI: −0.97, −0.03). However, the magnitude of the effect is small, and the clinical relevance remains uncertain.

Conjugated Linoleic Acid (CLA)

CLA represents a group of unsaturated fatty acid isomers with several biological effects seen in animals (reduces body fat accumulation, influences lipid and glucose metabolism) and it has been proposed that the trans10-cis12 isomer is the active isomer associated with the anti-obesity and insulin-sensitizing properties, although the metabolic effects in humans in general, and isomer-specific effects specifically, are not well characterized [94]. Interestingly, the gut microbiota has been suggested as a potential mediator of CLA effects on obesity.

Preliminary results showed that CLA may slightly decrease body fat in humans, particularly abdominal fat, but there was no effect on body weight or BMI, lipid or glucose metabolism [95]. However, recent studies indicate that although body weight and BMI were not significantly decreased, the body fat mass (p = 0.034), body fat percentage (p = 0.022), and truncal fat (p = 0.027) as well as serum leptin levels (p = 0.039) decreased significantly during intervention with CLA (3 g administered in 3 daily doses for 3 months) [96]. In addition, CLA (3 g/d for 12 weeks) significantly decreased hip circumference compared to placebo (p = 0.016), but again had no effect on body weight, BMI, or WC [97]. On the other hand, the t10c12-CLA isomer had been suggested as the bio-active isomer of CLA potentially influencing the body weight changes observed in subjects with T2DM [98]. One very recent meta-analysis indicates that CLA significantly reduced body weight (WMD −0.52 kg, 95% CI: −0.83, −0.21; I^2: 48.0%, p = 0.01), BMI (WMD −0.23 kg/m^2, 95% CI: −0.39, − 0.06; I^2: 64.7%, p = 0.0001) in overweight and obese subjects compared to the placebo, while the effects on WC was not significant [99]. Additionally, its impact on body weight in subjects older than 44 years (WMD −1.05 kg, 95% CI: −1.75, −0.35; I^2: 57.0%, p = 0.01), with longer duration (more than 12 weeks) (WMD −1.29 kg, 95% CI: −2.29, −0.29; I^2: 70.3%, p = 0.003) and dosage more than 3.4 g/day (WMD −0.77 kg, 95% CI: −1.28, −0.25; I^2: 62.7%, p = 0.004) were greater than comparator groups. Thus, the metabolic effects of CLA seems to be complex and future, longer studies, especially evaluating isomer-specific effects, are warranted.

Coleus Forskohlii Extract Supplementation

Coleus forskohlii extract (CFE) contains forskolin, which plays a major role in mediating the pharmacological action, and it is a popular ingredient of weight loss dietary supplements in Japan [100]. Increased cAMP synthesis by CFE may be associated with enhancement of cAMP-dependent lipolysis in adipose tissue.

The effects of supplementation with CFE (250 mg) on key markers of obesity and metabolic parameters in 30 overweight and obese individuals were investigated in an RCT for 12 weeks [101]. Significant reductions in waist and hip circumference (p = 0.02; p = 0.01, respectively) as well as HDL-cholesterol increases were recorded in both experimental and placebo groups, while the experimental group showed a favorable improvement in insulin concentration and insulin resistance (p = 0.001 and p = 0.01, respectively) compared to the placebo group. The results of another randomized, double blind study suggest that CFE (250 mg of 10% CFE two times per day for 12 weeks) does not appear to promote weight loss but may help mitigate weight gain in overweight women with apparently no clinically significant side effects [102]. However, further investigation is needed to validate the effects of CFE/forskolin in humans.

White Kidney Bean (*Phaseolus vulgaris* L.)

White kidney beans, mostly known as common beans (*Phaseolus vulgaris* L.), originate from South America. White kidney beans are important source of energy and vegetarians' proteins. White kidney beans are used as a nutraceutical due to their enrichment in bioactive peptides, polyphenols, resistant starch, and oligosaccharides [103]. One proposed mechanism of action of white kidney beans in weight loss is through its content of alpha-amylase inhibitor with ability to reduce spikes in blood sugar caused by dietary carbohydrates intake [104]. Consequently, after the consumption of white kidney bean extract (WKBE), the absorption of carbohydrates is lowered.

In clinical studies, including one meta-analysis, few products containing white kidney beans extract with high quantities of α-amylase inhibitors for weight loss have been investigated. A meta-analysis analyzed the effect of one single product containing white kidney beans extract (Phase2®) for weight loss [105]. After analyzing data from 11 studies (573 subjects), *Phaseolus vulgaris* supplementation lead to a reduction in body weight by −1.08 kg (95% CI: −0.42 kg to −1.16 kg, $p < 0.00001$), compared to placebo. Moreover, an important reduction in body fat of −3.26 kg (95% CI: −2.35 kg to −4.163 kg, $p = 0.02$) was reported [105]. Other WKBE formulations have been also studied in the context of RCTs in overweight and obese participants. At a dosage between 445 and 3000 mg for 28–84 days of follow-up period, the reported weight loss ranged from 1.8 to 3.5 kg [106]. When comparing high (450 mg) vs low (300 mg) doses of WKBE for 9 months, no difference was observed between the 2 groups, therefore, prolonged supplementation may be equally effective at high or low doses of WKBE supplementation [107]. To our knowledge only 2 studies by Udani et al. [108, 109] reported a significant difference in weight loss in obese participants supplemented with WKBE vs placebo. The first study investigated the effect of 3000 mg/d WKBE (2 × 1500 mg/d) for 56-days, while the second one evaluated the administration of 2000 mg/d for 28-days. These investigators found that those subjects with a greater intake of carbohydrates might benefit more from WKBE supplementation for weight loss with WKBE. Moreover, WKBE could have an impact on other health-related parameters such as blood glucose, insulin, triglycerides, total cholesterol, LDL-cholesterol, oxidative stress markers, gut and microbiota composition [106] as well as antihypertensive, anticancer, antioxidant and anti-inflammatory proprieties [103]. In conclusion, WKBE might be a useful nutraceutical for weight reduction, but more solid clinical evidence including a meta-analysis with all available RCTs is needed.

Prebiotics and Probiotics

Modulation of gut microbiota could be a potential target in the fight against obesity and obesity related disorders [110]. There are differences between lean vs overweight vs obese subjects in terms of gut microbiota composition. Intervention with probiotics could produce changes in gut microbiota composition and therefore could trigger some mechanisms causally related to body weight and body fat. Gut microbiota can change the expression of host genes that are involved in the development of adiposity, fat storage, and oxidation. Moreover, gut microbiota can play an important role in energy metabolism, gastrointestinal hormone modulation, as well as in obesity-related inflammation [111, 112]. The Food and Agriculture Organization of the United Nations (FAO) and World Health Organization (WHO) defined a probiotic as "*live microorganisms that, when administered in adequate amounts, confer a health benefit on the host*", while prebiotic is defined as "*a substrate that is selectively utilized by host microorganisms conferring a health benefit*" [113]. A synbiotic is a combination of both probiotics and prebiotics offering beneficial effect on the host microbiota. Supplementation with prebiotics, probiotics and synbiotics have been demonstrated to possess anti-inflammatory, immunomodulatory, antioxidant, anti-cancer, and anti-aging properties, as well an improvement in the responses to clinical treatment against several diseases [71, 114, 115].

Probiotics and prebiotics can indirectly lead to weight loss by influencing a number of mechanisms. Prebiotics could induce weight loss by modulating gut microbiota and the production of lipopolysaccharide (LPS), that hinders the process of low-grade inflammation and modulates the endocannabinoid (eCB) system. Furthermore, prebiotics are also involved in hunger promoting mechanisms by stimulating release of satiety peptides from L cells in the gut [18]. Probiotic supplementation could also induce beneficial changes in gut microbiota that impact body weight. Some of the proposed mechanism of action also includes production of bioactive compounds by probiotic strains, reduction in fat storage, induction of fatty acid oxidation genes, reduced expression of pro-inflammatory cytokines, and stimulating the production of satiety-inducing peptides [18]. Furthermore, probiotics could influence cholesterol metabolism by metabolizing both cholesterol and bile acids [116].

The inulin type of prebiotics could induce satiety, increase breath-hydrogen excretion, and modulate gut peptides involved in satiety regulation, and prompted the study of bifidobacteria and lactobacilli. *Lactobacillus* spp. and *Bifidobacterium* spp. are two extensively studied probiotics that have provided anti-obesity effects in animal models and human studies [18]. A growing body of literature has examined the administration of prebiotics, probiotics and synbiotics for weight management and the findings are contradictory. A recent review of the literature on this topic and data from a meta-analysis of 19 RCTs including a total of 1412 participants were analyzed. Investigators conclude that supplementation with probiotics or synbiotics had no effect on body weight or BMI and just a small effect in reducing WC [117]. However, this is a general conclusion, as several types of probiotics were investigated as capsules, yogurt, fermented milk, and cheese. Indeed, the biological effect is dependent on the specific prebiotic and probiotic used, and not every probiotic will perform the same role. In addition, the health-related benefit of probiotic supplements is species- and strain-specific [118]. A meta-analysis including 4 RCTs concluded that there is no significant effect of probiotics on body weight and BMI, but the authors reported that due to a low quality of the RCTs analyzed no definitive conclusion could be established [119]. On the other hand, a meta-analysis by Zang et al. [120] investigated the results of 25 studies including 1931 patients. The authors reported that probiotic supplementation could reduce body weight and BMI. Moreover, the effect was greater in overweight and obese subjects, when multiple species of probiotics were administrated, and the duration of intervention was longer than 2 months.

Other Nutraceuticals and Healthy Dietary Patterns

Compared with placebo (n = 25), the consumption of dietary supplements containing 125 mg green tea, 25 mg capsaicin and 50 mg ginger for 8 weeks led to a significant decrease in body weight (-1.8 ± 1.5 vs. $+0.4 \pm 1.2$ kg, respectively, p < 0.001) and BMI (-0.7 ± 0.5 vs. $+0.1 \pm 0.5$ kg/m^2, respectively, p < 0.001) in 25 overweight women. Also, beneficial effects were seen on markers of insulin metabolism and plasma glutathione (GSH) levels [121].

An increased consumption of vegetables, fruits, nuts, legumes, whole grain, but also of fish, eggs, poultry, red meat as well as low to moderate amounts of wine (characteristics of the Mediterranean Diet) has favorable effects on obesity as shown in clinical studies [122], but also in a meta-analysis (where a decrease in body weight (-2.2 kg; 95% CI: -3.9 to -0.6 kg) and BMI (0.6 kg/m^2; 95% CI: -1 to -0.1 kg/m^2) were reported [123]. It should be highlighted that the Mediterranean dietary model has been supported as a suitable model for T2DM (frequently associated with obesity) and that its beneficial health effects lie primarily in the synergy among various nutrients and foods rather than on any individual component [124]. Furthermore, in a parallel design study of 39 overweight hyperlipidaemic men and postmenopausal women advised to consume either a low-carbohydrate vegan diet (containing increased protein and fat from gluten and soy products, nuts and vegetable oils) or a high-carbohydrate lacto-ovo vegetarian diet for 6 months after completing 1 month metabolic (all foods provided) versions of these diets [125]. The metabolic treatment lead to an approximate 4 kg weight loss that was increased to −6.9 kg on low-carbohydrate and −5.8 kg on high-carbohydrate *ad libitum* treatments (treatment difference (95% CI) −1.1 kg (−2.1 to 0.0), $p = 0.047$). One meta-analysis of RCTs with 1369 participants assessed the effects of low-carbohydrate diets vs low-fat diets on weight loss and risk factors of CVD [126] and showed a greater reduction in body weight (WMD −2·17 kg; 95% CI −3·36, −0·99) in participants on low-carbohydrate diets.

A multi-ingredient supplement containing primarily raspberry ketone, caffeine, capsaicin, garlic, ginger and *Citrus aurantium* (Prograde Metabolism™ [METABO]) as an adjunct to an 8-week weight loss program, in a randomized, placebo-controlled, double-blind study resulted in significant differences vs. placebo in body weight (−2.0% vs. -0.5%, $p < 0.01$), but also fat mass (−7.8 vs. -2.8%, $p < 0.001$), lean mass (+3.4% vs. +0.8%, $p < 0.03$), waist girth (−2.0% vs. −0.2%, $p < 0.0007$), hip girth (−1.7% vs. −0.4%, $p < 0.003$), as well as energy levels [127].

Four-month treatment with a dietary supplement containing cinnamon, chromium and carnosine (1.2 g/day) had no significant effects on body weight and energy, but significantly decreased fasting plasma glucose and increased fat-free mass in overweight or obese pre-diabetic subjects [128]. These beneficial effects might open new avenues in the prevention of diabetes.

In conclusion, nutraceuticals and functional food have a beneficial effect on obesity and body weight. However, the current evidence is limited and still there are controversial findings, while the studies often differ among them (by the length of interventions, the dose used, the methodology, the population selected, etc). Consequently, their direct comparison is not possible. Future, well-designed, and longer-term studies are needed to further support the use of nutraceuticals in the prevention and/or management of obesity as well as obesity-related complications, but also to better understand their underlying mechanisms of action.

References

1. Martin-Rodriguez E, Guillen-Grima F, Marti A, Brugos-Larumbe A. Comorbidity associated with obesity in a large population: the APNA study. Obes Res Clin Pract. 2015;9:435–47.
2. Global BMIMC, Di Angelantonio E, Bhupathiraju Sh N, Wormser D, Gao P, Kaptoge S, et al. Body-mass index and all-cause mortality: individual-participant-data meta-analysis of 239 prospective studies in four continents. Lancet. 2016;388:776–86.

3. World Health Organization. Obesity and overweight. Available from: https://www.who.int/news-room/fact-sheets/detail/obesity-and-overweight
4. NHLBI Obesity education initiative expert panel on the identification, evaluation, and treatment of obesity in adults (US). Clinical guidelines on the identification, evaluation, and treatment of overweight and obesity in adults: the evidence report. Bethesda (MD): National Heart, Lung, and Blood Institute; 1998 Sep.. Available from: https://www.ncbi.nlm.nih.gov/books/NBK2003/
5. Jensen MD, Ryan DH, Apovian CM, Ard JD, Comuzzie AG, Donato KA, et al. 2013 AHA/ACC/TOS guideline for the management of overweight and obesity in adults: a report of the American College of Cardiology/American Heart Association Task Force on Practice Guidelines and The Obesity Society. J Am Coll Cardiol. 2014;63:2985–3023.
6. Garvey WT, Mechanick JI, Brett EM, Garber AJ, Hurley DL, Jastreboff AM, et al. American Association of Clinical Endocrinologists and American College of Endocrinology comprehensive clinical practice guidelines for medical care of patients with obesity. Endocr Pract. 2016;22(Suppl 3):1–203.
7. Valsamakis G, Konstantakou P, Mastorakos G. New targets for drug treatment of obesity. Annu Rev Pharmacol Toxicol. 2017;57:585–605.
8. Pillitteri JL, Shiffman S, Rohay JM, Harkins AM, Burton SL, Wadden TA. Use of dietary supplements for weight loss in the United States: results of a national survey. Obesity (Silver Spring). 2008;16:790–6.
9. Dikeman CL, Murphy MR, Fahey GC Jr. Dietary fibers affect viscosity of solutions and simulated human gastric and small intestinal digesta. J Nutr. 2006;136:913–9.
10. Howarth NC, Saltzman E, Roberts SB. Dietary fiber and weight regulation. Nutr Rev. 2001;59:129–39.
11. Wanders AJ, van den Borne JJ, de Graaf C, Hulshof T, Jonathan MC, Kristensen M, et al. Effects of dietary fibre on subjective appetite, energy intake and body weight: a systematic review of randomized controlled trials. Obes Rev. 2011;12:724–39.
12. Du H, van der Daphne A, Boshuizen HC, Forouhi NG, Wareham NJ, Halkjaer J, et al. Dietary fiber and subsequent changes in body weight and waist circumference in European men and women. Am J Clin Nutr. 2010;91:329–36.
13. Lairon D. Dietary fiber and control of body weight. Nutr Metab Cardiovasc Dis. 2007;17:1–5.
14. Slavin JL. Dietary fiber and body weight. Nutrition. 2005;21:411–8.
15. Thompson SV, Hannon BA, An R, Holscher HD. Effects of isolated soluble fiber supplementation on body weight, glycemia, and insulinemia in adults with overweight and obesity: a systematic review and meta-analysis of randomized controlled trials. Am J Clin Nutr. 2017;106:1514–28.
16. Pal S, McKay J, Jane M, Ho S. Chapter 19 – Using psyllium to prevent and treat obesity comorbidities. Nutrition in the prevention and treatment of abdominal obesity. 2nd ed. 2019. p. 245–260.
17. Masood R, Miraftab M. Psyllium: current and future applications. Medical and Healthcare Textiles 2010. p. 244-253.
18. Dahiya DK, Renuka, Puniya M, Shandilya UK, Dhewa T, Kumar N, et al. Gut microbiota modulation and its relationship with obesity using prebiotic fibers and probiotics: a review. Front Microbiol. 2017;8:563.
19. Darooghegi Mofrad M, Mozaffari H, Mousavi SM, Sheikhi A, Milajerdi A. The effects of psyllium supplementation on body weight, body mass index and waist circumference in adults: a systematic review and dose-response meta-analysis of randomized controlled trials. Crit Rev Food Sci Nutr. 2020;60:859–72.
20. Pal S, Radavelli-Bagatini S. Effects of psyllium on metabolic syndrome risk factors. Obes Rev. 2012;13:1034–47.
21. Ziai SA, Larijani B, Akhoondzadeh S, Fakhrzadeh H, Dastpak A, Bandarian F, et al. Psyllium decreased serum glucose and glycosylated hemoglobin significantly in diabetic outpatients. J Ethnopharmacol. 2005;102:202–7.

22. Kris-Etherton PM, Taylor DS, Smiciklas-Wright H, Mitchell DC, Bekhuis TC, Olson BH, et al. High-soluble-fiber foods in conjunction with a telephone-based, personalized behavior change support service result in favorable changes in lipids and lifestyles after 7 weeks. J Am Diet Assoc. 2002;102:503–10.
23. Pal S, Ho S, Gahler RJ, Wood S. Effect on body weight and composition in overweight/obese Australian adults over 12 months consumption of two different types of fibre supplementation in a randomized trial. Nutr Metab (Lond). 2016;13:82.
24. Jane M, McKay J, Pal S. Effects of daily consumption of psyllium, oat bran and polyGlycopleX on obesity-related disease risk factors: a critical review. Nutrition. 2019;57:84–91.
25. Khan K, Jovanovski E, Ho HVT, Marques ACR, Zurbau A, Mejia SB, et al. The effect of viscous soluble fiber on blood pressure: a systematic review and meta-analysis of randomized controlled trials. Nutr Metab Cardiovasc Dis. 2018;28:3–13.
26. Bernstein AM, Titgemeier B, Kirkpatrick K, Golubic M, Roizen MF. Major cereal grain fibers and psyllium in relation to cardiovascular health. Nutrients. 2013;5:1471–87.
27. Xiao Z, Chen H, Zhang Y, Deng H, Wang K, Bhagavathula AS, et al. The effect of psyllium consumption on weight, body mass index, lipid profile, and glucose metabolism in diabetic patients: a systematic review and dose-response meta-analysis of randomized controlled trials. Phytother Res. 2020;34:1237–47.
28. Whitehead A, Beck EJ, Tosh S, Wolever TM. Cholesterol-lowering effects of oat beta-glucan: a meta-analysis of randomized controlled trials. Am J Clin Nutr. 2014;100:1413–21.
29. Lazaridou A, Biliaderis CG. Molecular aspects of cereal β-glucan functionality: physical properties, technological applications and physiological effects. J Cereal Sci. 2007;46:101–18.
30. Ho HV, Sievenpiper JL, Zurbau A, Blanco Mejia S, Jovanovski E, Au-Yeung F, et al. The effect of oat beta-glucan on LDL-cholesterol, non-HDL-cholesterol and apoB for CVD risk reduction: a systematic review and meta-analysis of randomised-controlled trials. Br J Nutr. 2016;116:1369–82.
31. Beck EJ, Tosh SM, Batterham MJ, Tapsell LC, Huang XF. Oat beta-glucan increases post-prandial cholecystokinin levels, decreases insulin response and extends subjective satiety in overweight subjects. Mol Nutr Food Res. 2009;53:1343–51.
32. Beck EJ, Tapsell LC, Batterham MJ, Tosh SM, Huang XF. Oat beta-glucan supplementation does not enhance the effectiveness of an energy-restricted diet in overweight women. Br J Nutr. 2010;103:1212–22.
33. Kabir M, Oppert JM, Vidal H, Bruzzo F, Fiquet C, Wursch P, et al. Four-week low-glycemic index breakfast with a modest amount of soluble fibers in type 2 diabetic men. Metabolism. 2002;51:819–26.
34. Maki KC, Galant R, Samuel P, Tesser J, Witchger MS, Ribaya-Mercado JD, et al. Effects of consuming foods containing oat beta-glucan on blood pressure, carbohydrate metabolism and biomarkers of oxidative stress in men and women with elevated blood pressure. Eur J Clin Nutr. 2007;61:786–95.
35. Queenan KM, Stewart ML, Smith KN, Thomas W, Fulcher RG, Slavin JL. Concentrated oat beta-glucan, a fermentable fiber, lowers serum cholesterol in hypercholesterolemic adults in a randomized controlled trial. Nutr J. 2007;6:6.
36. Rahmani J, Miri A, Cerneviciute R, Thompson J, de Souza NN, Sultana R, et al. Effects of cereal beta-glucan consumption on body weight, body mass index, waist circumference and total energy intake: a meta-analysis of randomized controlled trials. Complement Ther Med. 2019;43:131–9.
37. Muanprasat C, Chatsudthipong V. Chitosan oligosaccharide: biological activities and potential therapeutic applications. Pharmacol Ther. 2017;170:80–97.
38. van Bennekum AM, Nguyen DV, Schulthess G, Hauser H, Phillips MC. Mechanisms of cholesterol-lowering effects of dietary insoluble fibres: relationships with intestinal and hepatic cholesterol parameters. Br J Nutr. 2005;94:331–7.
39. Rios-Hoyo A, Gutierrez-Salmean G. New dietary supplements for obesity: what we currently know. Curr Obes Rep. 2016;5:262–70.

40. Barrea L, Altieri B, Polese B, De Conno B, Muscogiuri G, Colao A, et al. Nutritionist and obesity: brief overview on efficacy, safety, and drug interactions of the main weight-loss dietary supplements. Int J Obes Suppl. 2019;9:32–49.
41. Tang D, Wang Y, Kang W, Zhou J, Dong R, Feng Q. Chitosan attenuates obesity by modifying the intestinal microbiota and increasing serum leptin levels in mice. J Funct Foods. 2020;64:103659.
42. Huang H, Liao D, Zou Y, Chi H. The effects of chitosan supplementation on body weight and body composition: a systematic review and meta-analysis of randomized controlled trials. Crit Rev Food Sci Nutr. 2019:1–11.
43. Moraru C, Mincea MM, Frandes M, Timar B, Ostafe V. A meta-analysis on randomised controlled clinical trials evaluating the effect of the dietary supplement chitosan on weight loss, lipid parameters and blood pressure. Medicina (Kaunas). 2018;54
44. Jull AB, Ni Mhurchu C, Bennett DA, Dunshea-Mooij CA, Rodgers A. Chitosan for overweight or obesity. Cochrane Database Syst Rev. 2008:CD003892.
45. EFSA Panel on Dietetic Products N, Allergies. Scientific Opinion on the substantiation of health claims related to chitosan and reduction in body weight (ID 679, 1499), maintenance of normal blood LDL-cholesterol concentrations (ID 4663), reduction of intestinal transit time (ID 4664) and reduction of inflammation (ID 1985) pursuant to Article 13(1) of Regulation (EC) No 1924/2006. 2011; 9: 2214.
46. Han Y, Zhang L, Liu XQ, Zhao ZJ, Lv LX. Effect of glucomannan on functional constipation in children: a systematic review and meta-analysis of randomised controlled trials. Asia Pac J Clin Nutr. 2017;26:471–7.
47. Janani F, Changaee F. The effect of glucomannan on pregnancy constipation. J Family Med Prim Care. 2018;7:903–6.
48. Zalewski BM, Chmielewska A, Szajewska H. The effect of glucomannan on body weight in overweight or obese children and adults: a systematic review of randomized controlled trials. Nutrition. 2015;31:437–42. e2
49. Sood N, Baker WL, Coleman CI. Effect of glucomannan on plasma lipid and glucose concentrations, body weight, and blood pressure: systematic review and meta-analysis. Am J Clin Nutr. 2008;88:1167–75.
50. Onakpoya I, Posadzki P, Ernst E. The efficacy of glucomannan supplementation in overweight and obesity: a systematic review and meta-analysis of randomized clinical trials. J Am Coll Nutr. 2014;33:70–8.
51. Solah VA, Kerr DA, Hunt WJ, Johnson SK, Boushey CJ, Delp EJ, et al. Effect of fibre supplementation on body weight and composition, frequency of eating and dietary choice in overweight individuals. Nutrients. 2017;9
52. Ross SM. African mango (IGOB131): a proprietary seed extract of Irvingia gabonensis is found to be effective in reducing body weight and improving metabolic parameters in overweight humans. Holist Nurs Pract. 2011;25:215–7.
53. Ngondi JL, Oben JE, Minka SR. The effect of Irvingia gabonensis seeds on body weight and blood lipids of obese subjects in Cameroon. Lipids Health Dis. 2005;4:12.
54. Oben JE, Ngondi JL, Momo CN, Agbor GA, Sobgui CS. The use of a Cissus quadrangularis/Irvingia gabonensis combination in the management of weight loss: a double-blind placebo-controlled study. Lipids Health Dis. 2008;7:12.
55. Ngondi JL, Etoundi BC, Nyangono CB, Mbofung CM, Oben JE. IGOB131, a novel seed extract of the West African plant Irvingia gabonensis, significantly reduces body weight and improves metabolic parameters in overweight humans in a randomized double-blind placebo controlled investigation. Lipids Health Dis. 2009;8:7.
56. Lee J, Chung M, Fu Z, Choi J, Lee HJ. The effects of Irvingia gabonensis seed extract supplementation on anthropometric and cardiovascular outcomes: a systematic review and meta-analysis. J Am Coll Nutr. 2019:1–9.
57. Gammone MA, D'Orazio N. Anti-obesity activity of the marine carotenoid fucoxanthin. Mar Drugs. 2015;13:2196–214.

58. Abidov M, Ramazanov Z, Seifulla R, Grachev S. The effects of Xanthigen in the weight man-
    agement of obese premenopausal women with non-alcoholic fatty liver disease and normal
    liver fat. Diabetes Obes Metab. 2010;12:72–81.
59. Guo B, Yang B, Pang X, Chen T, Chen F, Cheng KW. Fucoxanthin modulates cecal and fecal
    microbiota differently based on diet. Food Funct. 2019;10:5644–55.
60. Haber SL, Awwad O, Phillips A, Park AE, Pham TM. Garcinia cambogia for weight loss. Am
    J Health Syst Pharm. 2018;75:17–22.
61. Maia-Landim A, Ramirez JM, Lancho C, Poblador MS, Lancho JL. Long-term effects of
    Garcinia cambogia/Glucomannan on weight loss in people with obesity, PLIN4, FTO and
    Trp64Arg polymorphisms. BMC Complement Altern Med. 2018;18:26.
62. Pekala J, Patkowska-Sokola B, Bodkowski R, Jamroz D, Nowakowski P, Lochynski S,
    et al. L-carnitine--metabolic functions and meaning in humans life. Curr Drug Metab.
    2011;12:667–78.
63. Nazari M, Saberi A, Karandish M, Neisi N, Jalali MT, Makvandi M. Influence of L-carnitine
    on the expression level of adipose tissue miRNAs related to weight changes in obese rats. Pak
    J Biol Sci. 2016;19:227–32.
64. Karlic H, Lohninger A. Supplementation of L-carnitine in athletes: does it make sense?
    Nutrition. 2004;20:709–15.
65. Pooyandjoo M, Nouhi M, Shab-Bidar S, Djafarian K, Olyaeemanesh A. The effect of (L-)
    carnitine on weight loss in adults: a systematic review and meta-analysis of randomized con-
    trolled trials. Obes Rev. 2016;17:970–6.
66. Hursel R, Viechtbauer W, Westerterp-Plantenga MS. The effects of green tea on weight loss
    and weight maintenance: a meta-analysis. Int J Obes. 2009;33:956–61.
67. Lin JK, Lin CL, Liang YC, Lin-Shiau SY, Juan IM. Survey of catechins, gallic acid,
    and methylxanthines in green, oolong, pu-erh, and black teas. J Agric Food Chem.
    1998;46:3635–42.
68. Chacko SM, Thambi PT, Kuttan R, Nishigaki I. Beneficial effects of green tea: a literature
    review. Chin Med. 2010;5:13.
69. Wolfram S, Wang Y, Thielecke F. Anti-obesity effects of green tea: from bedside to bench.
    Mol Nutr Food Res. 2006;50:176–87.
70. Grove KA, Sae-tan S, Kennett MJ, Lambert JD. (−)-Epigallocatechin-3-gallate inhib-
    its pancreatic lipase and reduces body weight gain in high fat-fed obese mice. Obesity.
    2012;20:2311–3.
71. Venkatakrishnan K, Chiu HF, Wang CK. Extensive review of popular functional foods and
    nutraceuticals against obesity and its related complications with a special focus on random-
    ized clinical trials. Food Funct. 2019;10:2313–29.
72. Chen IJ, Liu CY, Chiu JP, Hsu CH. Therapeutic effect of high-dose green tea extract on
    weight reduction: a randomized, double-blind, placebo-controlled clinical trial. Clin Nutr.
    2016;35:592–9.
73. Zhang X, Zhang M, Ho CT, Guo X, Wu Z, Weng P, et al. Metagenomics analysis of gut
    microbiota modulatory effect of green tea polyphenols by high fat diet-induced obesity mice
    model. J Funct Foods. 2018;46:268–77.
74. Lin Y, Shi D, Su B, Wei J, Gaman MA, Sedanur Macit M, et al. The effect of green tea
    supplementation on obesity: a systematic review and dose-response meta-analysis of
    randomized controlled trials. Phytother Res. 2020;
75. Li X, Wang W, Hou L, Wu H, Wu Y, Xu R, et al. Does tea extract supplementation ben-
    efit metabolic syndrome and obesity? A systematic review and meta-analysis. Clin Nutr.
    2020;39:1049–58.
76. Jurgens TM, Whelan AM, Killian L, Doucette S, Kirk S, Foy E. Green tea for weight loss and
    weight maintenance in overweight or obese adults. Cochrane Database Syst Rev. 2012;
77. Smith C, Krygsman A. Hoodia gordonii: to eat, or not to eat. J Ethnopharmacol.
    2014;155:987–91.
78. Blom WA, Abrahamse SL, Bradford R, Duchateau GS, Theis W, Orsi A, et al. Effects of 15-d
    repeated consumption of Hoodia gordonii purified extract on safety, ad libitum energy intake,

and body weight in healthy, overweight women: a randomized controlled trial. Am J Clin Nutr. 2011;94:1171–81.

79. Landor M, Benami A, Segev N, Loberant B. Efficacy and acceptance of a commercial Hoodia parviflora product for support of appetite and weight control in a consumer trial. J Med Food. 2015;18:250–8.

80. Perna S, Infantino V, Peroni G, Gasparri C, Faliva MA, Naso M, et al. Effects of Hoodia Parviflora on satiety, abdominal obesity and weight in a group of overweight subjects: a randomized, blinded, placebo-controlled trial. Minerva Gastroenterol Dietol. 2020;

81. Onakpoya I, Hunt K, Wider B, Ernst E. Pyruvate supplementation for weight loss: a systematic review and meta-analysis of randomized clinical trials. Crit Rev Food Sci Nutr. 2014;54:17–23.

82. Ostojic SM, Ahmetovic Z. The effect of 4 weeks treatment with a 2-gram daily dose of pyruvate on body composition in healthy trained men. Int J Vitam Nutr Res. 2009;79:173–9.

83. Icken D, Feller S, Engeli S, Mayr A, Muller A, Hilbert A, et al. Caffeine intake is related to successful weight loss maintenance. Eur J Clin Nutr. 2016;70:532–4.

84. Tabrizi R, Saneei P, Lankarani KB, Akbari M, Kolahdooz F, Esmaillzadeh A, et al. The effects of caffeine intake on weight loss: a systematic review and dos-response meta-analysis of randomized controlled trials. Crit Rev Food Sci Nutr. 2019;59:2688–96.

85. Stohs SJ. Safety, efficacy, and mechanistic studies regarding Citrus aurantium (bitter orange) extract and p-Synephrine. Phytother Res. 2017;31:1463–74.

86. Capomolla AS, Janda E, Paone S, Parafati M, Sawicki T, Mollace R, et al. Atherogenic index reduction and weight loss in metabolic syndrome patients treated with a novel pectin-enriched formulation of bergamot polyphenols. Nutrients. 2019;11

87. Ribeiro C, Dourado G, Cesar T. Orange juice allied to a reduced-calorie diet results in weight loss and ameliorates obesity-related biomarkers: a randomized controlled trial. Nutrition. 2017;38:13–9.

88. Albarracin CA, Fuqua BC, Evans JL, Goldfine ID. Chromium picolinate and biotin combination improves glucose metabolism in treated, uncontrolled overweight to obese patients with type 2 diabetes. Diabetes Metab Res Rev. 2008;24:41–51.

89. Frauchiger MT, Wenk C, Colombani PC. Effects of acute chromium supplementation on postprandial metabolism in healthy young men. J Am Coll Nutr. 2004;23:351–7.

90. Hoffman JR, Kang J, Ratamess NA, Jennings PF, Mangine G, Faigenbaum AD. Thermogenic effect from nutritionally enriched coffee consumption. J Int Soc Sports Nutr. 2006;3:35–41.

91. National Institutes of HealthDietary Supplement Fact Sheet: Chromium Bethesda, MD: Office of Dietary Supplements, NIH ClinicalCenter, National Institutes of Health. 2007.

92. Tsang C, Taghizadeh M, Aghabagheri E, Asemi Z, Jafarnejad S. A meta-analysis of the effect of chromium supplementation on anthropometric indices of subjects with overweight or obesity. Clin Obes. 2019;9:e12313.

93. Onakpoya I, Posadzki P, Ernst E. Chromium supplementation in overweight and obesity: a systematic review and meta-analysis of randomized clinical trials. Obes Rev. 2013;14:496–507.

94. den Hartigh LJ. Conjugated linoleic acid effects on cancer, obesity, and atherosclerosis: a review of pre-clinical and human trials with current perspectives. Nutrients. 2019;11

95. Riserus U, Smedman A, Basu S, Vessby B. CLA and body weight regulation in humans. Lipids. 2003;38:133–7.

96. Esmaeili Shahmirzadi F, Ghavamzadeh S, Zamani T. The effect of conjugated linoleic acid supplementation on body composition, serum insulin and leptin in obese adults. Arch Iran Med. 2019;22:255–61.

97. Madry E, Chudzicka-Strugala I, Grabanska-Martynska K, Malikowska K, Grebowiec P, Lisowska A, et al. Twelve weeks CLA supplementation decreases the hip circumference in overweight and obese women. A double-blind, randomized, placebo-controlled trial. Acta Sci Pol Technol Aliment. 2016;15:107–13.

98. Belury MA, Mahon A, Banni S. The conjugated linoleic acid (CLA) isomer, t10c12-CLA, is inversely associated with changes in body weight and serum leptin in subjects with type 2 diabetes mellitus. J Nutr. 2003;133:257S–60S.

99. Namazi N, Irandoost P, Larijani B, Azadbakht L. The effects of supplementation with conjugated linoleic acid on anthropometric indices and body composition in overweight and obese subjects: a systematic review and meta-analysis. Crit Rev Food Sci Nutr. 2019;59:2720–33.
100. Suzuki S, Nishijima C, Sato Y, Umegaki K, Murata M, Chiba T. Coleus forskohlii extract attenuated the beneficial effect of diet-treatment on NASH in mouse model. J Nutr Sci Vitaminol (Tokyo). 2020;66:191–9.
101. Loftus HL, Astell KJ, Mathai ML, Su XQ. Coleus forskohlii extract supplementation in conjunction with a Hypocaloric diet reduces the risk factors of metabolic syndrome in overweight and obese subjects: a randomized controlled trial. Nutrients. 2015;7:9508–22.
102. Henderson S, Magu B, Rasmussen C, Lancaster S, Kerksick C, Smith P, et al. Effects of coleus forskohlii supplementation on body composition and hematological profiles in mildly overweight women. J Int Soc Sports Nutr. 2005;2:54–62.
103. Heredia-Rodríguez L, de la Garza AL, Garza-Juarez AJ, Vazquez-Rodriguez JA. Nutraceutical properties of bioactive peptides in common bean (Phaseolus vulgaris L.). J Food Nutri Diete. 2016;2:111.
104. Barrett ML, Udani JK. A proprietary alpha-amylase inhibitor from white bean (Phaseolus vulgaris): a review of clinical studies on weight loss and glycemic control. Nutr J. 2011;10:24.
105. Udani J, Tan O, Molina J. Systematic review and meta-analysis of a proprietary alpha-amylase inhibitor from white bean (Phaseolus vulgaris L.) on weight and fat loss in humans. Foods. 2018:7.
106. Nolan R, Shannon OM, Robinson N, Joel A, Houghton D, Malcomson FC. It's no has bean: a review of the effects of white kidney bean extract on body composition and metabolic health. Nutrients. 2020;12
107. Støa Birketvedt G, Langbakk B, Florholmen J. A dietary supplement with bean extract decreases body weight, body fat, waist circumference and blood pressure in over-weight and obese subjects. Curr Top Nutraceutical Res. 2005;3:137–42.
108. Udani J, Hardy M, Madsen DC. Blocking carbohydrate absorption and weight loss: a clinical trial using Phase 2 brand proprietary fractionated white bean extract. Altern Med Rev. 2004;9:63–9.
109. Udani J, Singh BB. Blocking carbohydrate absorption and weight loss: a clinical trial using a proprietary fractionated white bean extract. Altern Ther Health Med. 2007;13:32–7.
110. Davis CD. The gut microbiome and its role in obesity. Nutr Today. 2016;51:167–74.
111. Delzenne NM, Neyrinck AM, Backhed F, Cani PD. Targeting gut microbiota in obesity: effects of prebiotics and probiotics. Nat Rev Endocrinol. 2011;7:639–46.
112. Boulange CL, Neves AL, Chilloux J, Nicholson JK, Dumas ME. Impact of the gut microbiota on inflammation, obesity, and metabolic disease. Genome Med. 2016;8:42.
113. Hill C, Guarner F, Reid G, Gibson GR, Merenstein DJ, Pot B, et al. Expert consensus document. The international scientific Association for Probiotics and Prebiotics consensus statement on the scope and appropriate use of the term probiotic. Nat Rev Gastroenterol Hepatol. 2014;11:506–14.
114. George Kerry R, Patra JK, Gouda S, Park Y, Shin HS, Das G. Benefaction of probiotics for human health: a review. J Food Drug Anal. 2018;26:927–39.
115. Ctoi AF, Corina A, Katsiki N, Vodnar DC, Andreicut AD, Stoian AP, et al. Gut microbiota and aging – a focus on centenarians. Biochim Biophys Acta Mol basis Dis. 1866;2020:165765.
116. Hunter PM, Hegele RA. Functional foods and dietary supplements for the management of dyslipidaemia. Nat Rev Endocrinol. 2017;13:278–88.
117. Suzumura EA, Bersch-Ferreira AC, Torreglosa CR, da Silva JT, Coqueiro AY, Kuntz MGF, et al. Effects of oral supplementation with probiotics or synbiotics in overweight and obese adults: a systematic review and meta-analyses of randomized trials. Nutr Rev. 2019;77:430–50.
118. Ejtahed HS, Angoorani P, Soroush AR, Atlasi R, Hasani-Ranjbar S, Mortazavian AM, et al. Probiotics supplementation for the obesity management; a systematic review of animal studies and clinical trials. J Funct Foods. 2019;52:228–42.

119. Park S, Bae JH. Probiotics for weight loss: a systematic review and meta-analysis. Nutr Res. 2015;35:566–75.
120. Zhang Q, Wu Y, Fei X. Effect of probiotics on body weight and body-mass index: a systematic review and meta-analysis of randomized, controlled trials. Int J Food Sci Nutr. 2015;67:571–80.
121. Taghizadeh M, Farzin N, Taheri S, Mahlouji M, Akbari H, Karamali F, et al. The effect of dietary supplements containing green tea, capsaicin and ginger extracts on weight loss and metabolic profiles in overweight women: a randomized double-blind placebo-controlled clinical trial. Ann Nutr Metab. 2017;70:277–85.
122. Salvia R, D'Amore S, Graziano G, Capobianco C, Sangineto M, Paparella D, et al. Short-term benefits of an unrestricted-calorie traditional Mediterranean diet, modified with a reduced consumption of carbohydrates at evening, in overweight-obese patients. Int J Food Sci Nutr. 2017;68:234–48.
123. Nordmann AJ, Suter-Zimmermann K, Bucher HC, Shai I, Tuttle KR, Estruch R, et al. Meta-analysis comparing Mediterranean to low-fat diets for modification of cardiovascular risk factors. Am J Med. 2011;124:841–51. e2
124. Vitale M, Masulli M, Calabrese I, Rivellese AA, Bonora E, Signorini S, et al. Impact of a Mediterranean dietary pattern and its components on cardiovascular risk factors, glucose control, and body weight in people with type 2 diabetes: a real-life study. Nutrients. 2018;10
125. Jenkins DJ, Wong JM, Kendall CW, Esfahani A, Ng VW, Leong TC, et al. Effect of a 6-month vegan low-carbohydrate ('Eco-Atkins') diet on cardiovascular risk factors and body weight in hyperlipidaemic adults: a randomised controlled trial. BMJ Open. 2014;4:e003505.
126. Mansoor N, Vinknes KJ, Veierod MB, Retterstol K. Effects of low-carbohydrate diets v. low-fat diets on body weight and cardiovascular risk factors: a meta-analysis of randomised controlled trials. Br J Nutr. 2016;115:466–79.
127. Lopez HL, Ziegenfuss TN, Hofheins JE, Habowski SM, Arent SM, Weir JP, et al. Eight weeks of supplementation with a multi-ingredient weight loss product enhances body composition, reduces hip and waist girth, and increases energy levels in overweight men and women. J Int Soc Sports Nutr. 2013;10:22.
128. Liu Y, Cotillard A, Vatier C, Bastard JP, Fellahi S, Stevant M, et al. A dietary supplement containing cinnamon, chromium and Carnosine decreases fasting plasma glucose and increases lean mass in overweight or obese pre-diabetic subjects: a randomized, placebo-controlled trial. PLoS One. 2015;10:e0138646.

Chapter 9
Nutraceuticals for Non-alcoholic Fatty Liver Disease

Alper Sonmez, Cemal Nuri Ercin, Mustafa Cesur, and Teoman Dogru

Introduction and Definition

Nonalcoholic Fatty liver Disease (NAFLD) is a clinical spectrum of liver disorders characterized by increased fat storage in the hepatocytes without a history of excessive alcohol consumption. The disorders in the spectrum of NAFLD range from Nonalcoholic Fatty Liver (NAFL), namely steatosis without significant inflammation or fibrosis; to nonalcoholic steatohepatitis (NASH) with varying degrees of inflammation, injury or fibrosis; and finally, to Cirrhosis [1–3].

Epidemiology

Different reports from different geographical regions give the NAFLD incidence about 10–50 per 1000 person-years and a global prevalence around 25% [4–9]. The population data for NASH is quite few, as the gold standard diagnostic method, liver biopsy, cannot be performed for epidemiological purposes. However, it can be estimated that 7–30% of NAFLD patients who undergo liver biopsies have NASH. This

A. Sonmez (✉)
Department of Endocrinology and Metabolism, University of Health Sciences, Gulhane Faculty of Medicine, Ankara, Turkey

C. N. Ercin
Department of Gastroenterology, University of Health Sciences, Gulhane Faculty of Medicine, Ankara, Turkey

M. Cesur
Department of Endocrinology and Metabolism, Ankara Guven Hospital, Ankara, Turkey

T. Dogru
Department of Gastroenterology, Balıkesir University, Faculty of Medicine, Balıkesir, Turkey

© Springer Nature Switzerland AG 2021
A. F.G. Cicero, M. Rizzo (eds.), *Nutraceuticals and Cardiovascular Disease*, Contemporary Cardiology, https://doi.org/10.1007/978-3-030-62632-7_9

indicates that the overall prevalence of NASH is likely to be between 1.5% and 6.45% [4]. The prevalence of NAFLD become highest in the fourth to fifth decades [10, 11]. There are conflicting reports about the gender distribution of NAFLD. Some reports suggest that NAFLD is more prevalent in men [12, 13]. While others mention it is more common in women [14, 15]. Ethnicity may be a predictor for NAFLD [16–18]. The prevalence appears to be higher in Hispanics than the Caucasian and the African American population [17]. The high prevalence of obesity in the Hispanic population may be a reason for the ethnic variations in the NAFLD frequency. Some genetic modifiers of disease severity may also have role in the ethnic variations of NAFLD frequency [19].

The risk of NAFLD is significantly increased in patients with Metabolic Syndrome mainly in patients with obesity [20, 21]. The whole spectrum of visceral adiposity, from overweight to severe obesity, is associated with the increased risk of NAFLD. More than 95% of subjects who undergo bariatric surgery are reported to have NAFLD [22]. The prevalence is also high in subjects with type 2 diabetes. About one to two third of patients with type 2 diabetes are estimated to have NAFLD [23]. Finally, more than half of patients with dyslipidemia have NAFLD. Patients with high TG and low HDL Cholesterol levels are the ones with the highest frequency of NAFLD [24, 25]. The lipoprotein phenotypes are more atherogenic in patients with NASH than those with NAFL [26].

Diagnosis

NAFLD can only be diagnosed after ruling out several etiological factors such as chronic alcohol intake (>20 gr/day for woman and > 30 gr/day for man), long term use of steatogenic drugs and hereditary disorders [1]. Liver enzymes are often abnormal in NAFLD. However, liver enzyme elevation by itself is not sufficient for the diagnosis of NAFLD. There are many cases with normal liver enzyme levels and there are many different causes of liver enzyme elevation other than the NAFLD. Ultrasound imaging is the most common diagnostic test, which detects NAFLD when the 10% of the hepatocytes have fat deposits [27]. Proton magnetic resonance spectroscopy (HMRS) and quantitative fat/water selective magnetic resonance imaging (MRI) are among the other diagnostic tests [28] which are less frequently used. Vibration controlled transient elastography is a common method to grade fibrosis based on liver stiffness and is also developed to the severity of hepatic steatosis [29]. Liver histology is the gold standard test which can establish NAFLD when 5% of hepatocytes have fat depots. However, it is not necessary to perform liver biopsy for every case with an ultrasound finding consistent with NAFLD. When other etiologies of liver disease cannot be not ruled out, or when the patient is at high risk of cirrhosis, liver biopsy would be necessary for the definite diagnosis.

Pathogenesis

The pathogenesis of NAFLD involves both genetic and environmental factors which in combination cause the metabolic alterations in the hepatocyte. The so called 'Multiple Hit' theory puts forward the role of multiple etiopathological factors on a genetic background [30]. The genetic and epigenetic factors not only determine the transition period from NAFL to NASH but also cause inflammation and fibrosis from the very beginning of the process [30]. The main pathology is the TG deposition in the hepatocytes, which occurs due to the higher fatty acid intake than the consumption. The 75% of the total TG depot is exogenous, while only 25% is produced in liver by the de novo lipogenesis [31, 32]. The amount of lipogenesis is significantly increased, and fatty acid beta oxidation rate is impaired in patients with NAFLD. The TG transformation to the very low density lipoproteins (VLDL) is also decreased in patients with NAFLD [32]. It is estimated that one third of patients with NAFL progress to NASH. This progression occurs due to the maladaptation of liver to the increased fatty acid input and involves the sequences of lipotoxicity, inflammation, increased hepatocellular dysfunction and fibrosis [32, 33].

Clinical Picture

The clinical and pathological features of NAFLD are diverse. The spectrum starts from noninflammatory deposition of fatty acids and may progress to fibrosis and hepatocellular carcinoma (HCC) [34, 35]. NASH is the second leading cause of liver disease among adults awaiting liver transplantation [36]. Inflammation and fibrosis are the most important factors playing role in the liver related mortality and morbidity [37–39]. Genetic factors play significant role in the severity of inflammation [40]. The mechanism of the progression of NAFL to NASH is not clear. Prospective studies show that progression to NASH is observed in about 40% of cases with NAFLD, while progression to fibrosis without inflammation is reported in the 40% [41]. Mortality is significantly higher in patients with NAFLD which includes mostly the cardiovascular deaths [1, 42]. HCC may occur in every patient with cirrhosis. HCC patients with a background of NAFLD have shorter surveys when compared to HCC patients without NAFLD. They are older and they generally have cardiovascular comorbidities [43]. Interestingly, about half of these HCC patients do not have a significant clinical picture of cirrhosis [44]. Especially patients with metabolic syndrome may develop HCC without fibrosis [45].

Treatment Strategies in Patients with NAFLD

There are two major aims of managing patients with NAFLD. The first one is reducing the cardiovascular risk and the other is preventing the progression of liver disease. Therefore, a wise approach should always involve lifestyle modification while taking into account the comorbidities and the stage of the liver disease [46].

Lifestyle Modification

Living a healthy life is the first and foremost strategy to prevent NAFLD. Weight reduction significantly improves liver histology, liver enzymes, serum insulin levels and quality of life in patients with NAFLD [47–49]. Hepatic steatosis and NAFLD activity score (NAS) significantly improve in patients after a modest (>5%) weight loss [47, 50]. There is robust data showing that moderate to severe alcohol intake increase disease progression [51]. Although there is no evidence about the effect of light alcohol intake in NAFLD, it would be a prudent approach to recommend people to refrain from alcohol intake. Cardiorespiratory fitness has a strong relation with the risk of fatty liver, especially in the population with obesity [52]. Exercise increases fatty acid oxidation, reduce fatty acid synthesis, and prevents mitochondrial and hepatocellular damage [53]. Exercise programs of 2–3 sessions a week of 30–60 min over a period of 6–12 weeks are recommended for patients with NAFLD [1].

Treatment of the Components of Metabolic Syndrome

Metabolic syndrome grows on top of insulin resistance and obesity. Therefore, treatment regimens establishing insulin sensitivity and weight lose have the potential to improve metabolic syndrome and NAFLD [54–56]. Metformin is the most common insulin sensitizer. However, it's not effective in NAFLD treatment [57]. There is more robust data for Pioglitazone. Pioglitazone treatment significantly improves ballooning degeneration, lobular inflammation, steatosis and combined necroinflammation in patients with NASH [58].

If patients cannot lose enough weight with diet and exercise, medical treatment of obesity and bariatric surgery are considered as further strategies. Medical agents for weight loss may improve liver enzymes and liver histology. Orlistate improves biochemical indicators of liver damage, while it is far from being a first-choice drug for the management of NAFLD or NASH [59]. On the other hand, Liraglutide treatment may be a promising agent to prevent fibrosis progression and resolve NASH [60]. Patients can be referred for bariatric surgery, if they do not meet weight loss goals after 6 months of lifestyle interventions and medical treatment. Especially for patients with NASH or advanced fibrosis bariatric surgery is a promising treatment strategy. Bariatric surgery decreases steatosis and inflammation and improves fibrosis score [61].

Liver Specific Treatments in NAFLD

Numerous liver specific pharmacological agents with anti-inflammatory, antioxidant, antifibrotic or insulin sensitizing properties have been investigated for NAFLD treatment. However, there is so far no single pharmacological agent which is highly effective and safe. Therefore, pharmacotherapy should be reserved for patients with NASH and with significant fibrosis (stage ≥2) [28]. Current evidence shows that nondiabetic patients with biopsy proven NASH and fibrosis can be treated with vitamin E (800 IU/day) replacement [46, 62]. As there are reports about the increased all-cause mortality in patients taking high dosage vitamin E [63, 64], the risk and benefits of treatment should be discussed with the patient before the treatment. Pioglitazone or Liraglutide can be preferred on top of metformin treatment in patients with diabetes mellitus and biopsy proven NASH [58, 60].

Nutraceuticals for NAFLD Treatment

As there is no highly effective pharmacological treatment strategy for NAFLD, the effects of nutraceuticals on liver functions and histology have received much attention [65]. Numerous nutraceutical agents have been investigated for the treatment of NAFLD so far [66–68]. Phytochemicals, mono or Polyunsaturated fatty acids, antioxidant vitamins or minerals are the common bioactive molecules of nutraceuticals [69]. These active organic compounds are responsible for the protective effects of nutraceuticals by their positive effects on inflammation, oxidant stress and insulin resistance or by regulating the imbalance of the gut microbiota [67, 68]. Their effects on liver functions and liver histology have been observed in several clinical studies. Some nutraceuticals seem to have positive effects on liver enzymes and lower liver fat content [66]. However, despite the abundance of promising nutraceutical agents, the number of long-term, prospective randomized controlled clinical trials are not enough. The current evidence on the effects of nutraceuticals in NAFLD/NASH treatment is discussed below.

Silymarin

Silymarin, an ancient medicinal plant, is a flavonoid polyphenol, which is produced from the extracts of milk thistle or St. Mary's thistle (Silybum marianum). Silymarin and its active ingredient silybin have antioxidant, anti-inflammatory and anti-fibrotic effects [70, 71]. Silymarin reduces fibrogenesis, stimulates liver regeneration and inhibits hepatic stellate cell activation [71]. Because of its significant biological effects, silymarin is one of the most common nutraceuticals for liver disorders [72]. The oral bioavailability of silymarin is not high because of the poor intestinal absorption and fast first pass metabolism in liver. Several studies have been performed with silymarin with different follow up periods, different dosages and combinations. An observational study has shown that, 6 months treatment with a complex of silybin- vitamin E and phospholipids decreases liver enzymes, HOMA-IR levels and improves the ultrasound grade of NAFLD [73]. Silymarin and Vitamin E combination, implemented for 6 months, decreases transaminases, without significant improvements in the noninvasive markers, such as fatty liver index, lipid accumulation product and NAFLD-fibrosis Score [74]. Another report of 3 months long treatment with silymarin shows significant improvement in insulin resistance and the indirect markers of hepatosteatosis such as hepatic steatosis index and lipid accumulation product [75]. Combination of silymarin, phosphatidylcholine and vitamin E improved liver enzymes and ultrasonographical scoring of NAFLD in a 12 months long multicenter randomized double blind study in patients with histological diagnosis of NAFLD/NASH. Liver biopsies, performed in a subgroup both before and after the study period, showed significant improvements in the severity of steatosis, lobular inflammation, ballooning and fibrosis [76]. Another clinical study, twice daily intake of a food supplement containing vitamin E, L-glutation, L-systein, L-methionin and silybum marianum significantly improved liver enzyme levels and the ultrasonographical severity of NAFLD in 3 months [77]. Another placebo-controlled study of silymarin showed no improvement in liver enzymes but a significant improvement in biometric parameters such as waist circumference, body mass index and the sonographically measured size of right hepatic lobe [78]. A metanalysis which involves eight randomized controlled studies showed that silymarin has positive efficacy to reduce transaminases in patients with NAFLD [79].

In conclusion, according to the current data, silymarin supplementation appears to have beneficial effects on the NAFLD treatment. The high safety profile of silymarin may be an advantage in the long-term use of this product. Silymarin is mentioned as a potentially useful treatment for NASH in AsiaPacific guidelines [80]. However, in order to obtain a global approval, larger scientific evidence is warranted to find out optimal dose and duration and to implement silymarin in children and adult population with NAFLD.

Vitamin E

Vitamin E is a potent antioxidant fat soluble vitamin, abundantly found in sunflower oil, palm oil, rice bran oil, olive oil, nuts and grains [81]. Because oxidative stress has a significant role in the pathogenesis of NAFLD, vitamin E is largely investigated in NAFLD treatment. In comparison to the healthy population, Vitamin E levels are reported to be significantly lower in patients with NAFLD [82]. No difference is established between patients with simple steatosis or NASH [82]. Vitamin E replacement in patients with NAFLD show significant improvements in liver enzymes [83, 84].

There is also data about the effects of vitamin E replacement on liver histology. Significant improvement in fibrosis score without any change in inflammation is reported in a randomized, double blind, placebo-controlled study of adult patients with NASH [85]. PIVENS (Pioglitazone versus Vitamin E versus Placebo for the Treatment of Nondiabetic Patients with Nonalcoholic Steatohepatitis) was a multi-center, randomized, placebo controlled, double blind, phase 3 study. Vitamin E 800 IU daily was given to 84 nondiabetic patients with NASH for 96 weeks. The results of the PIVENS study show significant decreases in ALT levels and improvements in histopathological findings such as steatosis, lobular inflammation and ballooning degeneration in the Vitamin E arm when compared to placebo or pioglitazone arms [86]. TONIC (Effect of vitamin E or metformin for treatment of nonalcoholic fatty liver disease in children and adolescents) was a double-blind, double-dummy, placebo-controlled clinical trial performed in 173 children or adolescents with biopsy-confirmed NAFLD. Sustained reduction in ALT level were not established but significant histological improvements in hepatocellular ballooning scores and NAFLD activity scores were obtained after 96 weeks of treatment of Vitamin E (800 IU/day) when compared to metformin (1000 mg/day) or placebo [87]. A meta-nalysis of five randomized controlled studies has shown that vitamin E replacement significantly improves liver functions and liver histology in children and adult patients with NAFLD/NASH [88].

In conclusion, there is limited data on the effects of Vitamin E replacement in patients with NAFLD. In accordance to the results of PIVENS study, current guidelines recommend vitamin E (800 IU/day) replacement in nondiabetic patients with biopsy proven NASH [28, 89]. However, due to the unexpected data on increased all-cause mortality [63, 64] or prostate cancer risk [90], vitamin E replacement should not be unanimously recommended to all patients with NAFLD or NASH.

Vitamin D

Vitamin D is a steroid hormone playing role in bone mineral metabolism, immune response regulation, cell differentiation and inflammation. Only 10% of circulating vitamin D is derived from the food intake while the rest is de-novo synthesized by the epidermal effect of ultraviolet (UV) B radiation. The UV B effect converts 7-dehydrocholesterol to cholecalciferol which is sequentially hydroxylated in liver and kidney to its final active form 1,25-hydroxy-cholecalciferol or Calcitriol [91–93]. Vitamin D deficiency may have role in insulin resistance and increase the risk of Metabolic Syndrome and Type 2 diabetes. Several studies show increased prevalence of vitamin D deficiency in patients with metabolic syndrome. Also, people with biopsy diagnosed NASH have lower vitamin D levels with a negative correlation to the severity of liver fibrosis [94, 95]. Similar findings were also reported in patients with NAFLD and normal liver enzymes [96]. Vitamin receptors are expressed in hepatocytes and vitamin receptor interaction may have a role in the progression of NASH [97].

Despite the evidence about the role of vitamin D deficiency in NAFLD, there are controversial reports about the beneficial effects of vitamin D replacement in the improvement of fatty liver. In a double-blind randomized placebo controlled clinical study, vitamin D replacement (50,000 IU/weekly for 4 months to 53 patients) did not cause significant improvements in liver enzymes, insulin sensitivity or the severity of hepatosteatosis [98]. Another clinical study of vitamin D replacement (2000 IU daily) also did not show significant improvements on metabolic parameters and the severity of steatosis in 42 patients with NAFLD [99]. Likewise, vitamin D replacement (25,000 IU/weekly) for 24 weeks did not improve liver enzymes, insulin resistance and histological findings in biopsy proven patients with NASH [100]. Another randomized double-blind controlled study reported that there may be significant improvements in liver enzymes, lipid parameters and insulin sensitivity in patients with NAFLD when calcium is added to vitamin D replacement [101]. A metanalysis of 974 patients with NAFLD has shown that, the vitamin D levels were not different when patients with high and low NAS and patients with high and low fibrosis scores compared [102]. Therefore, although vitamin D deficiency appears to have role in the pathogenesis of NAFLD, it is not clear that vitamin D has a histopathological effect on NAFLD [102].

In summary, the data about the relationship between vitamin D deficiency and the pathogenesis of NAFLD is inconclusive. The inconsistencies between different reports may be related to the methodological differences between these studies. Therefore, larger and longer-term prospective studies are warranted to better understand the direct effects of vitamin D replacement on disease progression.

Carnitine

L-carnitine, is an endogenous precursor of the carnitine-palmitoyltransferase-1. L-carnitine plays critical roles in the transport of fatty acids into mitochondria, cell membrane stabilization, and lowering of serum lipid levels. It regulates the energy imbalance in cells where much of the energy is produced from the fatty acid oxidation. Also, L-carnitine regulates immune response. L-carnitine replacement is expected to have beneficial effects in several metabolic disorders such as obesity, type 2 diabetes and liver cirrhosis [103–105].

In a placebo controlled clinical study, oral L- carnitine replacement (2 g/daily for 24 weeks) significantly reduced liver enzymes, insulin resistance and inflammatory parameters in 24 weeks in patients with NASH. The control biopsy has shown that NASH activity index, defined by steatosis, parenchymal inflammation and hepatocellular injury and fibrosis score significantly improved [106]. However, another randomized controlled study reported that 52 weeks long L-carnitine replacement (500 mg twice daily) did not show significant alterations in liver enzymes and liver ultrasound findings about steatosis [107].

So far, the data about the effects of L-carnitine replacement on NAFLD pathogenesis is controversial. More data is warranted to better understand the effect of long-term L-carnitine replacement on liver pathology.

Omega-3 Fatty Acids

Adipose tissue has the ability to effectively deposit free fatty acids (FFA). Obesity is a major cause of lipotoxicity of FFA in liver and pancreas. The exposure to FFA activates inflammatory pathways, impairs cellular communication and results in cellular dysfunction. Metabolic disorders such as insulin resistance and type 2 diabetes ensue as a result of chronic lipotoxicity [108]. Omega-3 fatty acids are essential polyunsaturated fatty acids (PUFA), which are not produced in vivo or which are not derived from alfa-linolenic acid. The most common omega-3 FFAs are Docosahexaenoic acid (DHA) and Eicosapentaenoic acid (EPA). Fish oil is a suitable source for omega-3 fatty acids. The most important effect of omega-3 FFAs is the cellular regulation of the metabolism from lipogenesis and triacylglycerol deposition to the fatty acid oxidation. PUFAs regulate lipid metabolism by reducing lipogenesis via their effects on Peroxisome proliferator-activated receptor alfa (PPAR- α) and the transcription of sterol regulatory element binding protein 1c (SREMP-1). This mechanism facilitates FFA oxidation and reduces hepatosteatosis. Insulin resistance can be improved by the anti-inflammatory effects of PUFAs [109].

There are several studies about the role of PUFA replacement on the improvement of NAFLD. A clinical study about 12 months of PUFA replacement reports significant improvements in TG and ALT levels and the ultrasound grade of steatosis [110]. Similar findings were also reported in several randomized controlled studies of PUFA (2 g/daily) replacement [111, 112]. PUFA appears to lower serum TG levels without lowering liver TG content [113].

Another clinical study showed that DHA (250 mg/day and 500 mg/day) significantly lowered hepatosteatosis and serum triglycerides and improved insulin sensitivity in 60 children with NAFLD [114]. A metanalysis of 9 clinical studies showed that PUFA can significantly but modestly improve liver enzymes and hepatic fat content [115].

In conclusion there are well designed but heterogeneous clinical studies about the role of PUFAs in the pathogenesis of NAFLD. Also, the number of studies involving histopathological assessments are limited. Finally, the optimal dosage, treatment period and long-term safety data are not established.

Vitamin C

Vitamin C is a water-soluble antioxidant and a free radical scavenger which plays role in infection control and cellular development. Vitamin C is not synthesized in the body and taken mainly form the fruit and vegetables. Cross-sectional population studies have shown that about 10–20% of the western population may have Vitamin C deficiency [116, 117]. Low vitamin C levels are not only related to NAFLD but also the risk of hypertension, cancer and atherosclerotic cardiovascular diseases [118, 119].

Animal studies report that vitamin C deficiency results in elevation of plasma and liver lipids, and increased oxidative stress, inflammation and fibrosis in liver, and vitamin C replacement reduces hepatic oxidative stress [120]. There are controversial reports from the epidemiological studies about the relation between vitamin C intake and NAFLD. According to some reports people with NAFLD have low vitamin C intake [121, 122] while others do not report any relationship at all [123–125].

Direct examination of the effect of Vitamin C replacement in comparison to placebo has not been performed in patients with NAFLD so far. However, studies which combine Vitamin C in combination to other vitamins have been conducted. A 12 month, double-blinded, randomized controlled trial examined the differences between combined treatment with Vitamin C (500 mg/day) and vitamin E (600 IU/day) versus placebo in children [126]. The change in liver enzymes, lipid levels or the liver brightness in the ultrasound were not significantly different in the treatment groups [126].

Another study in patients with NASH with 6 months of treatment with vitamin C (1000 IU daily) and vitamin E (1 gr daily) caused significant histological improvements without any alteration in liver enzymes [85]. Another study, with 4 years treatment of combined vitamin C (1 gr/day) and vitamin E (1000 IU) showed improvements in hepatosteatosis [127]. However, it is not easy to discern whether these beneficial effects are due to Vitamin C itself or Vitamin E or the combination. In conclusion, the present data is not enough to recommend vitamin C replacement to patients with NAFLD.

Coenzyme Q10

Coenzyme Q10 is an antioxidant and anti-inflammatory molecule and a promising agent in NAFLD treatment. Coenzyme Q10 is abundant in striated muscle, heart and liver, but present in all cells of the organism [128]. Main limitation of Coenzyme Q10 treatment is its low bioavailability. Therefore, high dosages are necessary for the establishment of therapeutic effects. On the other side Coenzyme Q10 has high safety profile and low risk of drug interaction [129]. A 3 weeks long, randomized, double blind, placebo-controlled study of 100 mg Coenzyme Q10 has shown significant improvements in liver enzymes, and hsCRP levels in patients with NAFLD [130]. Also, Coenzyme Q10 replacement significantly improved lipid abnormalities in patients with NAFLD [131].

Berberine

Berberine, also called berberine hydrochloride, is an alkaloid extract of *Berberis vulgaris,* traditional Medicine from China and India. Studies have shown that berberine can improve blood glucose and lipid levels and regulate immune responses

[132, 133]. Animal studies have shown that berberine can decrease insulin resistance, lower hepatic and adipose tissue inflammation [134, 135]. Clinical studies with short term (2–4 months) berberine (500 mg/day) replacement has shown improvements in the indirect markers of hepatosteatosis such as Hepatic Steatosis Index and Lipid Accumulation Product [136]. A metanalysis of 6 randomized controlled studies has shown improvements in lipid parameters, insulin resistance and the grade of hepatic steatosis. However, these studies were performed with high dosages of berberine (1000–1500 mg/day) which caused significant intestinal side effects [137].

Curcumin

Curcumin is an extract of Curcuma longa. It improves insulin sensitivity, reduces oxidative stress and inflammation [138–141]. Curcumine has low bioavailability. Therefore, in most of the clinical studies of curcumin, piperine like molecules were added to improve its bioavailability. In patients with metabolic syndrome, curcumin reduced the serum levels of proinflammatory cytokines (TNF-α, IL-6, IL-1β, and MCP-1), increase anti-inflammatory adiponectine levels [139, 140] and improve Blood lipids [141]. Curcumin ingestion (1000 mg/day divided into two doses) for 8 weeks decrease, liver fat content, reduce liver enzyme levels, and increase hepatic vein flow with a reduction in portal vein diameter and liver volume [142].

Resveratrol

The natural nonflavonoid polyphenol compound resveratrol is an antioxidant, vasoprotective and insulin sensitizing agent abundant in nuts, berries and grape peel [143, 144]. Conflicting reports are present about the effects of resveratrol in patients with NAFLD. A placebo controlled double blind study of resveratrol replacement (500 mg/day for 12 months) did not result in any significant alteration in anthropometric measures, insulin sensitivity and lipid parameters, but reduced serum ALT levels and improved hepatic steatosis [145]. Another study of resveratrol replacement (600 mg/day for 3 months) resulted in decreased insulin resistance, blood glucose and lipids [146]. Furthermore, resveratrol improved the balance between important pro-inflammatory and anti-inflammatory cytokines [146]. On the contrary, another study of resveratrol replacement with much higher dosages (3000 mg/day for 8 weeks) did not reduce insulin resistance, steatosis, or abdominal fat distribution, but increased liver enzymes [147]. The discrepancies with the results of the clinical studies are probably related to differences between the resveratrol dosage and the study periods. As the previous reports are not consistent, long term clinical studies will be informative about the safety and efficacy of resveratrol in the treatment of NAFLD.

Salvia Miltiorrhiza

Salvia Miltiorrhiza is a traditional Asian herbal medication, which is used in China in the treatment of cardiovascular diseases for more than 2000 years. A metanalysis of 8 controlled studies has shown that, *Salvia miltiorrhiza* dry extract supplementation significantly improves plasma transaminases and radiological severity of hepatosteatosis [148].

Probiotics

The dysbiosis of gut microbiota can take part in the pathogenesis of liver diseases. Probiotics, Prebiotics and symbiotics modulate gut microbiota and they are potential therapeutic agents for NAFLD [149].

Several studies performed with probiotics or symbiotics have shown significant improvements in insulin resistance, liver enzymes and the severity of steatosis in patients with NAFLD. But different probiotics were used in different amounts with different periods in these studies. Therefore, it is not easy to discern a specific probiotic type, dosage and treatment period for [150].

Randomized controlled studies with L. Acidophilus, B. Lactis, L. Bulgaris, S. Thermophilus or L. rhamnosus showed significant improvements in liver enzymes in children and adults [151–153]. Another study in children has shown that 4 months long replacement of bifidobacteria, lactobacilli and S. thermophilus improves the severity of steatosis in liver [154].

In conclusion, probiotics can improve gut microbiota and liver pathology. However, there is problem in the standardization of results from different probiotics. The evidence is promising about the effect of agents targeting gut microbiota in NAFLD treatment.

Anthocyanins

Anthocyanins, are water soluble bioactive flavonoid compounds. Nutrients rich in Anthocyanins improve oxidative stress, dyslipidemia and hepatic steatosis in experimental NASH models. Replacement of purified anthocyanin (320 mg/day) significantly improved insulin resistance and liver enzymes in patients with NAFLD [155]. However, we need more data, especially on histological improvements, in order to get benefit of Anthocyanins on NAFLD [156].

Betaine

Betaine is an important methyl donor. It is either synthesized de novo or taken by the diet. Animal studies has shown that betaine replacement can prevent liver fat deposition [157, 158]. The effects of Betaine replacement were also investigated in a small number of clinical studies.

There appears to be a negative correlation between plasma betaine concentrations and the severity of NAFLD [159]. Eight weeks of Betaine replacement reduced 25% of liver steatosis and improved liver enzymes of patients with NASH [160]. However, another randomized controlled study of 12 months long oral betaine replacement did not show any significant effect on liver enzymes and liver histology [161].

Camellia Sinensis

Camellia Sinensis (Green Tea) is the leaf extract of the green tea plant Camellia Sinensis. Green Tea has been under scrutiny especially for its effects on cardiovascular diseases [162]. Green tea ingestion improves exercise performance, increase fat oxidation, and prevent obesity in mice [163, 164]. In recent years Green Tea is also investigated for the treatment of NAFLD. In two randomized controlled studies, Green Tea extract (500 mg/day for 12 weeks) significantly improved liver enzymes, insulin resistance and the ultrasound findings of liver steatosis when compared to the placebo arm [165, 166]. Another randomized controlled study with 12 weeks of green tea (700 ml/day) containing high density catechins improved liver fat content and inflammation by reducing oxidative stress in patients with NAFLD [167].

Coffee

Coffee consumption decreases insulin resistance and oxidative stress in hepatocytes and have anti-inflammatory and antifibrotic effects in animal models [168, 169]. The role of coffee consumption on NAFLD has been investigated in several clinical studies. A significant negative correlation between the amount of coffee consumption and fibrosis scores were established in patients with biopsy proven NAFLD [170]. A 7 years follow up study has shown that coffee consumption prevents the progression of liver fibrosis [171]. The real-life data also show that healthy patients have higher coffee consumption rates when compared to patients with NAFLD [172]. A metanalysis has shown that the risks of NAFLD and NASH are significantly lower in patients with regular daily coffee consumption [173].

Spirulina

Spirulina (Arthrospira platensis), is a cyanobacterium which has long been used as a food supplement. FDA approved Spirulina as a food supplement as it has a high safety profile and a rich source of proteins, vitamins, minerals, carotenoids, and phytocyanins. Spirulina has hypolipidemic, hypoglycemic, anti-viral, hepatoprotective, anti-inflammatory, anti-oxidant, anti-neoplastic, and immunomodulatory effects [174]. Spirulina replacement decreases liver enzymes and improves fibrosis in the animal models of NAFLD [175]. In a clinical study, 6 months of treatment with spirulina (6 gr/day) significantly improved lipid parameters, insulin resistance and liver enzymes, without any alteration in the severity of hepatosteatosis [176]. There is very limited data about the effect of spirulina in NAFLD treatment. Further studies with spirulina, especially on its effects on liver histology, are warranted.

S-adenosyl-L-methionine

S-adenosylmethionine (SAM), is an organic molecule unanimously found in every living cell. Current data about the effect of SAM in the pathogenesis of NAFLD are derived from experimental animal models. Chronic liver SAM deficiency may play role in the development of NASH, and SAM replacement may be effective in prevention of NAFLD in experimental animals [177]. There is however, limited clinical evidence about the role of SAM replacement on the pathogenesis of NAFLD [178].

Astaxanthin

Astaxanthin is an antioxidant caroten derivative, which inhibits lipid peroxidation more powerfully than vitamin E. It is regarded as a possible nutraceutical alternative to vitamin E [65]. Astaxanthin more significantly reduce lipogenesis, insulin resistance, liver inflammation and fibrogenesis when compared to vitamin E in the experimental models [179]. With the preliminary data, Astaxanthin appears to be the ideal antioxidant for the prevention of liver injury induced by NAFLD. However, there is insufficient human data about the effect of Astaxanthin in NAFLD [180].

Conclusion

In conclusion, numerous nutraceuticals are currently in use in different therapeutic forms such as food ingredients, dietary supplements, herbal teas or over the counter pills. Many clinical studies have been performed so far, to investigate the effects of nutraceuticals on NAFLD. There are several technical problems in quite a lot of these reports, such as small sample sizes, short study periods, lack of placebo arms or overestimation of the benefits. However, there is also high-quality evidence derived from randomized, placebo controlled prospective studies. According to these data at least some of these nutraceuticals such as *Silmarin, Curcumin, Green Tea or Vitamin E* have promising metabolic advantages and may improve liver functions or liver histology. However, there is hardly enough data about the optimal dosage, optimal treatment period and long-term safety data for most of these nutraceuticals. Therefore, time is needed to reproduce long term, randomized controlled studies before the widespread use of nutraceuticals for the NAFLD treatment.

References

1. Chalasani N, Younossi Z, Lavine JE, Charlton M, Cusi K, Rinella M, et al. The diagnosis and management of nonalcoholic fatty liver disease: practice guidance from the American Association for the Study of Liver Diseases. Hepatology. 2018;67:328–57. https://doi.org/10.1002/hep.29367.
2. Sheth S, Gordon F, Chopra S. Nonalcoholic steatohepatitis. Ann Intern Med. 1997;126:137. https://doi.org/10.7326/0003-4819-126-2-199701150-00008.
3. Caldwell SH, Crespo DM. The spectrum expanded: cryptogenic cirrhosis and the natural history of non-alcoholic fatty liver disease. Powell EE, Cooksley WGE, Hanson R, Searle J, Halliday JW, Powell LW. The natural history of nonalcoholic steatohepatitis: a follow-up study of forty-two patients for up to 21 years [Hepatology 1990; 11:74–80]. J Hepatol 2004;40:578–84. https://doi.org/10.1016/j.jhep.2004.02.013.
4. Younossi ZM, Koenig AB, Abdelatif D, Fazel Y, Henry L, Wymer M. Global epidemiology of nonalcoholic fatty liver disease—mcta-analytic assessment of prevalence, incidence, and outcomes. Hepatology. 2016;64:73–84. https://doi.org/10.1002/hep.28431.
5. Sung K-C, Wild SH, Byrne CD. Development of new fatty liver, or resolution of existing fatty liver, over five years of follow-up, and risk of incident hypertension. J Hepatol. 2014;60:1040–5. https://doi.org/10.1016/j.jhep.2014.01.009.
6. Tsuneto A, Hida A, Sera N, Imaizumi M, Ichimaru S, Nakashima E, et al. Fatty liver incidence and predictive variables. Hypertens Res. 2010;33:638. https://doi.org/10.1038/hr.2010.45.
7. Wong V, Wong G, Yeung D, Lau T, Chan C, Chim A, et al. Incidence of non-alcoholic fatty liver disease in Hong Kong: a population study with paired proton-magnetic resonance spectroscopy. J Hepatol. 2015;62:182–9. https://doi.org/10.1016/j.jhep.2014.08.041.
8. Whalley S, Puvanachandra P, Desai A, Kennedy H. Hepatology outpatient service provision in secondary care: a study of liver disease incidence and resource costs. Clin Med. 2007;7:119–24. https://doi.org/10.7861/clinmedicine.7-2-119.
9. Zelber-Sagi S, Lotan R, Shlomai A, Webb M, Harrari G, Buch A, et al. Predictors for incidence and remission of NAFLD in the general population during a seven-year prospective follow-up. J Hepatol. 2012;56:1145–51. https://doi.org/10.1016/j.jhep.2011.12.011.
10. Estes C, Razavi H, Loomba R, Younossi Z, Sanyal AJ. Modeling the epidemic of nonalcoholic fatty liver disease demonstrates an exponential increase in burden of disease. Hepatology. 2018;67:123–33. https://doi.org/10.1002/hep.29466.
11. Koehler EM, Schouten J, Hansen BE, van Rooij F, Hofman A, Stricker BH, et al. Prevalence and risk factors of non-alcoholic fatty liver disease in the elderly: results from the Rotterdam study. J Hepatol. 2012;57:1305–11. https://doi.org/10.1016/j.jhep.2012.07.028.
12. Arun J, Clements RH, Lazenby AJ, Leeth RR, Abrams GA. The prevalence of nonalcoholic steatohepatitis is greater in morbidly obese men compared to women. Obes Surg. 2006;16:1351–8. https://doi.org/10.1381/096089206778663715.

13. Zelber-Sagi S, Nitzan-Kaluski D, Halpern Z, Oren R. Prevalence of primary non-alcoholic fatty liver disease in a population-based study and its association with biochemical and anthropometric measures. Liver Int. 2006;26:856–63. https://doi.org/10.1111/j.1478-3231.2006.01311.x.
14. Ludwig J, Viggiano T, McGill D, Oh B. Nonalcoholic steatohepatitis: Mayo Clinic experiences with a hitherto unnamed disease. Mayo Clin Proc. 1980;55:434–8.
15. Angulo P, Keach JC, Batts KP, Lindor KD. Independent predictors of liver fibrosis in patients with nonalcoholic steatohepatitis. Hepatology. 1999;30:1356–62. https://doi.org/10.1002/hep.510300604.
16. Agbim U, Carr RM, Pickett-Blakely O, Dagogo-Jack S. Ethnic disparities in adiposity: focus on non-alcoholic fatty liver disease, visceral, and generalized obesity. Curr Obes Rep. 2019;8(3):1–12. https://doi.org/10.1007/s13679-019-00349-x.
17. Browning JD, Szczepaniak LS, Dobbins R, Nuremberg P, Horton JD, Cohen JC, et al. Prevalence of hepatic steatosis in an urban population in the United States: impact of ethnicity. Hepatology. 2004;40:1387–95. https://doi.org/10.1002/hep.20466.
18. Nazare J-A, Smith JD, Borel A-L, Haffner SM, Balkau B, Ross R, et al. Ethnic influences on the relations between abdominal subcutaneous and visceral adiposity, liver fat, and cardiometabolic risk profile: the International Study of Prediction of Intra-Abdominal Adiposity and Its Relationship With Cardiometabolic Risk/Intra-Abdominal Adiposity. Am J Clin Nutr. 2012;96:714–26. https://doi.org/10.3945/ajcn.112.035758.
19. Dongiovanni P, Anstee Q, Valenti L. Genetic predisposition in NAFLD and NASH: impact on severity of liver disease and response to treatment. Curr Pharm Design. 2013;19:5219–38. https://doi.org/10.2174/13816128113199990381.
20. Byrne CD, Targher G. NAFLD: a multisystem disease. J Hepatol. 2015;62:S47–64. https://doi.org/10.1016/j.jhep.2014.12.012.
21. Yki-Järvinen H. Non-alcoholic fatty liver disease as a cause and a consequence of metabolic syndrome. Lancet Diabetes Endocrinol. 2014;2:901–10. https://doi.org/10.1016/s2213-8587(14)70032-4.
22. Sasaki A, Nitta H, Otsuka K, Umemura A, Baba S, Obuchi T, et al. Bariatric surgery and non-alcoholic fatty liver disease: current and potential future treatments. Front Endocrinol. 2014;5:164. https://doi.org/10.3389/fendo.2014.00164.
23. Leite NC, Salles GF, Araujo AL, Villela-Nogueira CA, Cardoso CR. Prevalence and associated factors of non-alcoholic fatty liver disease in patients with type-2 diabetes mellitus. Liver Int. 2009;29:113–9. https://doi.org/10.1111/j.1478-3231.2008.01718.x.
24. Assy N, Kaita K, Mymin D, Levy C, Rosser B, Minuk G. Fatty infiltration of liver in hyperlipidemic patients. Dig Dis Sci. 2000;45:1929–34. https://doi.org/10.1023/a:1005661516165.
25. Wu K-T, Kuo P-L, Su S-B, Chen Y-Y, Yeh M-L, Huang C-I, et al. Nonalcoholic fatty liver disease severity is associated with the ratios of total cholesterol and triglycerides to high-density lipoprotein cholesterol. J Clin Lipidol. 2016;10:420–425.e1. https://doi.org/10.1016/j.jacl.2015.12.026.
26. Sonmez A, Nikolic D, Dogru T, Ercin C, Genc H, Cesur M, et al. Low- and high-density lipoprotein subclasses in subjects with nonalcoholic fatty liver disease. J Clin Lipidol. 2015;9:576–82. https://doi.org/10.1016/j.jacl.2015.03.010.
27. Ballestri S, Nascimbeni F, Baldelli E, Marrazzo A, Romagnoli D, Targher G, et al. Ultrasonographic fatty liver indicator detects mild steatosis and correlates with metabolic/histological parameters in various liver diseases. Metabolism. 2017;72:57–65. https://doi.org/10.1016/j.metabol.2017.04.003.
28. European Association for the Study of the Liver (EASL); European Association for the Study of Diabetes (EASD); European Association for the Study of Obesity (EASO). EASL–EASD–EASO Clinical Practice Guidelines for the management of non-alcoholic fatty liver disease. J Hepatol. 2016;64:1388–402. https://doi.org/10.1016/j.jhep.2015.11.004.
29. Shi K, Tang J, Zhu X, Ying L, Li D, Gao J, et al. Controlled attenuation parameter for the detection of steatosis severity in chronic liver disease: a meta-analysis of diagnostic accuracy. J Gastroenterol Hepatol. 2014;29:1149–58. https://doi.org/10.1111/jgh.12519.

30. Lonardo A, Nascimbeni F, Maurantonio M, Marrazzo A, Rinaldi L, Adinolfi L. Nonalcoholic fatty liver disease: evolving paradigms. World J Gastroenterol. 2017;23:6571–92. https://doi.org/10.3748/wjg.v23.i36.6571.
31. Donnelly KL, Smith CI, Schwarzenberg SJ, Jessurun J, Boldt MD, Parks EJ. Sources of fatty acids stored in liver and secreted via lipoproteins in patients with nonalcoholic fatty liver disease. J Clin Invest. 2005;115:1343–51. https://doi.org/10.1172/jci23621.
32. Arab J, Arrese M, Trauner M. Recent insights into the pathogenesis of nonalcoholic fatty liver disease. Annu Rev Pathol Mech Dis. 2018;13:321–50. https://doi.org/10.1146/annurev-pathol-020117-043617.
33. Trauner M, Arrese M, Wagner M. Fatty liver and lipotoxicity. Biochimica Et Biophysica Acta Bba – Mol Cell Biol Lipids. 2010;1801:299–310. https://doi.org/10.1016/j.bbalip.2009.10.007.
34. Lonardo A, Nascimbeni F, Targher G, Bernardi M, Bonino F, et al. AISF position paper on nonalcoholic fatty liver disease (NAFLD): updates and future directions. Dig Liver Dis. 2017;49:471–83. https://doi.org/10.1016/j.dld.2017.01.147.
35. Farrell GC, Larter CZ. Nonalcoholic fatty liver disease: from steatosis to cirrhosis. Hepatology. 2006;43:S99–112. https://doi.org/10.1002/hep.20973.
36. Satapathy SK, Sanyal AJ. Epidemiology and natural history of nonalcoholic fatty liver disease. Semin Liver Dis. 2015;35:221–35. https://doi.org/10.1055/s-0035-1562943.
37. Ekstedt M, Hagström H, Nasr P, Fredrikson M, Stål P, Kechagias S, et al. Fibrosis stage is the strongest predictor for disease-specific mortality in NAFLD after up to 33 years of follow-up. Hepatology. 2015;61:1547–54. https://doi.org/10.1002/hep.27368.
38. Younossi Z, Henry L. Contribution of alcoholic and nonalcoholic fatty liver disease to the burden of liver-related morbidity and mortality. Gastroenterology. 2016;150:1778–85. https://doi.org/10.1053/j.gastro.2016.03.005.
39. Angulo P, Kleiner DE, Dam-Larsen S, Adams LA, Bjornsson ES, Charatcharoenwitthaya P, et al. Liver fibrosis, but no other histologic features, is associated with long-term outcomes of patients with nonalcoholic fatty liver disease. Gastroenterology. 2015;149:389–397.e10. https://doi.org/10.1053/j.gastro.2015.04.043.
40. Pelusi S, Cespiati A, Rametta R, Pennisi G, Mannisto V, Rosso C, et al. Prevalence and risk factors if significant fibrosis in patients with nonalcoholic fatty liver without steatohepatitis. Clin Gastroenterol Hepatol. 2019;17(11):2310–2319.e6. https://doi.org/10.1016/j.cgh.2019.01.027.
41. McPherson S, Hardy T, Henderson E, Burt AD, Day CP, Anstee QM. Evidence of NAFLD progression from steatosis to fibrosing-steatohepatitis using paired biopsies: implications for prognosis and clinical management. J Hepatol. 2015;62:1148–55. https://doi.org/10.1016/j.jhep.2014.11.034.
42. Stahl EP, Dhindsa DS, Lee SK, Sandesara PB, Chalasani NP, Sperling LS. Nonalcoholic fatty liver disease and the heart JACC state-of-the-art review. J Am Coll Cardiol. 2019;73:948–63. https://doi.org/10.1016/j.jacc.2018.11.050.
43. Mohamad B, Shah V, Onyshchenko M, Elshamy M, Aucejo F, Lopez R, et al. Characterization of hepatocellular carcinoma (HCC) in non-alcoholic fatty liver disease (NAFLD) patients without cirrhosis. Hepatol Int. 2016;10:632–9. https://doi.org/10.1007/s12072-015-9679-0.
44. Piscaglia F, Svegliati-Baroni G, Barchetti A, Pecorelli A, Marinelli S, Tiribelli C, et al. Clinical patterns of hepatocellular carcinoma in nonalcoholic fatty liver disease: a multicenter prospective study. Hepatology. 2016;63:827–38. https://doi.org/10.1002/hep.28368.
45. Paradis V, Zalinski S, Chelbi E, Guedj N, Degos F, Vilgrain V, et al. Hepatocellular carcinomas in patients with metabolic syndrome often develop without significant liver fibrosis: a pathological analysis. Hepatology. 2009;49:851–9. https://doi.org/10.1002/hep.22734.
46. Dyson J, Anstee Q, McPherson S. Non-alcoholic fatty liver disease: a practical approach to treatment. Frontline Gastroenterol. 2014;5:277. https://doi.org/10.1136/flgastro-2013-100404.
47. Romero-Gómez M, Zelber-Sagi S, Trenell M. Treatment of NAFLD with diet, physical activity and exercise. J Hepatol. 2017;67:829–46. https://doi.org/10.1016/j.jhep.2017.05.016.

48. Petersen K, Dufour S, Befroy D, Lehrke M, Hendler RE, Shulman GI. Reversal of nonalcoholic hepatic steatosis, hepatic insulin resistance, and hyperglycemia by moderate weight reduction in patients with type 2 diabetes. Diabetes. 2005;54:603–8. https://doi.org/10.2337/diabetes.54.3.603.
49. Promrat K, Kleiner DE, Niemeier HM, Jackvony E, Kearns M, Wands JR, et al. Randomized controlled trial testing the effects of weight loss on nonalcoholic steatohepatitis. Hepatology. 2010;51:121–9. https://doi.org/10.1002/hep.23276.
50. Musso G, Cassader M, Rosina F, Gambino R. Impact of current treatments on liver disease, glucose metabolism and cardiovascular risk in non-alcoholic fatty liver disease (NAFLD): a systematic review and meta-analysis of randomised trials. Diabetologia. 2012;55:885–904. https://doi.org/10.1007/s00125-011-2446-4.
51. Ekstedt M, Franzén LE, Holmqvist M, Bendtsen P, Mathiesen UL, Bodemar G, et al. Alcohol consumption is associated with progression of hepatic fibrosis in non-alcoholic fatty liver disease. Scand J Gastroenterol. 2009;44:366–74. https://doi.org/10.1080/00365520802555991.
52. Pälve KS, Pahkala K, Suomela E, Aatola H, Hulkkonen J, Juonala M, et al. Cardiorespiratory fitness and risk of fatty liver. Med Sci Sports Exerc. 2017;49:1834–41. https://doi.org/10.1249/mss.0000000000001288.
53. van der Windt DJ, Sud V, Zhang H, Tsung A, Huang H. The effects of physical exercise on fatty liver disease. Van Der Wind Dirk J. 2017;18:89–101. https://doi.org/10.3727/105221617x15124844266408.
54. Benedict M, Zhang X. Non-alcoholic fatty liver disease: an expanded review. World J Hepatol. 2017;9:715–32. https://doi.org/10.4254/wjh.v9.i16.715.
55. Wong V. Obesity, fatty liver and liver cancer. Adv Exp Med Biol. 2018;1061:149–57. https://doi.org/10.1007/978-981-10-8684-7_12.
56. Hung C, Bodenheimer HC. Current treatment of nonalcoholic fatty liver disease/nonalcoholic steatohepatitis. Clin Liver Dis. 2018;22:175–87. https://doi.org/10.1016/j.cld.2017.08.012.
57. Said A, Akhter A. Meta-analysis of randomized controlled trials of pharmacologic agents in non-alcoholic steatohepatitis. Ann Hepatol. 2017;16:538–47. https://doi.org/10.5604/01.3001.0010.0284.
58. Boettcher E, Csako G, Pucino F, Wesley R, Loomba R. Meta-analysis: pioglitazone improves liver histology and fibrosis in patients with non-alcoholic steatohepatitis. Aliment Pharmacol Ther. 2012;35:66–75. https://doi.org/10.1111/j.1365-2036.2011.04912.x.
59. Wang H, Wang L, Cheng Y, Xia Z, Liao Y, Cao J. Efficacy of orlistat in non-alcoholic fatty liver disease: a systematic review and meta-analysis. Biomed Rep. 2018;9:90–6. https://doi.org/10.3892/br.2018.1100.
60. Armstrong M, Gaunt P, Aithal GP, Barton D, Hull D, Parker R, et al. Liraglutide safety and efficacy in patients with non-alcoholic steatohepatitis (LEAN): a multicentre, double-blind, randomised, placebo-controlled phase 2 study. Lancet. 2016;387:679–90. https://doi.org/10.1016/s0140-6736(15)00803-x.
61. Uehara D, Seki Y, Kakizaki S, Horiguchi N, Tojima H, Yamazaki Y, et al. Long-term results of bariatric surgery for non-alcoholic fatty liver disease/non-alcoholic steatohepatitis treatment in morbidly obese Japanese patients. Obes Surg. 2019;29:1195–201. https://doi.org/10.1007/s11695-018-03641-2.
62. Perazzo H, Dufour J. The therapeutic landscape of non-alcoholic steatohepatitis. Liver Int. 2017;37:634–47. https://doi.org/10.1111/liv.13270.
63. Bjelakovic G, Nikolova D, Gluud L, Simonetti RG, Gluud C. Mortality in randomized trials of antioxidant supplements for primary and secondary prevention: systematic review and meta-analysis. JAMA. 2007;297:842–57. https://doi.org/10.1001/jama.297.8.842.
64. Miller ER, Pastor-Barriuso R, Dalal D, Riemersma RA, Appel LJ, Guallar EL. Meta-analysis: high-dosage vitamin E supplementation may increase all-cause mortality. ACC Curr J Rev. 2005;14:17. https://doi.org/10.1016/j.accreview.2005.04.017.
65. Cicero AF, Colletti A, Bellentani S. Nutraceutical approach to non-alcoholic fatty liver disease (NAFLD): the available clinical evidence. Nutrients. 2018;10:1153. https://doi.org/10.3390/nu10091153.

66. Liu Z, Xie L, Zhu J, Li GQ, Grant SJ, Liu J. Herbal medicines for fatty liver diseases. Cochrane Database Syst Rev. 2013;8:CD009059. https://doi.org/10.1002/14651858.cd009059.pub2.
67. Ben M, Polimeni L, Baratta F, Pastori D, Angelico F. The role of nutraceuticals for the treatment of non-alcoholic fatty liver disease. Br J Clin Pharmacol. 2017;83:88–95. https://doi.org/10.1111/bcp.12899.
68. Figueiredo P, Inada A, Fernandes M, Arakaki D, de Freitas K, de Guimarães R, et al. An overview of novel dietary supplements and food ingredients in patients with metabolic syndrome and non-alcoholic fatty liver disease. Molecules. 2018;23:877. https://doi.org/10.3390/molecules23040877.
69. Bahadoran Z, Golzarand M, Mirmiran P, Saadati N, Azizi F. The association of dietary phytochemical index and cardiometabolic risk factors in adults: Tehran lipid and glucose study. J Hum Nutr Diet. 2013;26:145–53. https://doi.org/10.1111/jhn.12048.
70. Loguercio C, Festi D. Silybin and the liver: from basic research to clinical practice. World J Gastroenterol. 2011;17:2288–301. https://doi.org/10.3748/wjg.v17.i18.2288.
71. Trappoliere M, Caligiuri A, Schmid M, Bertolani C, Failli P, Vizzutti F, et al. Silybin, a component of sylimarin, exerts anti-inflammatory and anti-fibrogenic effects on human hepatic stellate cells. J Hepatol. 2009;50:1102–11. https://doi.org/10.1016/j.jhep.2009.02.023.
72. Abenavoli L, Capasso R, Milic N, Capasso F. Milk thistle in liver diseases: past, present, future. Phytother Res. 2010;24:1423–32. https://doi.org/10.1002/ptr.3207.
73. Federico A, Trappoliere M, Tuccillo C, de Sio I, Leva DA, Blanco DC, et al. A new silybin-vitamin E-phospholipid complex improves insulin resistance and liver damage in patients with non-alcoholic fatty liver disease: preliminary observations. Gut. 2006;55:901. https://doi.org/10.1136/gut.2006.091967.
74. Aller R, Laserna C, Rojo M, Mora N, Sánchez C, Pina M, et al. Role of the PNPLA3 polymorphism rs738409 on silymarin + vitamin E response in subjects with non-alcoholic fatty liver disease. Rev Esp Enferm Dig. 2018;110(10):634–40. https://doi.org/10.17235/reed.2018.5602/2018.
75. Surai PF. Silymarin as a natural antioxidant: an overview of the current evidence and perspectives. Antioxidants. 2015;4:204–47. https://doi.org/10.3390/antiox4010204.
76. Loguercio C, Andreone P, Brisc C, Brisc M, Bugianesi E, Chiaramonte M, et al. Silybin combined with phosphatidylcholine and vitamin E in patients with nonalcoholic fatty liver disease: a randomized controlled trial. Free Radic Biol Med. 2012;52:1658–65. https://doi.org/10.1016/j.freeradbiomed.2012.02.008.
77. Cacciapuoti F, Scognamiglio A, Palumbo R, Forte R, Cacciapuoti F. Silymarin in non alcoholic fatty liver disease. World J Hepatol. 2013;5:109–13. https://doi.org/10.4254/wjh.v5.i3.109.
78. Sorrentino G, Crispino P, Coppola D, Stefano G. Efficacy of lifestyle changes in subjects with non-alcoholic liver steatosis and metabolic syndrome may be improved with an antioxidant nutraceutical: a controlled clinical study. Drugs R&D. 2015;15:21–5. https://doi.org/10.1007/s40268-015-0084-x.
79. Zhong S, Fan Y, Yan Q, Fan X, Wu B, Han Y, et al. The therapeutic effect of silymarin in the treatment of nonalcoholic fatty disease. Medicine. 2017;96:e9061. https://doi.org/10.1097/md.0000000000009061.
80. Chitturi S, Wong V, Chan W, Wong G, Wong S, Sollano J, et al. The Asia–Pacific working party on non-alcoholic fatty liver disease guidelines 2017—part 2: management and special groups. Eur J Gastroenterol Hepatol. 2018;33:86–98. https://doi.org/10.1111/jgh.13856.
81. Wong S, Chin K-Y, Suhaimi F, Ahmad F, Ima-Nirwana S. Vitamin E as a potential interventional treatment for metabolic syndrome: evidence from animal and human studies. Front Pharmacol. 2017;8:444. https://doi.org/10.3389/fphar.2017.00444.
82. Pastori D, Baratta F, Carnevale R, Cangemi R, Ben M, Bucci T, et al. Similar reduction of cholesterol-adjusted vitamin E serum levels in simple steatosis and non-alcoholic steatohepatitis. Clin Transl Gastroenterol. 2015;6:e113. https://doi.org/10.1038/ctg.2015.43.
83. Kawanaka M, Mahmood S, Niiyama G, Izumi A, Kamel A, Ikeda H, et al. Control of oxidative stress and reduction in biochemical markers by vitamin E treatment in patients with nonal-

coholic steatohepatitis: a pilot study. Hepatol Res. 2004;29:39–41. https://doi.org/10.1016/j.hepres.2004.02.002.

84. Kim G, Chung J, Lee J, Ok K, Jang E, Kim J, et al. Effect of vitamin E in nonalcoholic fatty liver disease with metabolic syndrome: a propensity score-matched cohort study. Clin Mol Hepatol. 2015;21:379–86. https://doi.org/10.3350/cmh.2015.21.4.379.

85. Harrison SA, Torgerson S, Hayashi P, Ward J, Schenker S. Vitamin E and vitamin C treatment improves fibrosis in patients with nonalcoholic steatohepatitis. Am J Gastroenterol. 2003;98:ajg2003574. https://doi.org/10.1111/j.1572-0241.2003.08699.x.

86. Sanyal AJ, Chalasani N, Kowdley KV, McCullough A, Diehl A, Bass NM, et al. Pioglitazone, vitamin E, or placebo for nonalcoholic steatohepatitis. New Engl J Med. 2010;362:1675–85. https://doi.org/10.1056/nejmoa0907929.

87. Lavine JE, Schwimmer JB, Natta ML, Molleston JP, Murray KF, Rosenthal P, et al. Effect of vitamin E or metformin for treatment of nonalcoholic fatty liver disease in children and adolescents: the TONIC randomized controlled trial. JAMA. 2011;305:1659–68. https://doi.org/10.1001/jama.2011.520.

88. Sato K, Gosho M, Yamamoto T, Kobayashi Y, Ishii N, Ohashi T, et al. Vitamin E has a beneficial effect on nonalcoholic fatty liver disease: a meta-analysis of randomized controlled trials. Nutrition. 2015;31:923–30. https://doi.org/10.1016/j.nut.2014.11.018.

89. Blond E, Disse E, Cuerq C, Drai J, Valette P-J, Laville M, et al. EASL–EASD–EASO clinical practice guidelines for the management of non-alcoholic fatty liver disease in severely obese people: do they lead to over-referral? Diabetologia. 2017;60:1218–22. https://doi.org/10.1007/s00125-017-4264-9.

90. Klein EA, Thompson IM, Tangen CM, Crowley JJ, Lucia SM, Goodman PJ, et al. Vitamin E and the risk of prostate cancer: the selenium and vitamin E cancer prevention trial (SELECT). JAMA. 2011;306:1549–56. https://doi.org/10.1001/jama.2011.1437.

91. Pinelli NR, Jaber LA, Brown MB, Herman WH. Serum 25-Hydroxy vitamin D and insulin resistance, metabolic syndrome, and glucose intolerance among Arab Americans. Diabetes Care. 2010;33:1373–5. https://doi.org/10.2337/dc09-2199.

92. Eliades M, Spyrou E. Vitamin D: a new player in non-alcoholic fatty liver disease? World J Gastroenterol. 2015;21:1718–27. https://doi.org/10.3748/wjg.v21.i6.1718.

93. Targher G, Bertolini L, Scala L, Cigolini M, Zenari L, Falezza G, et al. Associations between serum 25-hydroxyvitamin D3 concentrations and liver histology in patients with non-alcoholic fatty liver disease. Nutr Metab Cardiovasc Dis. 2007;17:517–24. https://doi.org/10.1016/j.numecd.2006.04.002.

94. Keane JT, Elangovan H, Stokes RA, Gunton JE. Vitamin D and the liver—correlation or cause? Nutrients. 2018;10:496. https://doi.org/10.3390/nu10040496.

95. Salehpour A, Hosseinpanah F, Shidfar F, Vafa M, Razaghi M, Dehghani S, et al. A 12-week double-blind randomized clinical trial of vitamin D3supplementation on body fat mass in healthy overweight and obese women. Nutr J. 2012;11:78. https://doi.org/10.1186/1475-2891-11-78.

96. Barchetta I, Angelico F, Ben M, Baroni M, Pozzilli P, Morini S, et al. Strong association between non alcoholic fatty liver disease (NAFLD) and low 25(OH) vitamin D levels in an adult population with normal serum liver enzymes. BMC Med. 2011;9:85. https://doi.org/10.1186/1741-7015-9-85.

97. Barchetta I, Carotti S, Labbadia G, Gentilucci U, Muda A, Angelico F, et al. Liver vitamin D receptor, CYP2R1, and CYP27A1 expression: relationship with liver histology and vitamin D3 levels in patients with nonalcoholic steatohepatitis or hepatitis C virus. Hepatology. 2012;56:2180–7. https://doi.org/10.1002/hep.25930.

98. Sharifi N, Amani R, Hajiani E, Cheraghian B. Does vitamin D improve liver enzymes, oxidative stress, and inflammatory biomarkers in adults with non-alcoholic fatty liver disease? A randomized clinical trial. Endocrine. 2014;47:70–80. https://doi.org/10.1007/s12020-014-0336-5.

99. Barchetta I, Ben M, Angelico F, Martino M, Fraioli A, Torre G, et al. No effects of oral vitamin D supplementation on non-alcoholic fatty liver disease in patients with type 2 diabetes:

a randomized, double-blind, placebo-controlled trial. BMC Med. 2016;14:92. https://doi.org/10.1186/s12916-016-0638-y.

100. Kitson MT, Pham A, Gordon A, Kemp W, Roberts SK. High-dose vitamin D supplementation and liver histology in NASH. Gut. 2016;65:717. https://doi.org/10.1136/gutjnl-2015-310417.

101. Amiri H, Agah S, Azar J, Hosseini S, Shidfar F, Mousavi S. Effect of daily calcitriol supplementation with and without calcium on disease regression in non-alcoholic fatty liver patients following an energy-restricted diet: randomized, controlled, double-blind trial. Clin Nutr. 2017;36:1490–7. https://doi.org/10.1016/j.clnu.2016.09.020.

102. Jaruvongvanich V, Ahuja W, Sanguankeo A, Wijarnpreecha K, Upala S. Vitamin D and histologic severity of nonalcoholic fatty liver disease: a systematic review and meta-analysis. Dig Liver Dis. 2017;49:618–22. https://doi.org/10.1016/j.dld.2017.02.003.

103. Gülçin İ. Antioxidant and antiradical activities of l-carnitine. Life Sci. 2006;78:803–11. https://doi.org/10.1016/j.lfs.2005.05.103.

104. Cuturic M, Abramson RK, Moran RR, Hardin JW, Frank EM, Sellers AA. Serum carnitine levels and levocarnitine supplementation in institutionalized Huntington's disease patients. Neurol Sci. 2013;34:93–8. https://doi.org/10.1007/s10072-012-0952-x.

105. Flanagan JL, Simmons PA, Vehige J, Willcox MD, Garrett Q. Role of carnitine in disease. Nutr Metab. 2010;7:30. https://doi.org/10.1186/1743-7075-7-30.

106. Malaguarnera M, Gargante M, Russo C, Antic T, Vacante M, Malaguarnera M, et al. L-carnitine supplementation to diet: a new tool in treatment of nonalcoholic Steatohepatitis—a randomized and controlled clinical trial. Am J Gastroenterol. 2010;105:1338. https://doi.org/10.1038/ajg.2009.719.

107. Somi MH, Fatahi E, Panahi J, Havasian MR, Judaki A. Data from a randomized and controlled trial of LCarnitine prescription for the treatment for non- alcoholic fatty liver disease. Bioinformation. 2014;10:575–9. https://doi.org/10.6026/97320630010575.

108. van Herpen NA, Schrauwen-Hinderling VB. Lipid accumulation in non-adipose tissue and lipotoxicity. Physiol Behav. 2008;94:231–41. https://doi.org/10.1016/j.physbeh.2007.11.049.

109. Shahidi F, Ambigaipalan P. Omega-3 Polyunsaturated Fatty Acids and Their Health Benefits. Annu Rev Food Sci Technol. 2018;9:345–381.

110. Capanni M, Calella F, Ini M, Genise S, Raimondi L, Bedogni G, et al. Prolonged n-3 polyunsaturated fatty acid supplementation ameliorates hepatic steatosis in patients with non-alcoholic fatty liver disease: a pilot study. Aliment Pharmacol Ther. 2006;23:1143–51. https://doi.org/10.1111/j.1365-2036.2006.02885.x.

111. Spadaro L, Magliocco O, Spampinato D, Piro S, Oliveri C, Alagona C, et al. Effects of n-3 polyunsaturated fatty acids in subjects with nonalcoholic fatty liver disease. Dig Liver Dis. 2008;40:194–9. https://doi.org/10.1016/j.dld.2007.10.003.

112. Sofi F, Giangrandi I, Cesari F, Corsani I, Abbate R, Gensini G, et al. Effects of a 1-year dietary intervention with n-3 polyunsaturated fatty acid-enriched olive oil on non-alcoholic fatty liver disease patients: a preliminary study. Int J Food Sci Nutr. 2010;61:792–802. https://doi.org/10.3109/09637486.2010.487480.

113. Vega G, Chandalia M, Szczepaniak LS, Grundy SM. Effects of N-3 fatty acids on hepatic triglyceride content in humans. J Investig Med. 2008;56:780. https://doi.org/10.2310/jim.0b013e318177024d.

114. Nobili V, Bedogni G, Alisi A, Pietrobattista A, Risé P, Galli C, et al. Docosahexaenoic acid supplementation decreases liver fat content in children with non-alcoholic fatty liver disease: double-blind randomised controlled clinical trial. Arch Dis Child. 2011;96:350. https://doi.org/10.1136/adc.2010.192401.

115. Parker HM, Johnson NA, Burdon CA, Cohn JS, O'Connor HT, George J. Omega-3 supplementation and non-alcoholic fatty liver disease: a systematic review and meta-analysis. J Hepatol. 2012;56:944–51. https://doi.org/10.1016/j.jhep.2011.08.018.

116. Wrieden WL, Hannah MK, Bolton-Smith C, Tavendale R, Morrison C, Tunstall-Pedoe H. Plasma vitamin C and food choice in the third Glasgow MONICA population survey. J Epidemiol Commun H. 2000;54:355. https://doi.org/10.1136/jech.54.5.355.

117. Hampl JS, Taylor CA, Johnston CS. Vitamin C deficiency and depletion in the United States: the third national health and nutrition examination survey, 1988 to 1994. Am J Public Health. 2004;94:870–5. https://doi.org/10.2105/ajph.94.5.870.

118. Chen G, Lu D, Pang Z, Liu Q. Vitamin C intake, circulating vitamin C and risk of stroke: a meta-analysis of prospective studies. J Am Heart Assoc. 2013;2:e000329. https://doi.org/10.1161/jaha.113.000329.

119. Moser MA, Chun OK. Vitamin C and heart health: a review based on findings from epidemiologic studies. Int J Mol Sci. 2016;17:1328. https://doi.org/10.3390/ijms17081328.

120. Ipsen D, Tveden-Nyborg P, Lykkesfeldt J. Does vitamin C deficiency promote fatty liver disease development? Nutrients. 2014;6:5473–99. https://doi.org/10.3390/nu6125473.

121. Ferolla S, Ferrari T, Lima M, Reis T, Tavares W Jr, Couto O, et al. Dietary patterns in Brazilian patients with non-alcoholic fatty liver disease: a cross-sectional study. Clinics. 2013;68:11–7. https://doi.org/10.6061/clinics/2013(01)oa03.

122. Musso G, Gambino R, Michieli F, Cassader M, Rizzetto M, Durazzo M, et al. Dietary habits and their relations to insulin resistance and postprandial lipemia in nonalcoholic steatohepatitis. Hepatology. 2003;37:909–16. https://doi.org/10.1053/jhep.2003.50132.

123. Mager D, Patterson C, So S, Rogenstein C, Wykes L, Roberts E. Dietary and physical activity patterns in children with fatty liver. Eur J Clin Nutr. 2010;64:628. https://doi.org/10.1038/ejcn.2010.35.

124. Silva HE, Arendt BM, Noureldin SA, Therapondos G, Guindi M, Allard JP. A cross-sectional study assessing dietary intake and physical activity in Canadian patients with nonalcoholic fatty liver disease vs healthy controls. J Acad Nutr Diet. 2014;114:1181–94. https://doi.org/10.1016/j.jand.2014.01.009.

125. Madan K, Bhardwaj P, Thareja S, Gupta SD, Saraya A. Oxidant stress and antioxidant status among patients with nonalcoholic fatty liver disease (NAFLD). J Clin Gastroenterol. 2006;40:930–5. https://doi.org/10.1097/01.mcg.0000212608.59090.08.

126. Nobili V, Manco M, Devito R, Ciampalini P, Piemonte F, Marcellini M. Effect of vitamin E on aminotransferase levels and insulin resistance in children with non-alcoholic fatty liver disease. Aliment Pharmacol Ther. 2006;24:1553–61. https://doi.org/10.1111/j.1365-2036.2006.03161.x.

127. Arad Y, Spadaro LA, Roth M, Newstein D, Guerci AD. Treatment of asymptomatic adults with elevated coronary calcium scores with atorvastatin, vitamin C, and vitamin E: the St. Francis heart study randomized clinical trial. ACC Curr J Rev. 2005;14:10. https://doi.org/10.1016/j.accreview.2005.09.028.

128. Ayers J, Cook J, Koenig RA, Sisson EM, Dixon DL. Recent developments in the role of coenzyme Q10 for coronary heart disease: a systematic review. Curr Atheroscler Rep. 2018;20:29. https://doi.org/10.1007/s11883-018-0730-1.

129. Gutierrez-Mariscal FM, Yubero-Serrano EM, Villalba JM, Lopez-Miranda J. Coenzyme Q10: from bench to clinic in aging diseases, a translational review. Crit Rev Food Sci. 2018;2018:1–63. https://doi.org/10.1080/10408398.2018.1442316.

130. Farsi F, Mohammadshahi M, Alavinejad P, Rezazadeh A, Zarei M, Engali K. Functions of coenzyme Q10 supplementation on liver enzymes, markers of systemic inflammation, and adipokines in patients affected by nonalcoholic fatty liver disease: a double-blind, placebo-controlled, randomized clinical trial. J Am Coll Nutr. 2015;35:346–53. https://doi.org/10.1080/07315724.2015.1021057.

131. Sharifi N, Tabrizi R, Moosazadeh M, Mirhosseini N, Lankarani KB, Akbari M, et al. The effects of coenzyme Q10 supplementation on lipid profiles among patients with metabolic diseases: a systematic review and meta-analysis of randomized controlled trials. Curr Pharm Design. 2018;17(1):123. https://doi.org/10.2174/1381612824666180406104516.

132. Wei S, Zhang M, Yu Y, Lan X, Yao F, Yan X, et al. Berberine attenuates development of the hepatic gluconeogenesis and lipid metabolism disorder in type 2 diabetic mice and in palmitate-incubated HepG2 cells through suppression of the HNF-4α miR122 pathway. PLoS One. 2016;11:e0152097. https://doi.org/10.1371/journal.pone.0152097.

133. Vuddanda P, Chakraborty S, Singh S. Berberine: a potential phytochemical with multispectrum therapeutic activities. Expert Opin Investig Drugs. 2010;19:1297–307. https://doi.org/10.1517/13543784.2010.517745.
134. Guo T, Woo S-L, Guo X, Li H, Zheng J, Botchlett R, et al. Berberine ameliorates hepatic steatosis and suppresses liver and adipose tissue inflammation in mice with diet-induced obesity. Sci Rep-Uk. 2016;6:22612. https://doi.org/10.1038/srep22612.
135. Cao Y, Pan Q, Cai W, Shen F, Chen G-Y, Xu L-M, et al. Modulation of gut microbiota by berberine improves steatohepatitis in high-fat diet-fed BALB/C mice. Arch Iran Med. 2016;19:197–203.
136. Cicero AF, Baggioni A. Anti-inflammatory nutraceuticals and chronic diseases. Adv Exp Med Biol. 2016;928:27–45. https://doi.org/10.1007/978-3-319-41334-1_2.
137. Wei X, Wang C, Hao S, Song H, Yang L. The therapeutic effect of Berberine in the treatment of nonalcoholic fatty liver disease: a meta-analysis. Evid Based Complement Alternat Med. 2016;2016:3593951. https://doi.org/10.1155/2016/3593951.
138. Panahi Y, Hosseini M, Khalili N, Naimi E, Majeed M, Sahebkar A. Antioxidant and anti-inflammatory effects of curcuminoid-piperine combination in subjects with metabolic syndrome: a randomized controlled trial and an updated meta-analysis. Clin Nutr. 2015;34:1101–8. https://doi.org/10.1016/j.clnu.2014.12.019.
139. Panahi Y, Hosseini M, Khalili N, Naimi E, Simental-Mendía LE, Majeed M, et al. Effects of curcumin on serum cytokine concentrations in subjects with metabolic syndrome: a post-hoc analysis of a randomized controlled trial. Biomed Pharmacother. 2016;82:578–82. https://doi.org/10.1016/j.biopha.2016.05.037.
140. Panahi Y, Hosseini M, Khalili N, Naimi E, Soflaei S, Majeed M, et al. Effects of supplementation with curcumin on serum adipokine concentrations: a randomized controlled trial. Nutrition. 2016;32:1116–22. https://doi.org/10.1016/j.nut.2016.03.018.
141. Panahi Y, Khalili N, Hosseini M, Abbasinazari M, Sahebkar A. Lipid-modifying effects of adjunctive therapy with curcuminoids–piperine combination in patients with metabolic syndrome: results of a randomized controlled trial. Complement Ther Med. 2014;22:851–7. https://doi.org/10.1016/j.ctim.2014.07.006.
142. Panahi Y, Kianpour P, Mohtashami R, Jafari R, Simental-Mendía LE, Sahebkar A. Efficacy and safety of phytosomal curcumin in non-alcoholic fatty liver disease: a randomized controlled trial. Drug Res. 2017;67:244–51. https://doi.org/10.1055/s-0043-100019.
143. Sivaprakasapillai B, Edirisinghe I, Randolph J, Steinberg F, Kappagoda T. Effect of grape seed extract on blood pressure in subjects with the metabolic syndrome. Metabolism. 2009;58:1743–6. https://doi.org/10.1016/j.metabol.2009.05.030.
144. Zhao L, Guo X, Wang O, Zhang H, Wang Y, Zhou F, et al. Fructose and glucose combined with free fatty acids induce metabolic disorders in HepG2 cell: a new model to study the impacts of high-fructose/sucrose and high-fat diets in vitro. Mol Nutr Food Res. 2016;60:909–21. https://doi.org/10.1002/mnfr.201500635.
145. Faghihzadeh F, Adibi P, Hekmatdoost A. The effects of resveratrol supplementation on cardiovascular risk factors in patients with non-alcoholic fatty liver disease: a randomised, double-blind, placebo-controlled study. Br J Nutr. 2015;114:796–803. https://doi.org/10.1017/s0007114515002433.
146. Chen S, Zhao X, Ran L, Wan J, Wang X, Qin Y, et al. Resveratrol improves insulin resistance, glucose and lipid metabolism in patients with non-alcoholic fatty liver disease: a randomized controlled trial. Dig Liver Dis. 2015;47:226–32. https://doi.org/10.1016/j.dld.2014.11.015.
147. Chachay VS, Macdonald GA, Martin JH, Whitehead JP, O'Moore–Sullivan TM, Lee P, et al. Resveratrol does not benefit patients with nonalcoholic fatty liver disease. Clin Gastroenterol Hepatol. 2014;12:2092–2103.e6. https://doi.org/10.1016/j.cgh.2014.02.024.
148. Peng H, He Y, Zheng G, Zhang W, Yao Z, Xie W. Meta-analysis of traditional herbal medicine in the treatment of nonalcoholic fatty liver disease. Cell Mol Biol (Noisy-le-Grand). 2016;62:88–95.
149. Ma J, Zhou Q, Li H. Gut microbiota and nonalcoholic fatty liver disease: insights on mechanisms and therapy. Nutrients. 2017;9:1124. https://doi.org/10.3390/nu9101124.

150. Lavekar AS, Raje DV, Manohar T, Lavekar AA. Role of probiotics in the treatment of nonalcoholic fatty liver disease: a meta-analysis. Euroasian J Hepato-Gastroenterol. 2017;7:130–7. https://doi.org/10.5005/jp-journals-10018-1233.
151. Aller R, Luis DD, Izaola O, Conde R, Sagrado GM, Primo D, et al. Effect of a probiotic on liver aminotransferases in nonalcoholic fatty liver disease patients: a double blind randomized clinical trial. Eur Rev Med Pharmacol Sci. 2011;15:1090–5.
152. Vajro P, Mandato C, Licenziati M, Franzese A, Vitale D, Lenta S, et al. Effects of Lactobacillus rhamnosus strain GG in pediatric obesity-related liver disease. J Pediatr Gastroenterol Nutr. 2011;52:740–3. https://doi.org/10.1097/mpg.0b013e31821f9b85.
153. Nabavi S, Rafraf M, Somi MH, Homayouni-Rad A, Asghari-Jafarabadi M. Effects of probiotic yogurt consumption on metabolic factors in individuals with nonalcoholic fatty liver disease. J Dairy Sci. 2014;97:7386–93. https://doi.org/10.3168/jds.2014-8500.
154. Alisi A, Bedogni G, Baviera G, Giorgio V, Porro E, Paris C, et al. Randomised clinical trial: the beneficial effects of VSL#3 in obese children with non-alcoholic steatohepatitis. Aliment Pharmacol Ther. 2014;39:1276–85. https://doi.org/10.1111/apt.12758.
155. Suda I, Ishikawa F, Hatakeyama M, Miyawaki M, Kudo T, Hirano K, et al. Intake of purple sweet potato beverage affects on serum hepatic biomarker levels of healthy adult men with borderline hepatitis. Eur J Clin Nutr. 2007;62:1602674. https://doi.org/10.1038/sj.ejcn.1602674.
156. Zhang P-W, Chen F-X, Li D, Ling W-H, Guo H-H. A CONSORT-compliant, randomized, double-blind, placebo-controlled pilot trial of purified anthocyanin in patients with nonalcoholic fatty liver disease. Medicine. 2015;94:e758. https://doi.org/10.1097/md.0000000000000758.
157. Deminice R, da Silva RP, Lamarre SG, Kelly KB, Jacobs RL, Brosnan ME, et al. Betaine supplementation prevents fatty liver induced by a high-fat diet: effects on one-carbon metabolism. Amino Acids. 2015;47:839–46. https://doi.org/10.1007/s00726-014-1913-x.
158. Kawakami S, Han K-H, Nakamura Y, Shi K, Kitano T, Aritsuka T, et al. Effects of dietary supplementation with betaine on a nonalcoholic steatohepatitis (NASH) mouse model. J Nutr Sci Vitaminol. 2012;58:371–5. https://doi.org/10.3177/jnsv.58.371.
159. Chen Y, Liu Y, Zhou R, Chen X, Wang C, Tan X, et al. Associations of gut-flora-dependent metabolite trimethylamine-N-oxide, betaine and choline with non-alcoholic fatty liver disease in adults. Sci Rep-Uk. 2016;6:19076. https://doi.org/10.1038/srep19076.
160. Miglio F, Rovati L, Santoro A, Setnikar I. Efficacy and safety of oral betaine glucuronate in non-alcoholic steatohepatitis. Arzneimittelforschung. 2011;50:722–7. https://doi.org/10.1055/s-0031-1300279.
161. Abdelmalek MF, Sanderson SO, Angulo P, Soldevila-Pico C, Liu C, Peter J, et al. Betaine for nonalcoholic fatty liver disease: results of a randomized placebo-controlled trial. Hepatology. 2009;50:1818–26. https://doi.org/10.1002/hep.23239.
162. Venables MC, Hulston CJ, Cox HR, Jeukendrup AE. Green tea extract ingestion, fat oxidation, and glucose tolerance in healthy humans. Am J Clin Nutr. 2008;87:778–84. https://doi.org/10.1093/ajcn/87.3.778.
163. Shimotoyodome A, Haramizu S, Inaba K, Murase T, Tokimitsu I. Exercise and green tea extract stimulate fat oxidation and prevent obesity in mice. Med Sci Sports Exerc. 2005;37:1884–92. https://doi.org/10.1249/01.mss.0000178062.66981.a8.
164. Murase T, Haramizu S, Shimotoyodome A, Nagasawa A, Tokimitsu I. Green tea extract improves endurance capacity and increases muscle lipid oxidation in mice. Am J Phys Regul Integr Comp Phys. 2005;288:R708–15. https://doi.org/10.1152/ajpregu.00693.2004.
165. Pezeshki A, Safi S, Feizi A, Askari G, Karami F. The effect of green tea extract supplementation on liver enzymes in patients with nonalcoholic fatty liver disease. Int J Prev Med. 2015;6:131. https://doi.org/10.4103/2008-7802.173051.
166. Hussain M, Habib-Ur-Rehman AL. Therapeutic benefits of green tea extract on various parameters in non-alcoholic fatty liver disease patients. Pak J Med Sci. 2017;33:931–6. https://doi.org/10.12669/pjms.334.12571.

167. Sakata R, Nakamura T, Torimura T, Ueno T, Sata M. Green tea with high-density catechins improves liver function and fat infiltration in non-alcoholic fatty liver disease (NAFLD) patients: a double-blind placebo-controlled study. Int J Mol Med. 2013;32:989–94. https://doi.org/10.3892/ijmm.2013.1503.
168. Salomone F, Volti G, Vitaglione P, Morisco F, Fogliano V, Zappalà A, et al. Coffee enhances the expression of chaperones and antioxidant proteins in rats with nonalcoholic fatty liver disease. Transl Res. 2014;163:593–602. https://doi.org/10.1016/j.trsl.2013.12.001.
169. Watanabe S, Takahashi T, Ogawa H, Uehara H, Tsunematsu T, Baba H, et al. Daily coffee intake inhibits pancreatic beta cell damage and nonalcoholic steatohepatitis in a mouse model of spontaneous metabolic syndrome, Tsumura-Suzuki obese diabetic mice. Metab Syndr Relat Disord. 2017;15:170–7. https://doi.org/10.1089/met.2016.0114.
170. Bambha K, Wilson LA, Unalp A, Loomba R, Neuschwander-Tetri BA, Brunt EM, et al. Coffee consumption in NAFLD patients with lower insulin resistance is associated with lower risk of severe fibrosis. Liver Int. 2014;34:1250–8. https://doi.org/10.1111/liv.12379.
171. Zelber-Sagi S, Salomone F, Webb M, Lotan R, Yeshua H, Halpern Z, et al. Coffee consumption and nonalcoholic fatty liver onset: a prospective study in the general population. Transl Res. 2015;165:428–36. https://doi.org/10.1016/j.trsl.2014.10.008.
172. Gutiérrez-Grobe Y, Chávez-Tapia N, Sánchez-Valle V, Gavilanes-Espinar J, Ponciano-Rodríguez G, Uribe M, et al. High coffee intake is associated with lower grade nonalcoholic fatty liver disease: the role of peripheral antioxidant activity. Ann Hepatol. 2012;11:350–5. https://doi.org/10.1016/s1665-2681(19)30931-7.
173. Wijarnpreecha K, Thongprayoon C, Ungprasert P. Coffee consumption and risk of nonalcoholic fatty liver disease. Eur J Gastroenterol Hepatol. 2017;29:e8–12. https://doi.org/10.1097/meg.0000000000000776.
174. Karkos P, Leong S, Karkos C, Sivaji N, Assimakopoulos D. Spirulina in clinical practice: evidence-based human applications. Evid Based Complement Alternat Med. 2011;2011:531053. https://doi.org/10.1093/ecam/nen058.
175. Coué M, Tesse A, Falewée J, Aguesse A, Croyal M, Fizanne L, et al. Spirulina liquid extract protects against fibrosis related to non-alcoholic steatohepatitis and increases ursodeoxycholic acid. Nutrients. 2019;11:194. https://doi.org/10.3390/nu11010194.
176. Mazokopakis EE, Papadomanolaki MG, Fousteris AA, Kotsiris DA, Lampadakis IM, Ganotakis ES. The hepatoprotective and hypolipidemic effects of Spirulina (Arthrospira platensis) supplementation in a Cretan population with non-alcoholic fatty liver disease: a prospective pilot study. Ann Gastroenterol. 2014;27:387–94.
177. Mora SI, García-Román J, Gómez-Ñañez I, García-Román R. Chronic liver diseases and the potential use of S-adenosyl-L-methionine as a hepatoprotector. Eur J Gastroenterol Hepatol. 2018;30:893–900. https://doi.org/10.1097/meg.0000000000001141.
178. Zubiete-Franco I, García-Rodríguez J, Martínez-Uña M, Martínez-Lopez N, Woodhoo A, Juan V, et al. Methionine and S-adenosylmethionine levels are critical regulators of PP2A activity modulating lipophagy during steatosis. J Hepatol. 2016;64:409–18. https://doi.org/10.1016/j.jhep.2015.08.037.
179. Ni Y, Nagashimada M, Zhuge F, Zhan L, Nagata N, Tsutsui A, et al. Astaxanthin prevents and reverses diet-induced insulin resistance and steatohepatitis in mice: a comparison with vitamin E. Sci Rep-Uk. 2015;5:srep17192. https://doi.org/10.1038/srep17192.
180. Chen G, Ni Y, Nagata N, Xu L, Ota T. Micronutrient antioxidants and nonalcoholic fatty liver disease. Int J Mol Sci. 2016;17:1379. https://doi.org/10.3390/ijms17091379.

Chapter 10
Nutraceuticals Supporting Cognitive Function in Mild Cognitive Impairment

Larysa Strilchuk

Introduction

Dementia is a chronic condition characterized by the decreased cognitive capacity, which is more severe than in case of normal aging. The most common types of dementia include Alzheimer's disease (AD) and vascular dementia (VD), which often coexist [1, 2]. Neurodegeneration can also accompany such disorders as amyotrophic lateral sclerosis, Huntington's disease, frontotemporal dementia, and Parkinson's disease (PD) [3].

Cognitive impairment is a major social and economic problem of modern society [4–6]. World Health Organization states that dementia affects about 47 million people worldwide, and 9.9 million of new cases emerge each year [7]. Advances in general quality of life and medical science had shifted the population towards older people, so the incidence of dementia is predicted to increase dramatically [8]. So-called non-infectious pandemia of diabetes mellitus may accelerate this increase [9].

The first stage of dementia is defined as mild cognitive impairment (MCI) [10]. Characteristics of MCI include decline of memory, executive function, attention, visuospatial skills and speech [11, 12]. Pathogenic links of cognitive impairment are represented by neuroinflammation, excessive amyloid-β protein (ABP) production and deposition, formation of neurofibrillary tangles, oxidative stress and free radical damage, hyperphosphorylation of the tau protein, changes in the cholinergic system, cellular senescence, genome instability and proteostasis dysregulation [1, 13–17].

In the recent years, the interest of scientists and consumers in natural plant-derived compounds for the treatment of dementia and MCI has increased [18].

L. Strilchuk (✉)
Department of Therapy, Medical Diagnostics and Hematology and Transfusiology,
Lviv National Medical University named after Danylo Halytsky,
Lviv, Ukraine

© Springer Nature Switzerland AG 2021
A. F.G. Cicero, M. Rizzo (eds.), *Nutraceuticals and Cardiovascular Disease*,
Contemporary Cardiology, https://doi.org/10.1007/978-3-030-62632-7_10

It can be partly explained by the desire to receive effective, but safe non-drug therapy [19]. In this chapter, we summarize the available evidence supporting the benevolent action of some botanicals and phytochemicals on cognitive function.

Ginkgo biloba (Gb)

Gb is a widely used plant for the prevention and treatment of memory loss, depression, tinnitus and confusion [20]. Spectrum of Gb chemical constituents is very wide and includes terpene trilactones, flavonol glycosides, isoflavonoids, biflavones, proanthocyanidins, alkylphenols, carboxylic acids, 4-O-methylpyridoxine and polyprenols [21–23]. Preclinical evidence suggests that flavonol glycosides are mostly responsible for the antioxidant activity of ginkgo [24], whereas terpene trilactones like bilobalide provide neuroprotective effect and promote nerve regeneration [25] by the means of counteracting the decrease of brain-derived neurotropic factor (BDNF), norepinephrine transporter and dopamine transporter [26–28].

The most widely studied Gb extract called EGb761 was approved as a drug in 1967 [29]. EGb761 contains ≈24% flavone glycosides (quercetin, kaempferol, and isorhamnetin), 6% terpene lactones (ginkgolides A, B and C; bilobalide), 0.8% ginkgolide B [30]. These chemical constituents seem to have either separate or synergistic actions, which contribute to the global Ginkgo effect [31–34].

Neuroprotective and cognition-enhancing action of Gb are mostly attributed to its property to improve cerebral blood flow (CBF). This could be related to inhibition of platelet-activating factor (PAF), enhancing of nitric oxide (NO) production in vessels, and suppression of the acetylcholinesterase (AChE) activity [35–37]. EGb761 stabilizes cell membranes, reduces vascular permeability, promotes neurogenesis, and improves synaptic plasticity [38, 39]. Then, EGb761 has direct (free radicals scavenging) and indirect (stimulation of cytochrome P450 enzyme systems) antioxidative effect [40]. Gb extract also may counteract inflammation in microglial cells due to its property to inhibit production of prostaglandin E_2, tumor necrosis factor α (TNF), interleukins (IL)-6, and -1β [41].

One of the AD pathogenesis theories suggests that AD is mediated by mitochondrial dysfunction, which is associated with the oxidative stress and decreased energy metabolism. W.E. Müller et al. (2017) attribute Gb procognitive effect to the inhibition of mitochondrial dysfunction cascade [42].

Gb has been extensively investigated in a large number of preclinical studies, especially, different dementia models in rodents. In galactose-induced dementia in rats Gb extract attenuated memory impairment and neuron apoptosis [43]. In a vascular dementia model in gerbils, it induced recovery of spatial memory, protected the hippocampal CA1 neurons and counteracted the decrease in plasma superoxide dismutase (SOD) activity [44]. Gb pretreatment significantly improved cognitive function in rats exposed to bisphenol A. Authors explain this by increasing hippocampal levels of estrogen-dependent biogenic amines and controlling oxidative stress [45]. In aged rodents, Gb extracts improved spatial learning and memory, producing favorable effects on synaptic efficacy and plasticity in the hippocampus CA1 area [46, 47]. Gb extracts were also shown to activate cell proliferation in the hippocampus of mice [28]. In animal models of AD, Gb extract inhibits ABP aggregation, ABP_{1-42}-induced dysfunction and death of hippocampal neurons [48]. It also inhibits the formation of ABP-derived neurotoxic ligands, decreases mitochondrial-initiated apoptosis and caspase-3 activity [49, 50], suppresses formation of amyloid fibrils [51, 52], and modulates phosphorylation of tau protein – the main component of neurofibrillary tangles and one of the key neuropathological characteristic of AD [53].

Gb is extremely widely studied in clinical trials, which, however, had showed heterogeneous results. For instance, in the GuidAge trial [54] and the Ginkgo Evaluation of Memory trial [55] EGb761 (240 mg/day) had been administered to participants with no cognitive impairment for 4–6 years. Authors did not reveal any positive effect of Gb extract on dementia incidence. Such conclusions were supported by the meta-analysis of eight trials of non-cognitively impaired participants treated with Gb for up to 13 weeks [56].

On the other side, a meta-analysis of 21 trials including 2608 patients with dementia or MCI showed that combination of Gb and conventional medicine taken for 24 weeks was superior in improving Mini-Mental State Examination (MMSE) score above the conventional medicine alone [48]. These results have been confirmed by the meta-analysis, concluding that Gb extract at doses >200 mg/day for at least 5 months has potentially beneficial effects for people with dementia [57]. In some studies EGb761 was significantly more effective above placebo in enhancing cognition according to Syndrom-Kurz test evaluating memory and attention [58–60], whereas in others it was not [61, 62].

Single administration of Gb extract (600 mg) had been demonstrated to improve short-term memory in volunteers with [63, 64] and without cognitive impairment [65]. A large meta-analysis showed that a long-time treatment with Gb extract (240 mg/day for 22–26 weeks) may stabilize or slow down the cognitive decline in patients with neuropsychiatric symptoms [66]. Other analytic paper states the Gb extract has sufficient evidence of beneficial effect only in doses above 200 mg/day given longer than 22 weeks [57]. Accordingly, a 20-year long follow-up population-based study has revealed that EGb761 prevented cognitive decline in a non-demented elderly population in comparison to non-users [67].

The guidelines of World Federation of Societies of Biological Psychiatry for the biological treatment of AD and other dementias state that EGb761 has the same strength of evidence as AChE inhibitors and N-methyl-D-aspartate (NMDA) antagonists (Grade 3 recommendation; Level B evidence) [68]. EGb761 showed efficacy equal to donepezil (5 mg/day) according to MMSE in a small (n = 76) randomized controlled trial [69]. Authors of other comparison of EGb761 and donepezil agreed that these agents had a comparable therapeutic effect on cognitive symptoms in elderly AD patients and underlined the better safety of the former [70].

EGb761 has a positive risk-benefit profile according to an in-depth analysis [71] and European Medicines Agency report [72]. Once existing concerns regarding a possibility of bleeding risk increase due to the inhibition of platelet aggregation and

PAF function were not supported by several randomized trials and meta-analyses [73]. From 1966 to 2004 the association between GB extract and bleeding events was described in 15 case reports, but some of these patients had major bleeding risk factors (liver cirrhosis, hypertension and warfarin or high dose aspirin consumption) [74]. Nevertheless, a large study based on the Veterans Administration Informatics and Computing Infrastructure database (USA, n = 807,399) showed that Gb extract significantly increased risk of bleeding when taken together with warfarin in comparison to warfarin alone [75].

Despite some authors state that Gb extracts do not have any drug-drug interactions [29, 32, 71], other ones note that this herbal drug may interact with aspirin, warfarin, trazodone, omeprazole, antihypertensive and antihyperglycaemic medications [76, 77].

To sum up, Gb is potentially beneficial for the improvement of cognitive function in patients with MCI or AD when given in doses of >200 mg/day for >22 weeks. It should be noted that active compounds of Gb extract have short half-lives, so this nutraceutical should be taken more than once daily [78, 79].

Vitis vinifera

Seeds and berry peels of grape (*Vitis vinifera*) are well-known nutraceuticals. Beneficial properties of grape are usually attributed to its polyphenolic compounds [80]. Grape polyphenols are represented by proanthocyanidins, which are the polymers of flavan-3-ol links like catechin, catechin gallate, epicatechin, and epicatechin gallate [81]. Polyphenolic compounds of grape can improve memory and cognition decreased in aging process [82] due to their antioxidant activity, which was proven in animal models of AD [83, 84]. This effect is in part realized via inhibiting the depletion of antioxidant enzymes in hippocampal regions involved in short-term memory [85]. Other mechanisms of procognitive and neuroprotective action of grape polyphenols include promotion of synaptic transmission in the hippocampus, enhancement of the synaptic plasticity, suppression of ABP oligomer aggregation, epigenetic regulation of BDNF, anti-inflammatory and antiapoptotic effects [86–91]. Apart from that, grape induces increase of SOD, hemeoxygenase-1 (HO-1), and glutathione peroxidase activities, decreases levels of toxic malondialdehyde (MDA) and activates the nuclear factor (erythroid-derived 2)-like 2 (Nrf2)/ARE pathway [92].

In preclinical models, *Vitis vinifera* extract dose-dependently attenuated aluminum-induced impairment in learning and memory, by modifying the biochemical cascades as a central cholinomimetic agent, inhibiting the mRNA expression of amyloid precursor protein and tau protein, and suppressing the activity of myeloperoxidase (anti-inflammatory effect) [93].

Chronic treatment with grape-derived polyphenolic supplements results in the increase in bioactive neurometabolites able to antagonize pathological mechanisms and restore neuronal function [94]. In a randomized, double-blind, placebo-controlled clinical trial a food supplement based on grape extract (250 mg/day for 12 weeks) led to the significant improvement of MMSE score in comparison to placebo. Among the Repeatable Battery for the Assessment of Neuropsychological Status (RBANS) parameters, *Vitis vinifera* supplementation significantly enhanced attention, language, immediate and delayed memory without having any superiority above placebo in terms of visuospatial/constructional abilities [95].

Resveratrol (3,5,4'-trihydroxystilbene) [96, 97] is one of the most studied grape polyphenols [98]. It exists in two isomeric forms: the trans-isomer is present in the berry skins of most grape cultivars and cis-isomer is formed from the trans-isomer under UV exposure [99]. Most research on resveratrol describes the effects of more stable trans-isomer [100]. As a potent antioxidant, resveratrol can prevent the oxidative stress and, subsequently, senile plaques formation and AD development [101, 102]. Resveratrol also protects neurons and microglia [103, 104], attenuates the ABP-induced accumulation of intracellular reactive oxygen species (ROS) [105], restores the normal levels of glutathione depleted by the ABP_{1-42} [106], protects cell components against electrophilic injury [107], and strengthens the HO-1 pathway [108]. Resveratrol can counteract the neuroinflammation [109] via suppression of astrocytes and microglia activation [110, 111], and the inhibition of p38 mitogen-activated protein kinase (MAPK) phosphorylation and nuclear factor (NF)-κB activation, eventually reducing production of TNF and NO [112]. Resveratrol was also shown to inhibit IL-1β and IL-6 expression [113], and signal transducer and activator of transcription 1 (STAT1) and STAT3 phosphorylation [114]. Resveratrol or grape seed extract coadministration along with bisphenol A attenuated the negative dementia-inducing effects of the latter in rats [115].

Even single doses of resveratrol (250 or 500 mg per os) increased CBF in healthy volunteers [116]. Dietary supplementation with resveratrol (200 mg/day) and quercetin (320 mg/day) led to the memory retention and improved the functional connectivity between hippocampus and frontal, parietal, and occipital areas of brain [117, 118]. Resveratrol also improves the cerebral vasodilatory responsiveness, which is associated with cognitive function [119, 120].

In general, neuroprotective and cognition-enhancing effects of resveratrol may be mostly explained by its antioxidant and vasoactive action, whereas mechanisms of grape extract effects may be more diverse.

Camellia sinensis

Tea is produced from the leaves, buds, and young stems of *Camellia sinensis* plant [121]. Daily tea intake might be associated to a significant reduction in the risk of cognitive impairment, cognitive decline, and ungrouped cognitive disorders [122–125]. Green tea consumption (2–4 cups/day for 3 months) improved cognitive status in subjects with already established cognitive dysfunction [126]. Acute supplementation of green tea also improves working memory (according to the reading span and N-back task paradigm) in healthy women aged 50–63 years, whereas it did not have any effect on younger counterparts [127].

Neuroprotective effects of tea may include antioxidant action, metal-chelating properties, and modulation of cell signaling and cell survival pathways [128–130]. Metal-chelating effect are of extreme importance, because iron can take part in the generation of harmful hydroxyl radicals [131], and copper forms complexes with ABP, promoting its neurotoxicity [132].

Different kinds of tea have different chemical composition due to fermentation process [133, 134] and, consequently, may have different efficacy. Some authors postulate that any kind of tea (green, black, or oolong) can be a procognitive agent [135–137], whereas other scientists report positive effects of green tea only [138–140], explaining this differences by the smaller amount of catechins in black and oolong tea as compared to green tea [135, 141]. Indeed, green tea main compounds belong to catechin family, whereas black tea principally contains tannins [142].

Green tea enhances memory formation in the fresh water pond snail, *Lymnaea stagnalis* [143], whereas black tea prevents long-term memory formation [144]. There is a hypothesis that higher content of flavan-3-ols in black tea may alter cognition [145]. In contrast, a Chinese cross-sectional study (n = 9375) found a positive correlation with cognitive function for black tea, whereas green tea showed no significant effect [146]. Procognitive effects of black tea seems to be associated with attention improvement [147–149].

Xu et al. (2018) found that black tea and oolong tea were not linked to the decreased risk of amnestic MCI. At the same time, green tea may be a protective factor for amnestic MCI in males aged 60–70 years, though this effect was not evident in males aged over 70 years. Females did not benefit from green tea at any age [150].

In general, the evidence of protective effects of any tea remains controversial [151, 152]. There are even studies showing negative effect of tea on cognition [153].

Main active substances of green tea, namely, epigallocatechin gallate (EGCG), epicatechin gallate (ECG), epicatechin and epigallocatechin (EGC), belong to catechin family and exert a potent antioxidant effect [154]. EGCG, ECG, and EGC constitute 80% of the total tea catechins [155]. Exposition of transgenic AD mice to catechins resulted in the decrease of ABP levels and plaques quantity associated with stimulation of non-amyloidogenic α-secretase pathway [156]. Tea also contains other phenolic compounds such as gallic, caffeic, and chlorogenic acids, quercetin, proanthocyanidols, caffeine, theophylline, l-theanine and minerals (fluorine, manganese, chromium) [157]. A systematic meta-analysis of 21 studies concluded that green tea may improve memory and attention due to synergetic action of its components. It is proved, for instance, by the fact that the most beneficial effects on cognition are observed under the influence of both caffeine and L-theanine, whereas separate administration of either agent has a smaller positive impact [158].

Green tea polyphenols can improve ethanol-induced impairment of spatial learning and memory in rats. This phenomenon is explained by the upregulation of pyramidal layer neurons density, expression of NMDA-receptor 1 subunit, and cAMP response element-binding protein (CREB) phosphorylation in the hippocampus [159]. These polyphenols amplify the cholinergic neurotransmission via the inhibition of AChE and butyrylcholinesterase [160].

It should be noted that excessive intake of green tea can be harmful, because abundant polyphenols can induce autooxidative reactions [161]. There also sporadic case reports describing liver toxicity of tea extracts [162]. Green tea may interact with some medications. For instance, it may lower the exposure to rosuvastatin (without clinically significant results), nadolol (significantly suppressing the systolic blood pressure-lowering effect) and tacrolimus or increase the exposure to sildenafil. There also reports considering green tea interaction with simvastatin and warfarin in clinical studies and with diltiazem, verapamil and nicardipine in animal experiments [163, 164].

EGCG ((2R,3R)-5,7-dihydroxy-2-(3,4,5-trihydroxyphenyl)-3,4-dihydro-2H-1-benzopyran-3-yl 3,4,5-trihydroxybenzoate) is the most abundant tea polyphenol, representing 50–80% of the total catechins [165–167]. This hydrophilic catechin is a potent antioxidant, metal chelator and anti-inflammatory agent, which has the ability to cross the blood-brain barrier [168, 169].

Animal studies on models of neurodegenerative disorders showed that EGCG may protect neurons and other cells from oxidative stress. EGCG also promotes the formation of non-cytotoxic spherical protein aggregates. The latter do not catalyze the formation of fibrils and, consequently, decrease the neurotoxicity of α-synuclein and ABP_{1-42} peptides [170, 171]. Molecular mechanisms of this effect include activation of the glycogen synthase kinase-3β (GSK-3β) and the inhibition of c-Abl/FE65 nuclear translocation [172]. Other mechanisms of antioxidant and anti-inflammatory action of EGCG are represented by its ability to suppress the expression of TNFα, IL-1β, IL-6, and inducible nitric oxide synthase (iNOS) and to restore the intracellular antioxidants' level in microglia [173].

Anti-neuroinflammatory effects of EGCG have been proven on different cells lines, namely, including MC65, EOC 13.31, SweAPP N2a, N2a/APP695, DIV8, CHO, and M146 L cells [174]. Results from these studies showed that the anti-neuroinflammatory capacity of EGCG is mainly associated to the inhibition of microglia-induced cytotoxicity via reducing NF-κB activation and MAPK signaling, including c-Jun N-terminal kinase (JNK) and p38 signaling [175].

In a D-galactose AD mouse model [175] and TgCRND8 transgenic AD mouse model [176] EGCG significantly reduced the ABP accumulation, attenuated hippocampal neuronal injury, and exerted beneficial effects on cognition. For instance, in one experiment EGCG showed the capacity to reduce ABP deposits by 60% in the frontal cortex and by 52% in the hippocampus. It also lowered the concentration of CD45 – a marker of microglial activation [177]. Other animal experiments showed that EGCG could prevent lipopolysaccharide-induced memory impairment [178] and streptozocin-induced cognitive deficit [179].

L-theanine is a major aminoacid of green tea, able to improve cognition and facilitate the long-lasting attention [180–182], presumably increasing brain serotonin, dopamine and gamma-aminobutyric acid (GABA) levels [183]. Task-related recordings of electroencephalography demonstrated that L-theanine may enhance cognition [184].

Tea leaves can contain between 2% and 5% of caffeine, depending on the age of the leaf (older leaves have a smaller concentration) [185]. Procognitive and neuroprotective effects of caffeine were shown in animal models of PD [186] and in patients with AD [187]. Three to five cups of coffee per day at midlife may reduce the AD or dementia risk by 65% [188]. Caffeine can block adenosine receptors and, consequently, induce their upregulation, which improves the function of blood-brain barrier and protects brain against AD [189]. Other mechanisms of caffeine beneficial action on brain include regulation of CBF [190–192] and increase of oxygen consumption [193]. Chronic caffeine intake is associated with the significantly lower risk to develop cognitive impairment [194, 195]. Nevertheless, a large meta-analysis (total n = 31,479) [196] and the Manitoba Study of Health and Ageing of Canada [197] failed to prove any link of caffeine intake from coffee or tea and risk of cognitive disorders. It is speculated that only long-term caffeine consumption (about 20 years) may inversely associate with AD risk [186]. Some studies state that caffeine consumption is associated with reduced cognitive decline in women only [198], whereas others find procognitive benefits of tea, but not coffee [199]. Oral contraceptive steroids and estrogen have a major impact on caffeine metabolism [200], so its effects should be studied separately in men and women.

In general, green tea and its compounds (mainly EGCG) exert antioxidant effect, modulate cell signaling and apoptosis, counteract neuroinflammation, and inhibit protein aggregation. Nevertheless, the results of clinical trials vary significantly. These discrepancies may be explained by various confounding factors (study design, beverage temperature, presence of harmful habits, differences in genetic and environmental factors). So, further clinical studies are needed to establish its doses, administration frequency, efficacy and safety in humans.

Theobroma cacao

Many authors state that regular consumption of cacao (*Theobroma cacao*), coffee and dark chocolate can have a positive influence on the brain, including diminishing the risks of age-related neurodegeneration [201]. Chocolate intake was associated with a 40% lower risk of cognitive decline in healthy individuals. It is interesting that this effect was observed only among subjects with low daily consumption of caffeine (<75 mg, about one average espresso) [202]. Chocolate drinks (daily for 8 weeks) improves cognitive performance in patients with MCI [203] and cognitively intact elderly [204]. Cacao extracts also appear to prevent the oligomerization of ABP [205] and improve cognitive performance according to MMSE, Trail Making Test A and B (TMT-A and -B), and verbal fluency test [203]. Cacao polyphenolic extract counteracts heat-induced cognitive impairment [206] and improves spatial memory, short-term and long-term learning in aged rats [207]. Nevertheless, some human studies failed to find any association between chocolate or cacao seed extract intake and cognitive performance [208].

The cocoa flavanols have a procognitive effect [209] by the means of direct action on neurons, enhancement of dentate gyrus function [210] and CBF improvement [211]. Apart from flavanols, cacao and coffee contain methylxanthines, namely, caffeine (1,3,7-trimethylxanthine), theobromine (3,7-dimethylxanthine) and theophylline (1,3-dimethylxanthine) [212, 213]. These compounds are also present in tea, yerba mate and cola drinks [214]. Methylxanthines intake may prevent PD and AD [215, 216]. Caffeine is the most studied methylxanthine; its effects have been discussed earlier (See section "*Camellia sinensis*").

Coadministration of theobromine and caffeine increased alertness (according to Simple Reaction Time task), working memory (Rapid Visual Information Processing task) and manual dexterity (Thurstone tapping task) [217]. Nevertheless, in other studies it failed to increase vigilance or enhance cognitive performance [218, 219]. Diet, rich in theobromine, polyphenols, and polyunsaturated fatty acids, improved age-induced memory decline, which can be explained by the means of enhancement of cholinergic and adrenergic neurotransmission [220].

Theobromine may reduce ABP-mediated neurotoxicity in a dose-dependent manner [221], improve CBF [222] and decrease the release of proinflammatory factors [223].

Other from caffeine cacao compounds and its whole extract are, in general, poorly studied, so there is a need to continue investigations.

Bacopa monnieri

Bacopa monnieri or water hyssop, belongs to the Scrophulariaceae family [180]. It is a perennial creeping herb that thrives in damp soils. BM had been known as a cognitive and memory enhancer [224]. The main active components of BM are represented by steroidal saponines (bacoside A and B) and various alkaloids (brahmin, herpestine, monierin, hersapunin) [225–228]. Among these substances, bacoside A is thought to be the most active [229].

Principal mechanisms of Bacopa action are related to anti-inflammatory, antioxidant, metal-chelating, anti-amyloid and cholinergic effects [230–233]. Bacopa also antagonizes serotonin-6 and -2A receptors, which influence neurological pathways associated with memory and learning disorders [234]. Administration of bacoside can lead to a significant decrease of proinflammatory cytokines (IL-1β and TNF), a significant induction of iNOS expression, and a reduction of total nitrite and lipofuscin content in the brain cortex [235]. Bacopa extract was shown to increase long-term potentiation magnitude, which can partly explain its beneficial mnemonic effect [236]. Water hyssop extract reversed cognitive impairment in various rodent models of AD and memory decline including phenytoin- [237], diazepam- [238], colchicine- [239], and scopolamine-induced [240] ones. It was also shown in a rat experiment to increase CBF by 25% [241].

According to numerous and animal studies, Bacopa can improve motor learning, acquisition and retention [242], reverse cognitive deficits [232], reduce ABP fibrils formations and stimulate segregation of previously formed ones [243], decrease inflammatory and oxidative stress markers [244], normalize the concentrations of major neurotransmitters (acetylcholine, glutamate, 5-hydroxytryptamine, dopamine, 3,4 dihydroxyphenylacetic acid, norepinephrine), down-regulate AChE and upregulate muscarinic M1 receptor and CREB expression in hippocampus [245]. Administration of Bacopa extract improves novel object recognition in mice by increasing the cell proliferation and differentiation in the dentate gyrus together with elevation of BDNF phosphorylation [246]. Bacopa extract had a procognitive action in rodent models of type 2 diabetes [247], AD [248], and amnesia [238].

In some human trials, consumption of Bacopa extract improved working memory and cognition in elderly individuals [249–251] and children/adolescents [252], enhanced logical memory in children with attention deficit hyperactivity disorder [253], increased information-retaining capacity [250], whereas in others it did not produce any positive effect [254]. One meta-analysis of clinical trials (total n = 437) showed that Bacopa improved cognition according to TMT-B test and decreased choice reaction time [255].

Interventions with separate compounds of Bacopa, namely, bacosides A and B, also show memory improvement [256], possibly, mediated by cholinergic density modulation [257] and ABP-scavenging effect [258].

In general, Bacopa has a multi-faceted action including direct pro-cholinergic, antioxidant, metal chelating, anti-inflammatory, pro-circulatory, adaptogenic and anti-amyloid effects.

Crocus sativus

Crocus sativus is a perennial herb of the Iridaceae family. Stigmata of Crocus are used to obtained the famous spice named saffron [259, 260]. They were shown to have neuroprotective properties [261].

Saffron stigma contains crocetin, crocin, picrocrocin and safranal [262]. Other saffron components include flavonoids, anthocyanins, vitamins (riboflavin, thiamine), proteins, starch, and aminoacids [262]. Crocin – the main compound of saffron – is a water-soluble carotenoid known to improve learning and memory [259, 260]. Mechanism of action of crocin is based on the antioxidant effect and inhibition of AChE activity [263].

Crocin or whole saffron extract can also antagonize the cognitive deficits caused by neurotoxic agents like streptozocin [264] or aflatoxin [265].

A trial including subjects with moderate AD symptoms showed that the 16 weeks of supplementation with 30 mg saffron per day was able to significantly improve the AD assessment scale-cognitive subscale (ADAS-cog) when compared to placebo [266]. The same authors demonstrated that one-year supplementation with 30 mg saffron per day improved the Severe Cognitive Impairment Rating Scale (SCIRS) and Functional Assessment Staging (FAST) in moderate to severe AD [267]. In all available trials on saffron, the incidence of adverse events was similar to that of placebo [268].

Saffron crocins could counteract natural forgetting (according to novel object-recognition task in rats) and may modulate recognition memory, so the combination of crocins and memantine can be an innovative strategy to treat memory disorders [269].

In general, saffron extract and crocin itself need to be studied in further experiments and trials.

Panax ginseng

Ginseng is a perennial plant belonging to the Aralliaceae family [270]. Its root contains triterpene saponins, polysaccharides, peptidoglycans, polyacetylenes, sesquiterpenes, nitrogen-containing and phenolic compounds [271]. Ginsenosides (ginseng-specific saponins) are the major active components of ginseng [272]. They are usually classified into three groups based on the chemical structure: the panaxadiol (Rb1, Rb2, Rb3, Rc, Rd, Rg3, Rh2, and Rs1), panaxatriol (Re, Rf, Rg1, Rg2, and Rh1), and oleanolic acid groups (Ro) [273].

Preclinical studies have revealed that ginseng and its compounds are pharmacologically efficacious in different models of cognitive impairment. In a VD model in rats ginseng extract reduced the number of glial fibrillary acidic protein-immunoreactive cells, decreased apoptosis, ameliorated cholinergic system performance, improved blood circulation in the brain and alleviated the learning and memory impairment [274]. In scopolamine-induced memory impairment ginseng was as effective as memantine in restoring memory [275].

Ginseng positively influenced memory in healthy volunteers [276, 277] and in AD patients (according the frontal assessment battery) [278]. Addition of ginseng to pharmacological AD preparations increased procognitive efficacy of the latter according to MMSE and ADAS-Cog [278]. Adjuvant therapy of AD by ginseng or its separate components may improve safety and tolerability of pharmacological preparations, enhance neuroprotection and delay disease progression [279].

On the contrary, some studies failed to prove ginseng effectiveness in AD [280, 281], so clinical application of ginseng is still limited [282].

Ginsenoside Rb1 enhanced cognition and reverse memory loss in various rodent models of cognitive impairment, namely, cisplatin-, isoflurane-, trymethillin and surgery-induced [283–285]. Rb1 intake was also accompanied by inhibition of neuronal loss, normalization of the cholinergic neuron function, antioxidant and anti-inflammatory effects [284, 285]. Ginsenoside Rd enhances learning and memory function and activate nonamyloidogenic cascade through estrogen receptors [279]. Ginsenoside Re improves the learning and memory in rats by the means of enhancing synaptic transmission and increasing the magnitude of the long-term potentiation in the dentate gyrus of hippocampus [286]. In other animal experiments, it attenuated diabetes-associated cognitive decline [287] and controlled the antioxidant systems via regulating the JNK pathway [288]. Ginsenoside Rg1 also has procognitive and antioxidant properties proven in the numerous animal experiments and dementia models [289–292], including isoflurane- [293], lipopolysaccharide- [294] and dexamethasone-induced [295]. Similar effects were demonstrated for ginsenosides Rg2 and Rg3 [296–299], Rh1, Rh2 and Rh3 [300–302]. Other widely investigated ginseng compounds with procognitive, memory-stimulating and neuro-protective action include pseudoginsenoside-F11, notoginsenoside R1, gintonin, and compound K [303]. Then, oral gintonin treatment decreases amyloid plaque deposits in the brain cortex and hippocampus [304].

Korean ginseng has been shown to increase cognitive performance in AD patients according to the ADAS-cog and the MMSE score, but after discontinuation of ginseng intake, these parameters returned to control group values [305]. Similar results were obtained in other studies for both Korean [306, 307] and American ginseng [308, 309]. Ginsenoside profile of American ginseng (*Panax quinquefolius*) differs from *Panax ginseng* [308], but both of them show beneficial effects on cognition.

Investigation of influence of lifetime ginseng intake on cognitive function showed that high ginseng use group was characterized by higher Consortium to Establish a Registry for AD Assessment Packet neuropsychological battery (CERAD) total score even after controlling for possible confounding factors (age, sex, education years, socioeconomic status, smoking, alcohol intake, presence of hypertension, stroke history, Geriatric Depression Scale, Cumulative Illness Rating Scale, and presence of the APOE e4 allele) [310].

Therapeutic potential of ginseng compounds is limited by their low bioavailability because of poor solubility in water, instability in the digestive system and extensive metabolism [311]. Moreover, ginsenosides function like prodrugs and are activated upon deglycosylation by colonic microbiota and further esterification [312]. Given these facts, it can be assumed that ginseng effects are characterized by high inter-individual variability.

Overall, ginseng is extremely widely studied as a cognition enhancer. It is worth noting that the majority of studies involve Asian population, where dietary intake of ginseng is quite high, so trials in other populations are needed.

Curcuma longa

Turmeric (*Curcuma longa*) is an herbaceous perennial plant, which belongs to Zingiberaceae family [313]. Some studies attribute lower dementia rates in Asia to higher curry (turmeric) consumption [314]. Curcuma contains three major compounds, namely, curcumin (60–70%), demethoxycurcumin (20–27%), and bisdemethoxycurcumin (10–15%) [315]. Curcumin is a hydrophobic polyphenol with low bioavailability in humans, which is able to cross the blood-brain barrier [316]. According to existing literature, curcumin has the antioxidant, anti-inflammatory, and amyloid-disaggregating properties [317, 318]. It can also decrease inflammation induced by ABP and moderately inhibits AChE activity [319, 320].

Curcumin pretreatment can effectively reduce H_2O_2-induced neurotoxicity by decreasing caspase activation, poly-(ADP-ribose)-polymerase cleavage, DNA damage, accumulation of ROS and reactive nitrogen species, and counteracting dys-regulation of the MAPK and Akt pathways [321–323]. These effects allow cur-cumin to reduce inflammation in microglial cells [324] and, consequently, enhance memory [325]. Curcumin alleviates ABP-induced neuroinflammation [326] and counteracts memory deficit [327] in the rat models of AD. In the experimental model of chronic stress curcumin supplementation enhanced memory and normal-ized redox state indicators (glutathione, SOD, MDA etc.) [328]. It is also able to inhibit JNK phosporylation, which is a link of ABP toxicity [327].

In numerous animal experiments, curcumin improved spatial memory and learn-ing [329], inhibited ABP generation [330], improved the quantity and structure of the synapse [331], normalized BDNF levels in hippocampus [332, 333], inhibited pro-inflammatory cytokines through the suppression of NF-kB and Activator Protein 1 in BV2 microglial cells [334, 335], enhanced cell proliferation in the den-tate gyrus [336], and decreased expression of oxidative stress biomarkers (MDA and SOD) [337]. However, in other study high intake of curcumin was accompanied by increased levels of MDA. [338].

Chronic administration of curcuma improves the dendritic arborization and, con-sequently, communication among neurons, reflected in long-term memory enhance-ment [339]. Curcumin (treatment or pre-treatment) attenuated streptozocin- [340], homocysteine- [341], and lipopolysaccharide-induced [342] cognitive impairment in rodents and cigarette smoke extract-induced neurocognitive impairment in zebrafish [343]. On the other side, some studies failed to reveal any link between curcumin and spatial memory enhancement in streptozocin model of aging [344]. It should be noted that these studies used different doses and different methods of analyzing memory, which could influence the results.

Clinical studies of curcumin in humans have received conflicting results [345]. This discrepancy may be partly related to the low bioavailability or the insufficient doses of tested product [346]. A small trial including non-demented adults showed that standardized curcumin intake (90 mg twice daily for 18 months) resulted in memory and attention enhancement [347]. Curcumin supplementation was associ-ated with better performance according to Montreal Cognitive Assessment scale in 24 weeks of treatment, but in 48 weeks, this benefit disappeared [348]. Some clini-cal trials have shown complete lack of curcumin efficacy in cognition enhancement [349, 350].

In general, preclinical studies state that curcumin is a promising agent able to counteract neurodegenerative disease by improving glucose and lipid homeostasis, inhibiting ABP aggregation and suppressing inflammation. Human studies now are not as convincing as animal experiments, so there is a need in clinical trials.

Paullinia cupana

Guaranà (*Paullinia cupana*) is a climbing plant of the Sapindaceae family, which increases alertness, calmness and memory performance [351]. Guarana contains caffeine, flavonoids [352], saponins and tannins [353, 354], which may improve cognition [355–357]. Single doses of guarana extract have been shown to improve memory performance and response speed [356], and this effect cannot be attributed to caffeine only, because its level in guarana is too low (4–8%) [351, 356]. Caffeine procognitive effects were discussed earlier (see section "*Camellia sinensis*").

Pretreatment by guarana powder prevented memory impairment caused by poloxamer-407-induced hyperlipidemia in rats [358]. Authors explain this by various procognitive effects of methylxanthines including adenosine blocking, enhancement of long-term potentiation in hippocampal neurons, increase of acetylcholine release into synapses.

Dried extract of guarana and its combination with ginseng extract stimulate attention, speed up the memory task performance, and improve serial subtraction task performance in healthy volunteers [356]. Complex multivitamin drinks and mouth rinses enriched by guarana extract increased the speed of information processing and decision making in athletes according to Simon task and a duration-production task [359, 360]. Functional magnetic resonance imaging during a Rapid Visual Information Processing and Inspection Time tasks proved that different multivitamin supplements increased activation in brain areas involved in cognition, but the activation was greater after intake of guarana-containing multivitamins [361].

Although guarana is often shown to be a potent procognitive agent, it is mostly investigated as a component of complex preparations, which assesses its own immanent properties inaccurate. Guarana effects are often attributed to its caffeine content, so, future trials are needed to distinguish between the action of whole guarana extract and its single components.

Glycine max

Soybean (*Glycine max*) belongs to Leguminosae family [362]. Soy peptides prevent aging-associated cognitive impairment in normal and accelerated aging mice [363]. Soy isoflavones (SI), which are the major phytochemicals of soybean, may improve the cognitive function, activate cholinergic system and decrease oxidative stress in mice with scopolamine- [364], ABP- [365, 366] and ovariectomy-induced [367, 368] memory impairment. Furthermore, SI upregulate the phosphorylation levels of extracellular signal-regulated kinase (ERK) and CREB, and increase BDNF expression levels in the hippocampus [364].

Treatment of healthy older adults with SI was associated with improved nonverbal memory, construction, and verbal fluency compared to placebo [369]. Nevertheless, in the Women's Isoflavone Soy Health trial including 350 healthy postmenopausal women 25 g of isoflavone-rich soy protein failed to enhance cognitive function. Moreover, increase of isoflavonoids intake was associated with general intelligence decrement [370].

Results of clinical trials of soybean are extremely controversial and show benefits for cognitive function [371–373], partial benefits [374], no effect [375–379] and even potential harm [380]. SI could exert a beneficial effect on cognitive function only in individuals able to metabolize them to equol [373]. It should be noted that in live organisms SI undergo hydrolysis with subsequent release of bioactive substances including daidzein, genistein and glycitein. Equol is a nonsteroidal soy estrogen synthesized from daidzein be intestinal microbiota [381]. Intestinal metabolism of soy is highly variable [382] and only about 1/5 – ¼ of adult Westerners can produce equol [383]. Moreover, this proportion decreases with age [384]. These facts can partially explain discrepancy in human trials' results.

As a source of phytoestrogens, soy is much largely studied in women than in men. Intake of soy protein isolate (50 g daily) improved reasoning speed, verbal working memory, numeric working memory and reaction time in older females [385]. Beneficial effect of SI on cognitive function in post-menopausal women was also noted in other studies [386, 387] and a large meta-analysis of 10 placebo-controlled trials of SI supplementation (total n = 1024). The latter revealed that SI intake was associated with increase of cognitive function test scores and visual memory improvement. Authors found out that age of starting supplementation, geographical region and treatment duration could influence the results [388]. Apart from age, gender, menopausal status and dosage, procognitive effects of soy phytoestrogens may be influenced by type of product – fermented or non-fermented [389] and menstrual cycle phase [390].

Gender-specific difference in soy procognitive effect may prove the hypothesis that the main mechanism of this action is represented by direct neuroprotection via estrogenic receptor pathways [391, 392] including both estrogen-agonist and antagonist actions [393]. Non-estrogenic mechanisms include antioxidant effect [394–396], reduction of ABP fibril accumulation [397], inhibition of tyrosine kinase [391], regulation of CBF, and beneficial effects on various neurotransmitter systems (cholinergic, dopaminergic, and GABAergic) [398].

Genistein is a major SI with multiple beneficial effects, attenuating spatial recognition, discrimination, and memory deficits in a dose-dependent manner [399]. Genistein acts as an antioxidant, lowering hippocampal level of MDA and increasing activity of SOD. Apart from that, genistein lowers hippocampal levels of IL-6, NF-κB p65, toll-like receptor 4 (TLR4), TNF, cyclooxygenase-2, iNOS and increases concentration of antioxidant Nrf2 [399]. Soy-derived glyceollins attenuate scopolamine-induced cognitive impairment in mice, but not in Nrf2 knockout animals, so it is suggested that the memory-enhancing effect of soy is mediated by the Nrf2 signaling pathway [400].

Pueraria lobata

Pueraria (lobata, mirifica) belongs to Fabaceae family. Puerarin is an isoflavone glycoside of the Pueraria root, which can protect neurons from apoptosis, induced by oxidative stress [401]. It is widely investigated in various animal experiments as a potentially neuroprotective agent.

Seo et al. (2018) state that a diet containing a mixture of *Pueraria lobata* and red ginseng extracts reverses learning and memory impairments caused by trimethyltin-induced neurodegeneration in mice [402]. A study in rats with ovariectomy-induced cognitive impairment showed that treatment by *Pueraria mirifica* extract and pure puerarin elicited neurotherapeutic effects. Authors report that the earlier treatment is optimal [403]. Beneficial effect of dietary puerarin on memory was also shown in D-galactose model of aging and cognitive decrease [404].

In a mice model of AD, puerarin decreased the escape latency of the Morris water maze in comparison to the model group. It also normalized the levels of BDNF, phosphorylated tau protein, MDA, AChE, GSK-3β, and the activity of SOD in the hippocampus and cerebral cortex. Authors concluded that puerarin might provide protection against cognitive decline, oxidative stress, and neurodegeneration in case of AD [401]. Puerarin attenuates ABP-induced cognitive decline and reverses the enhanced apoptosis of hippocampal neurons, so it can be perceived as an anti-AD candidate drug [405].

Therefore, puerarin seems to be a promising procognitive agent in preclinical studies, but more human trials are awaited to make final decision on its efficacy.

Pinus Maritima

A standardized extract of the bark of French maritime pine (*Pinus maritima*) in a dose 150 mg/day for 8 weeks can improve the cognitive function in healthy subjects assessed with the help of MMSE [406] and Informant Questionnaire on Cognitive Decline in the Elderly (IQ Code) [407]. Three months of taking this supplement resulted in improving of working memory and decrease of F2-isoprostanes level relative to the control group [408]. An animal experiment on ß-amyloidosis mouse model showed that French maritime pine bark extract significantly decreased the number of amyloid plaques and improved the spatial memory [409]. Authors propose to use this extract in the prevention or at the early stages of MCI or AD.

The mechanisms of pine bark positive influence on cognitive function include inhibition of the NF-κB and AP-1 pathway, which suppresses the activation of microglia [410, 411]; modulation of NO production by means of inhibition of NO synthase [411]; protection of neurons against glutamate-induced cytotoxicity [412]; inhibition of ABP-mediated apoptosis [413, 414]. Taking everything into account, pine bark extract reduces oxidative stress, diminishes neuroinflammation, and counteracts the synaptic dysfunction in brain cortex and hippocampus [415–417].

There are also sporadic reports on potential memory-enhancing or procognitive action of *Centella asiatica* [418], *Withania somnifera* [419], *Nardostachys jatamansi* [420], *Embelia ribes* [421], *Celastrus paniculatus* [422], *Foeniculum vulgare* [423], *Convolvulous pluricaulis* [424, 425], red clover [426], *Mellissa officinalis* [427], blueberry [428], various compounds of plant origin (astaxanthin [429–431], sesamin [432–434] and polyherbal remedies (combination of *Bacopa monniera* and *Sideritis scardica* [435]).

Conclusions

To sum up, it is quite difficult to make a definite conclusion on the preventive and therapeutic effects of nutraceuticals on cognitive decline. Whereas in vitro studies and animal experiments are very promising, human trials show significant discrepancies. The inconsistent results of clinical studies can be explained by different inclusion criteria and study designs, different doses and treatment duration, high inter-individual difference in plant-derived components bioavailability, lack of standardized scores used to evaluate cognitive function. Anyway, a lack of scientific evidence does not necessarily mean that the treatment is absolutely ineffective [436]. Maybe, future studies will be able to unveil all unsolved mysteries of phytobotanicals. It seems to us that ginkgo, green tea and ginseng are the most promising procognitive nutraceuticals. Known active substances and major effects of each listed above plant are represented in Table 10.1.

Table 10.1 Active substances and major effects of the most extensively studied plants that may improve cognition

Plant	Known active substances	Procognitive effects
Ginkgo biloba	Terpene trilactones (ginkgolides A, B, C; bilobalide), flavonol glycosides (quercetin, kaempferol, isorhamnetin), isoflavonoids, biflavones, proanthocyanidins, alkylphenols, carboxylic acids, 4-O-methylpyridoxine, polyprenols	Direct and indirect antioxidant, anti-inflammatory, anti-amyloid, promotion of nerve regeneration
Vitis vinifera	Polyphenols (proanthocyanidins), resveratrol	Antioxidant, anti-inflammatory, anti-amyloid, antiapoptotic, cholinomimetic, vasodilating, promotion of synaptic transmission
Camellia sinensis	Catechins (epicatechin, epigallocatechin, epigallocatechin and epicatechin gallate), other phenolic compounds (gallic, caffeic, and chlorogenic acids, quercetin, proanthocyanidols, caffeine, theophylline, l-theanine), minerals (fluorine, manganese, chromium), caffeine	Antioxidant, anti-inflammatory, anti-amyloid, metal-chelating, modulation of cell signaling and cell survival pathways, inhibition of AChE and butyrylcholinesterase
Theobroma cacao	Flavanols, methylxanthines (caffeine, theobromine, theophylline)	Anti-inflammatory, anti-amyloid
Bacopa monnieri	Steroidal saponines (bacoside A and B), alkaloids (brahmin, herpestine, monierin, hersaponin)	Antioxidant, anti-inflammatory, anti-amyloid, metal-chelating, cholinergic, pro-circulatory, adaptogenic
Crocus sativus	Crocin, crocetin, picrocrocin, safranal, flavonoids, anthocyanins, vitamins (riboflavin, thiamine)	Antioxidant, inhibition of acetylcholinesterase

(continued)

Table 10.1 (continued)

Plant	Known active substances	Procognitive effects
Panax ginseng	Triterpene saponins (ginsenosides), polysaccharides, peptidoglycans, polyacetylenes, sesquiterpenes, nitrogen-containing and phenolic compounds	Antioxidant, anti-inflammatory, anti-amyloid, anti-apoptotic, cholinergic, pro-circulatory
Curcuma longa	Curcumin, demethoxycurcumin, bisdemethoxycurcumin	Antioxidant, anti-inflammatory, amyloid-disaggregating, acetylcholinesterase inhibition
Paullinia cupana	Caffeine, flavonoids, saponins, tannins	Adenosine-blocking, enhancement of long-term potentiation in hippocampal neurons, cholinergic
Glycine max	Soy isoflavones (genistein)	Antioxidant, anti-amyloid, cholinergic
Pueraria lobata	Puerarin	Antioxidant, anti-apoptotic, anti-amyloid
Pinus maritima	Polyphenols	Antioxidant, anti-inflammatory, anti-amyloid, anti-apoptotic

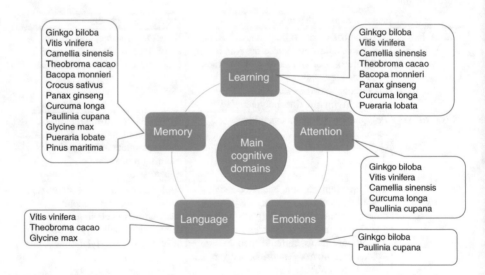

Fig. 10.1 Influence of various nutraceuticals on main cognitive domains

Talking about separate cognitive domains, it can be said that the majority of nutraceuticals positively affect memory and learning (Fig. 10.1), having less action on attention, language and emotions. On the other side, it may be explained by the fact that language and emotions cannot be investigated in animal experiments. Anyway, in future it may become possible to create targeted procognitive medications, aimed at separate domains of their combinations.

References

1. Sanabria-Castro A, Alvarado-Echeverria I, Monge-Bonilla C. Molecular pathogenesis of Alzheimer's disease: an update. Ann Neurosci. 2017;24(1):46–54.
2. Fotuhi M, Hachinski V, Whitehouse PJ. Changing perspectives regarding late-life dementia. Nat Rev Neurol. 2009;5(12):649–58. https://doi.org/10.1038/nrneurol.2009.175.
3. Chung CG, Lee H, Lee SB. Mechanisms of protein toxicity in neurodegenerative diseases. Cell Mol Life Sci. 2018;75:3159–80. https://doi.org/10.1007/s00018-018-2854-4.
4. Hugo J, Ganguli M. Dementia and cognitive impairment: epidemiology, diagnosis, and treatment. Clin Geriatr Med. 2014;30:421–42. https://doi.org/10.1016/j.cger.2014.04.001.
5. Hill NL, Mogle JM, Munoz E, Wion R, Colancecco EM. Assessment of subjective cognitive impairment among older adults. J Gerontol Nurs. 2015;41:28–35. https://doi.org/10.3928/00989134-20150309-01.
6. Prince M, Wimo A, Guerchet M, Gemma-Claire A, Wu YT, Prina M. Data from: World Alzheimer Report 2015: the global impact of dementia. London: Alzheimer's Disease International (ADI). Available online at: http://www.alz.co.uk/research/world-report-2015. Accessed 14 May 2019.
7. World Health Organization, Medical centre, Fact sheets, Dementia. http://www.who.int/mediacentre/factsheets/fs362/en. Last updated 2017. Accessed 11 May 2019.
8. Jaul E, Barron J. Age-related diseases and clinical and public health implications for the 85 years old and over population. Front Public Health. 2017;5:335.
9. Yaffe K, Falvey C, Hamilton N, et al. Diabetes, glucose control and 9 year cognitive decline among non-demented older adults. Arch Neurol. 2012;69:1170–5. https://doi.org/10.1001/archneurol.2012.1117.
10. Petersen RC. Mild cognitive impairment: transition between aging and Alzheimer's disease. Neurologia. 2000;15:93–101.
11. Janoutová J, Šerý O, Hosák L, Janout V. Is mild cognitive impairment a precursor of Alzheimer's disease? Short review. Cent Eur J Public Health. 2015;23:365–7.
12. Hadjichrysanthou C, McRae-McKee K, Evans S, Wolf F. Potential factors associated with cognitive improvement of individuals diagnosed with mild cognitive impairment or dementia in longitudinal studies. J Alzheimers Dis. 2018;66:587–600. https://doi.org/10.3233/JAD-180101.
13. Franceschi C, Capri M, Monti D, Giunta S, Olivieri F, Sevini F, et al. Inflammaging and anti-inflammaging: a systemic perspective on aging and longevity emerged from studies in humans. Mech Ageing Dev. 2007;128:92–105. https://doi.org/10.1016/j.mad.2006.11.016.
14. Niranjan R. Recent advances in the mechanisms of neuroinflammation and their roles in neurodegeneration. Neurochem Int. 2018;120:13–20. https://doi.org/10.1016/j.neuint.2018.07.003.
15. Kar S, Slowikowski S, Westaway D, et al. Interactions between β-amyloid and central cholinergic neurons: implications for Alzheimer's disease. J Psychiatry Neurosci. 2004;29(6):427–41.
16. Packer L. Free radical scavengers and antioxidants in prophylaxy and treatment of brain diseases. In: Packer L, Prilipko L, Christen Y, editors. Free radicals in the brain. New York: Springer; 1992.
17. Stough CK, Pase MP, Cropley V, Myers S, Karen N, King R, et al. A randomized controlled trial investigating the effect of Pycnogenol and *Bacopa* CDRI08 herbal medicines on cognitive, cardiovascular, and biochemical functioning in cognitively healthy elderly people: the Australian Research Council Longevity Intervention (ARCLI) study protocol (ANZCTR12611000487910). Nutr J. 2012;11:11. https://doi.org/10.1186/1475-2891-11-11.
18. Wasik A, Antkiewicz-Michaluk L. The mechanism of neuroprotective action of natural compounds. Pharmacol Rep. 2017;69(5):851–60.

19. Carlson S, Peng N, Prasain JK, Wyss JM. The effects of botanical dietary supplements on cardiovascular, cognitive and metabolic function in males and females. Gender Med. 2008;5(Suppl A):S76–90. https://doi.org/10.1016/j.genm.2008.03.008.
20. Charemboon T, Jaisin K. Ginkgo biloba for prevention of dementia: a systematic review and meta-analysis. J Med Assoc Thail. 2015;98:508–13.
21. van Beek TA, Montoro P. Chemical analysis and quality control of Ginkgo biloba leaves, extracts, and phytopharmaceuticals. J Chromatogr A. 2009;1216:2002–32. https://doi.org/10.1016/j.chroma.2009.01.013.
22. Li L, Zhao Y, Du F, et al. Intestinal absorption and presystemic elimination of various chemical constituents present in GBE50 extract, a standardized extract of Ginkgo biloba leaves. Curr Drug Metab. 2012;13:494–509. https://doi.org/10.2174/1389200211209050494.
23. Cao J, Yang M, Cao F, et al. Tailor-made hydrophobic deep eutectic solvents for cleaner extraction of polyprenyl acetates from Ginkgo biloba leaves. J Clean Prod. 2017;152:399–405. https://doi.org/10.1016/j.jclepro.2017.03.140.
24. Pilija V, Mirjana R, Brenesel MD, et al. Inhibitory effect of ginkgo biloba extract on the tonus of the small intestine and the colon of rabbits. Molecules. 2010;15:2079–86. https://doi.org/10.3390/molecules15042079.
25. Singh S, Barreto G, Aliev G, et al. Ginkgo biloba as an alternative medicine in the treatment of anxiety in dementia and other psychiatric disorders. Curr Drug Metab. 2017;18:112–9. https://doi.org/10.2174/1389200217666161201112206.
26. Nam Y, Shin E-J, Shin SW, et al. YY162 prevents ADHD-like behavioral side effects and cytotoxicity induced by Aroclor1254 via interactive signaling between antioxidant potential, BDNF/TrkB, DAT and NET. Food Chem Toxicol. 2014;65:280–92. https://doi.org/10.1016/j.fct.2013.12.046.
27. Tchantchou F, Pncao L. Stimulation of neurogenesis and synaptogenesis by bilobalide and quercetin via common final pathway in hippocampal neurons. J Alzheimers Dis. 2009;18:787–98.
28. Tchantchou F, Xu Y, Wu Y, Christen Y, Luo Y. EGb 761 enhances adult hippocampal neurogenesis and phosphorylation of CREB in transgenic mouse model of Alzheimer's disease. FASEB J. 2007;21:2400–8.
29. Kleijnen J, Knipschild P. Ginkgo biloba. Lancet. 1992;340:1136–9.
30. Guang Y. The reconsideration of the importance on Ginkgo resource research. Beijing J Tradit Chin Med. 2008;27:463–5.
31. Maclennan KM, Darlington CL, Smith PF. The CNS effects of *Ginkgo biloba* extracts and ginkgolide B. Prog Neurobiol. 2002;67(3):235–57.
32. De Feudis FV, Drieu K. *Ginkgo biloba* extract (EGb 761) and CNS functions: basic studies and clinical applications. Curr Drug Targets. 2000;1(1):25–58.
33. Ahlemeyer B, Krieglstein J. Neuroprotective effects of *Ginkgo biloba* extract. Cell Mol Life Sci. 2003;60(9):1779–92.
34. De Feudis F. Bilobalide and neuroprotection. Pharmacol Res. 2002;46(6):565–8.
35. Mansour SM, Bahgat AK, El-Khatib AS, et al. Ginkgo biloba extract (EGb 761) normalizes hypertension in 2K, 1C hypertensive rats: role of antioxidant mechanisms, ACE inhibiting activity and improvement of endothelial dysfunction. Phytomedicine. 2011;18:641–7.
36. Zhang P, Liao L, Deng Z, Tan Y. Research progress of pharmacological effects and clinical application of ginkgo biloba extract. Jinzhou Yike Daxue Xuebao. 2017:426–9.
37. Hirsch GE, Viecili PR, de Almeida AS, Nascimento S, Porto FG, Otero J, et al. Natural products with antiplatelet action. Curr Pharm Des. 2017;23(8):1228–46. https://doi.org/10.2174/1381612823666161123151611.
38. Ren C, Ji YQ, Liu H, Wang Z, Wang JH, Zhang CY, et al. Effects of *Ginkgo biloba* extract EGb761 on neural differentiation of stem cells offer new hope for neurological disease treatment. Neural Regen Res. 2019;14:1152–7.
39. Diamond BJ, Shiflett SC, Feiwel N, Matheis RJ, Noskin O, Richards JA, Schoenberger NE. Ginkgo biloba extract: mechanisms and clinical indications. Arch Phys Med Rehabil. 2000;81:668–78.

40. Logani S, Chen MC, Tran T, Le T, Raffa RB. Actions of Ginkgo biloba related to potential utility for the treatment of conditions involving cerebral hypoxia. Life Sci. 2000;67:1389–96.

41. Gargouri B, Carstensen J, Bhatia HS, Huell M, Dietz GPH, Fiebich BL. Anti-neuroinflammatory effects of *Ginkgo biloba* extract EGb761 in LPS-activated primary microglial cells. Phytomedicine. 2018;44:45–55. https://doi.org/10.1016/j.phymed.2018.04.009.

42. Müller WE, Eckert A, Eckert GP, Fink H, Friedland K, Gauthier S, et al. Therapeutic efficacy of the Ginkgo special extract EGb761® within the framework of the mitochondrial cascade hypothesis of Alzheimer's disease. World J Biol Psychiatry. 2017;20(3):1–17. https://doi.org/10.1080/15622975.2017.1308552.

43. Wang N, Chen X, Geng D, et al. *Ginkgo biloba* leaf extract improves the cognitive abilities of rats with D-galactose induced dementia. J Biomed Res. 2013;27(1):29–36.

44. Rocher MN, Carre D, Spinnewyn B, et al. Long-term treatment with standardized *Ginkgo biloba* extract (EGb 761) attenuates cognitive deficits and hippocampal neuron loss in a gerbil model of vascular dementia. Fitoterapia. 2011;82(7):1075–80.

45. El Tabaa MM, Sokkar SS, Ramadan ES, Abd El Salam IZ, Zaid A. Neuroprotective role of Ginkgo biloba against cognitive deficits associated with Bisphenol A exposure: an animal model study. Neurochem Int. 2017;108:199–212. https://doi.org/10.1016/j.neuint.2017.03.019.

46. Wang Y, Wang L, Wu J, et al. The in vivo synaptic plasticity mechanism of EGb 761-induced enhancement of spatial learning and memory in aged rats. Br J Pharmacol. 2006;148(2):147–53.

47. Williams B, Watanabe CMH, Schultz PG, et al. Age-related effects of *Ginkgo biloba* extract on synaptic plasticity and excitability. Neurobiol Aging. 2004;25(7):955–62.

48. Suliman NA, Mat Taib CN, Mohd Moklas MA, Adenan MI, Hidayat Baharuldin MT, Basir R. Establishing natural nootropics: recent molecular enhancement influenced by natural nootropic. Evid Based Complement Alternat Med. 2016;2016:4391375. https://doi.org/10.1155/2016/4391375.

49. Yao Z, Drieu K, Papadopoulos V. The *Ginkgo biloba* extract EGb 761 rescues the PC12 neuronal cells from beta-amyloid-induced cell death by inhibiting the formation of beta-amyloid-derived diffusible neurotoxic ligands. Brain Res. 2001;889(1–2):181–90.

50. Luo Y, Smith JV, Paramasivam V, et al. Inhibition of amyloid-beta aggregation and caspase-3 activation by the *Ginkgo biloba* extract EGb761. Proc Natl Acad Sci U S A. 2002;99(19):12197–202.

51. Colciaghi F, Borroni B, Zimmermann M, et al. Amyloid precursor protein metabolism is regulated toward alpha-secretase pathway by *Ginkgo biloba* extracts. Neurobiol Dis. 2004;16(2):454–60.

52. Longpré F, Garneau P, Christen Y, et al. Protection by EGb 761 against β-amyloid-induced neurotoxicity: involvement of NF-κB, SIRT1, and MAPKs pathways and inhibition of amyloid fibril formation. Free Radic Biol Med. 2006;41(12):1781–94.

53. Kwon KJ, Lee EJ, Cho KS, et al. *Ginkgo biloba* extract (Egb761) attenuates zinc-induced tau phosphorylation at Ser262 by regulating GSK3beta activity in rat primary cortical neurons. Food Funct. 2015;6(6):2058–67.

54. Vellas B, Coley N, Ousset PJ, et al. Long-term use of standardised Ginkgo biloba extract for the prevention of Alzheimer's disease (GuidAge): a randomised placebo-controlled trial. Lancet Neurol. 2012;11:851–9. https://doi.org/10.1016/S1474-4422(12)70206-5.

55. DeKosky ST, Williamson JD, Fitzpatrick AL, Kronmal RA, Ives DG, Saxton JA, et al. Ginkgo biloba for prevention of dementia: a randomized controlled trial. JAMA. 2008;300:2253–62.

56. Canter PH, Ernst E. Ginkgo biloba is not a smart drug: an updated systematic review of randomised clinical trials testing the nootropic effects of G. biloba extracts in healthy people. Hum Psychopharmacol. 2007;22:265–78.

57. Yuan Q, Wang CW, Shi J, Lin ZX. Effects of Ginkgo biloba on dementia: an overview of systematic reviews. J Ethnopharmacol. 2017;195:1–9. https://doi.org/10.1016/j.jep.2016.12.005.

58. Kanowski S, Hoerr R. *Ginkgo biloba* extract EGb 761 in dementia: intent-to-treat analyses of a 24-week, multi-center, double-blind, placebo-controlled, randomized trial. Pharmacopsychiatry. 2003;36(6):297–303.
59. Herrschaft H, Nacu A, Likhachev S, et al. *Ginkgo biloba* extract EGb 761® in dementia with neuropsychiatric features: a randomised, placebo-controlled trial to confirm the efficacy and safety of a daily dose of 240 mg. J Psychiatr Res. 2012;46(6):716–23.
60. Napryeyenko O, Borzenko I. *Ginkgo biloba* special extract in dementia with neuropsychiatric features: a randomised, placebo-controlled, double-blind clinical trial. Arzneimittelforschung. 2007;57(1):4–11.
61. van Dongen M, van Rossum E, Kessels A, et al. *Ginkgo* for elderly people with dementia and age-associated memory impairment: a randomized clinical trial. J Clin Epidemiol. 2003;56(4):367–76.
62. Nikolova G, Yancheva S, Raychev I, et al. *Ginkgo biloba* extract in dementia: a 22-week randomised, placebo-controlled, double-blind trial [in Bulgarian]. Bulg Neurol. 2013;14(3):139–43.
63. Allain H, Raoul P, Lieury A, LeCoz F, Gandon JM, d'Arbigny P. Effect of two doses of *Ginkgo biloba* extract (EGb 761) on the dual-coding test in elderly subjects. Clin Ther. 1993;15:549–58.
64. Le Bars PL, Kastelan J. Efficacy and safety of a *Ginkgo biloba* extract. Public Health Nutr. 2000;3:495–9. https://doi.org/10.1017/S1368980000000574.
65. Subhan Z, Hindmarch I. The psychopharmacological effects of *Ginkgo biloba* in normal healthy volunteers. Int J Clin Pharmacol Res. 1984;4:89–93.
66. Tan MS, Yu JT, Tan CC, Wang HF, Meng XF, Wang C, et al. Efficacy and adverse effects of *Ginkgo biloba* for cognitive impairment and dementia: a systematic review and meta-analysis. J Alzheimers Dis. 2015;43:589–603. https://doi.org/10.3233/JAD-140837.
67. Amieva H, Meillon C, Helmer C, Barberger-Gateau P, Dartigues JF. *Ginkgo biloba* extract and long-term cognitive decline: a 20-year follow-up population-based study. PLoS One. 2013;8:e52755. https://doi.org/10.1371/journal.pone.0052755.
68. Ihl R, Frolich L, Winblad B, Schneider L, Burns A, Moller HJ, et al. World Federation of Societies of biological psychiatry (WFSBP) guidelines for the biological treatment of Alzheimer's disease and other dementias. World J Biol Psychiatry. 2011;12:2–32. https://doi.org/10.3109/15622975.2010.538083.
69. Mazza M, Capuano A, Bria P, et al. *Ginkgo biloba* and donepezil: a comparison in the treatment of Alzheimer's dementia in a randomized placebo-controlled double-blind study. Eur J Neurol. 2006;13(9):981–5.
70. Rapp M, Burkart M, Kohlmann T, Bohlken J. Similar treatment outcomes with *Ginkgo biloba* extract EGb 761 and donepezil in Alzheimer's dementia in very old age: a retrospective observational study. Int J Clin Pharmacol Ther. 2018;56(3):130–3.
71. Heinonen T, Gaus W. Cross matching observations on toxicological and clinical data for the assessment of tolerability and safety of *Ginkgo biloba* leaf extract. Toxicology. 2015;327:95–115.
72. European Union herbal monograph on *Ginkgo biloba* L., folium. London: European Medicines Agency; 2015.
73. Kandiah N, Ong PA, Yuda T, Ng LL, Mamun K, Merchant RA, et al. Treatment of dementia and mild cognitive impairment with or without cerebrovascular disease: expert consensus on the use of Ginkgo biloba extract, EGb 761®. CNS Neurosci Ther. 2019;25(2):288–98. https://doi.org/10.1111/cns.13095.
74. Bent S, Goldberg H, Padula A, et al. Spontaneous bleeding associated with ginkgo biloba: a case report and systematic review of the literature. J Gen Intern Med. 2005;20:657–61.
75. Stoddard GJ, Archer M, Shane-McWhorter L, Bray BE, Redd DF, Proulx J, Zeng-Treitler Q. Ginkgo and warfarin interaction in a large veterans administration population. AMIA Annu Symp Proc. 2015:1174–83.

76. Hu Z, Yang X, Ho PC, Chan SY, Heng PW, Chan E, Duan W, Koh HL, Zhou S. Herb-drug interactions: a literature review. Drugs. 2005;65:1239–82.
77. Izzo AA, Ernst E. Interactions between herbal medicines and prescribed drugs: a systematic review. Drugs. 2001;61:2163–75.
78. Tanakan [standardized ginkgo biloba extract (EGb 761)] 40 mg film-coated tablets and 40 mg/ml oral solution: summary of product characteristics (Czech Republic). Boulogne-Billancourt: Ipsen Pharma; 2016.
79. Ude C, Schubert-Zsilavecz M, Wurglics M. *Ginkgo biloba* extracts: a review of the pharmacokinetics of the active ingredients. Clin Pharmacokinet. 2013;52(9):727–49.
80. Patki G, Ali Q, Pokkunuri I, Asghar M, Salim S. Grape powder treatment prevents anxiety-like behavior in a rat model of aging. Nutr Res. 2015;35:504–11. https://doi.org/10.1016/j.nutres.2015.05.005.
81. Sharma V, Zhang C, Pasinetti G, Dixon R. Fractionation of grape seed proanthocyanidins for bioactivity assessment. In: Gang DR, editor. The biological activity of phytochemicals. New York: Springer; 2011. p. 33–46.
82. Fuhrman B, Volkova N, Coleman R, Aviram M. Grape powder polyphenols attenuate atherosclerosis development in apolipoprotein E deficient (E0) mice and reduce macrophage atherogenicity. J Nutr. 2005;135:722–8.
83. Rezai-Zadeh K, Shytle D, Sun N, Mori T, Hou H, Jeanniton D, et al. Green tea epigallocatechin-3-gallate (EGCG) modulates amyloid precursor protein cleavage and reduces cerebral amyloidosis in Alzheimer transgenic mice. J Neurosci. 2005;25:8807–14. https://doi.org/10.1523/JNEUROSCI.1521-05.2005.
84. Hartman RE, Shah A, Fagan AM, Schwetye KE, Parsadanian M, Schulman RN, et al. Pomegranate juice decreases amyloid load and improves behavior in a mouse model of Alzheimer's disease. Neurobiol Dis. 2006;24:506–15. https://doi.org/10.1016/j.nbd.2006.08.006.
85. Assuncao M, Santos-Marques MJ, De Freitas V, Carvalho F, Andrade JP, Lukoyanov NV, et al. Red wine antioxidants protect hippocampal neurons against ethanol-induced damage: a biochemical, morphological and behavioral. Neuroscience. 2007;146:1581–92. https://doi.org/10.1016/j.neuroscience.2007.03.040.
86. Ma L, Xiao H, Wen J, Liu Z, He Y, Yuan F. Possible mechanism of *Vitis vinifera* L. flavones on neurotransmitters, synaptic transmission and related learning and memory in Alzheimer model rats. Lipids Health Dis. 2018;17(1):152. https://doi.org/10.1186/s12944-018-0708-6.
87. Yousuf S, Atif F, Ahmad M, Hoda N, Ishrat T, Khan B, et al. Resveratrol exerts its neuroprotective effect by modulating mitochondrial dysfunctions and associated cell death during cerebral ischemia. Brain Res. 2009;1250:242–53. https://doi.org/10.1016/j.brainres.2008.10.068.
88. Salim S, Asghar M, Taneja M, Hovatta I, Chugh G, Vollert C, et al. Potential contribution of oxidative stress and inflammation to anxiety and hypertension. Brain Res. 2011;1404:63–71. https://doi.org/10.1016/j.brainres.2011.06.024.
89. Solanki N, Alkadhi I, Atrooz F, Patki G, Salim S. Grape powder prevents cognitive, behavioral, and biochemical impairments in a rat model of posttraumatic stress disorder. Nutr Res. 2015;35:65–75. https://doi.org/10.1016/j.nutres.2014.11.008.
90. Wang YJ, Thomas P, Zhong JH, Bi FF, Kosaraju S, Pollard A, et al. Consumption of grape seed extract prevents amyloid-beta deposition and attenuates inflammation in brain of an Alzheimer's disease mouse. Neurotox Res. 2009;15:3–14. https://doi.org/10.1007/s12640-009-9000-x.
91. He Q, Yang SY, Wang W, Wu ZJ, Ma HL, Lu Y. Proanthocyanidins affects the neurotoxicity of Aβ25-35 on C57/bl6 mice. Eur Rev Med Pharmacol Sci. 2016;20:679–84.
92. Tabeshpour J, Mehri S, Shaebani Behbahani F, Hosseinzadeh H. Protective effects of Vitis vinifera (grapes) and one of its biologically active constituents, resveratrol, against natural and chemical toxicities: a comprehensive review. Phytother Res. 2018;32(11):2164–90. https://doi.org/10.1002/ptr.6168.

93. Rapaka D, Bitra VR, Vishala TC, Akula A. *Vitis vinifera* acts as anti-Alzheimer's agent by modulating biochemical parameters implicated in cognition and memory. J Ayurveda Integr Med. 2018. pii: S0975-9476(17)30060-8. https://doi.org/10.1016/j.jaim.2017.06.013. [Epub ahead of print].

94. Wang J, Ferruzzi MG, Ho L, Blount J, Janle EM, Gong B, et al. Brain-targeted proanthocyanidin metabolites for Alzheimer's disease treatment. J Neurosci. 2012;32:5144–50. https://doi.org/10.1523/JNEUROSCI.6437-11.2012.

95. Calapai G, Bonina F, Bonina A, Rizza L, Mannucci C, Arcoraci V, et al. Randomized, double-blinded, clinical trial on effects of a *Vitis vinifera* extract on cognitive function in healthy older adults. Front Pharmacol. 2017;8:776.

96. Shi J, He M, Cao J, Wang H, Ding J, Jiao Y, Li R, He J, Wang D, Wang Y. The comparative analysis of the potential relationship between resveratrol and stilbene synthase gene family in the development stages of grapes (Vitis quinquangularis and Vitis vinifera). Plant Physiol Biochem. 2014;74:24–32.

97. Sahebkar A, Serban C, Ursoniu S, Wong ND, Muntner P, Graham IM, Mikhailidis DP, Rizzo M, Rysz J, Sperling LS, Lip GY, Banach M, Lipid and Blood Pressure Meta-analysis Collaboration Group. Lack of efficacy of resveratrol on C-reactive protein and selected cardiovascular risk factors – Results from a systematic review and meta-analysis of randomized controlled trials. Int J Cardiol. 2015;189:47–55. https://doi.org/10.1016/j.ijcard.2015.04.008.

98. Lee J, Torosyan N, Silverman DH. Examining the impact of grape consumption on brain metabolism and cognitive function in patients with mild decline in cognition: a double-blinded placebo controlled pilot study. Exp Gerontol. 2017;87(Pt A):121–8. https://doi.org/10.1016/j.exger.2016.10.004.

99. Moreno M, Castro E, Falqué E. Evolution oftrans- andcis- resveratrol content in red grapes (Vitis vinifera L. cv Menciá, Albarello and Merenzao) during ripening. Eur Food Res Technol. 2008;227:667–74.

100. Trela BC, Waterhouse AL. Resveratrol: isomeric molar absorptivities and stability. J Agric Food Chem. 1996;44:1253–7.

101. Wahlster L, Arimon M, Nasser-Ghodsi N, Post KL, Serrano-Pozo A, Uemura K, Berezovska O. Presenilin-1 adopts pathogenic conformation in normal aging and in sporadic Alzheimer's disease. Acta Neuropathol. 2013;125:187–99.

102. Kim J, Lee HJ, Lee KW. Naturally occurring phytochemicals for the prevention of Alzheimer's disease. J Neurochem. 2010;112:1415–30.

103. Zhuang H, Kim YS, Koehler RC, Dore S. Potential mechanism by which resveratrol, a red wine constituent, protects neurons. Ann N Y Acad Sci. 2003;993:276–86.

104. Candelario-Jalil E, de Oliveira AC, Graf S, Bhatia HS, Hull M, Munoz E, Fiebich BL. Resveratrol potently reduces prostaglandin E2production and free radical formation in lipopolysaccharide-activated primary rat microglia. J Neuroinflammation. 2007;4:25.

105. Jang JH, Surh YJ. Protective effect of resveratrol on β-amyloid- induced oxidative PC12 cell death. Free Radic Biol Med. 2003;34:1100–10.

106. Kwon KJ, Kim HJ, Shin CY, Han SH. Melatonin potentiates the neuroprotective properties of resveratrol against beta amyloid-induced neurodegeneration by modulating AMP activated protein kinase pathways. J Clin Neurol. 2010;6:127–37.

107. Cao Z, Li Y. Potent induction of cellular antioxidants and phase 2 enzymes by resveratrol in cardiomyocytes: protection against oxidative and electrophilic injury. Eur J Pharmacol. 2004;489:39–48.

108. Kwon KJ, Kim JN, Kim MK, Lee J, Ignarro LJ, Kim HJ, Shin CY, Han SH. Melatonin synergistically increases resveratrol induced heme oxygenase-1 expression through the inhibition of ubiquitin-dependent proteasome pathway: a possible role in neuroprotection. J Pineal Res. 2011;50:110–23.

109. Venigalla M, Sonego S, Gyengesi E, Sharman MJ, Münch G. Novel promising therapeutics against chronic neuroinflammation and neurodegeneration in Alzheimer's disease. Neurochem Int. 2016;95:63–74.

110. Wang Q, Xu J, Rottinghaus GE, Simonyi A, Lubahn D, Sun GY, Sun AY. Resveratrol protects against global cerebral ischemic injury in gerbils. Brain Res. 2002;958:439–47.
111. Bi XL, Yang JY, Dong YX, Wang JM, Cui YH, Ikeshima T, Zhao YQ, Wu CF. Resveratrol inhibits nitric oxide and TNF-α production by lipopolysaccharide-activated microglia. Int Immunopharmacol. 2005;5:185–93.
112. Cheng X, Wang Q, Li N, Zhao H. Effects of resveratrol on hippocampal astrocytes and expression of TNF-α in Alzheimer's disease model rate. J Hyg Res. 2015;44:610–4.
113. Yao Y, Li J, Niu Y, Yu JQ, Yan L, Miao ZH, Zhao XX, Li YJ, Yao WX, Zheng P, et al. Resveratrol inhibits oligomeric Aβ-induced microglial activation via NADPH oxidase. Mol Med Rep. 2015;12:6133–9.
114. Capiralla H, Vingtdeux V, Zhao H, Sankowski R, Al-Abed Y, Davies P, Marambaud P. Resveratrol mitigates lipopolysaccharide- and Aβ-mediated microglial inflammation by inhibiting the TLR4/NF-κB/STAT signaling cascade. J Neurochem. 2012;120:461–72.
115. Rameshrad M, Razavi BM, Imenshahidi M, Hosseinzadeh H. *Vitis vinifera* (grape) seed extract and resveratrol alleviate bisphenol-A-induced metabolic syndrome: biochemical and molecular evidences. Phytother Res. 2019;33:832–44. https://doi.org/10.1002/ptr.6276.
116. Kennedy D, Wightman EL, Reay JL, Lietz G, Okello EJ, Wilde A, Haskell CF. Effects of resveratrol on cerebral blood flow variables and cognitive performance in humans: a double-blind, placebo-controlled, crossover investigation. Am J Clin Nutr. 2010;91:1590–7.
117. Witte AV, Kerti L, Margulies DS, Flöel A. Effects of resveratrol on memory performance, hippocampal functional connectivity, and glucose metabolism in healthy older adults. J Neurosci. 2014;34:7862–70.
118. Serban MC, Sahebkar A, Zanchetti A, Mikhailidis DP, Howard G, Antal D, Andrica F, Ahmed A, Aronow WS, Muntner P, Lip GY, Graham I, Wong N, Rysz J, Banach M, Lipid and Blood Pressure Meta-analysis Collaboration (LBPMC) Group. Effects of quercetin on blood pressure: a systematic review and meta-analysis of randomized controlled trials. J Am Heart Assoc. 2016;5(7):pii: e002713. https://doi.org/10.1161/JAHA.115.002713.
119. Wong RH, Nealon RS, Scholey A, Howe PR. Low dose resveratrol improves cerebrovascular function in type 2 diabetes mellitus. Nutr Metab Cardiovasc Dis. 2016;26:393–9.
120. Evans HM, Howe PR, Wong RH. Effects of resveratrol on cognitive performance, mood and cerebrovascular function in post-menopausal women; a 14-week randomised placebo-controlled intervention trial. Nutrients. 2017;9(1):pii: E27. https://doi.org/10.3390/nu9010027.
121. Gardner EJ, Ruxton CH, Leeds AR. Black tea – helpful or harmful? A review of the evidence. Eur J Clin Nutr. 2007;61:3–18.
122. Ma QP, Huang C, Cui QY, Yang DJ, Sun K, Chen X, Li XH. Meta-analysis of the association between tea intake and the risk of cognitive disorders. PLoS One. 2016;11(11):e0165861. https://doi.org/10.1371/journal.pone.0165861.
123. Yang L, Jin X, Yan J, Jin Y, Yu W, Wu H, Xu S. Prevalence of dementia, cognitive status and associated risk factors among elderly of Zhejiang province, China in 2014. Age Ageing. 2016;45:708–12. https://doi.org/10.1093/ageing/afw088.
124. Kuriyama S, Hozawa A, Ohmori K, Shimazu T, Matsui T, Ebihara S, et al. Green tea consumption and cognitive function: a cross-sectional study from the Tsurugaya project 1. Am J Clin Nutr. 2006;83:355–61.
125. Ng TP, Feng L, Niti M, Kua EH, Yap KB. Tea consumption and cognitive impairment and decline in older Chinese adults. Am J Clin Nutr. 2008;88(1):224–31.
126. Ide K, Yamada H, Takuma N, Park M, Wakamiya N, Nakase J, et al. Green tea consumption affects cognitive dysfunction in the elderly: a pilot study. Nutrients. 2014;6(10):4032–42. https://doi.org/10.3390/nu6104032.
127. Liu Y, Fly AD, Wang Z, Klaunig JE. The effects of green tea extract on working memory in healthy women. J Nutr Health Aging. 2018;22(3):446–50. https://doi.org/10.1007/s12603-017-0962-8.

128. Weinreb O, Mandel S, Amit T, Youdim MB. Neurological mechanisms of green tea polyphenols in Alzheimer's and Parkinson's diseases. J Nutr Biochem. 2004;15(9):506–16.
129. Mandel S, Youdim MB. Catechin polyphenols: neurodegeneration and neuroprotection in neurodegenerative diseases. Free Radic Biol Med. 2004;37(3):304–17.
130. Hou RR, Chen JZ, Chen H, Kang XG, Li MG, Wang BR. Neuroprotective effects of (−)-epigallocatechin-3-gallate (EGCG) on paraquat-induced apoptosis in PC12 cells. Cell Biol Int. 2008;32(1):22–30.
131. Kell DB. Towards a unifying, systems biology understanding of large-scale cellular death and destruction caused by poorly liganded iron: Parkinson's, Huntington's, Alzheimer's, prions, bactericides, chemical toxicology and others as examples. Arch Toxicol. 2010;84:825–89. https://doi.org/10.1007/s00204-010-0577-x.
132. Jomova K, Baros S, Valko M. Redox active metal-induced oxidative stress in biological systems. Transit Met Chem. 2012;37:127–34. https://doi.org/10.1007/s11243-012-9583-6.
133. Graham HN. Green tea composition, consumption, and polyphenol chemistry. Prev Med. 1992;21:334–50.
134. Yamamoto T, Juneja LR, Chu D, Kim M. Chemistry and applications of green tea. Boca Raton: CRC Press; 1997. p. 6–34.
135. Luczaj W, Skrzydlewska E. Antioxidative properties of black tea. Prev Med. 2005;40(6):910–8.
136. Bastianetto S, Yao ZX, Papadopoulos V, Quirion R. Neuroprotective effects of green and black teas and their catechin gallate esters against beta-amyloid-induced toxicity. Eur J Neurosci. 2006;23(1):55–64.
137. Grelle G, Otto A, Lorenz M, Frank RF, Wanker EE, Bieschke J. Black tea theaflavins inhibit formation of toxic amyloid-beta and alpha-synuclein fibrils. Biochemistry. 2011;50(49):10624–36.
138. Noguchi-Shinohara M, Yuki S, Dohmoto C, et al. Consumption of green tea, but not black tea or coffee, is associated with reduced risk of cognitive decline. PLoS One. 2014;9(5):e96013.
139. Martins A, Schimidt HL, Garcia A, et al. Supplementation with different teas from Camellia sinensis prevents memory deficits and hippocampus oxidative stress in ischemia-reperfusion. Neurochem Int. 2017;108:287–95. https://doi.org/10.1016/j.neuint.2017.04.019.
140. Schimidt HL, Garcia A, Martins A, Mello-Carpes PB, Carpes FP. Green tea supplementation produces better neuroprotective effects than red and black tea in Alzheimer-like rat model. Food Res Int. 2017;100(Part 1):442–8. https://doi.org/10.1016/j.foodres.2017.07.026.
141. Henning SM, Niu Y, Lee NH, et al. Bioavailability and antioxidant activity of tea flavanols after consumption of green tea, black tea, or a green tea extract supplement. Am J Clin Nutr. 2004;80(6):1558–64.
142. Wierzejska R. Tea and health – a review of the current state of knowledge. Przegl Epidemiol. 2014;68:595–9.
143. Swinton E, de Freitas E, Swinton C, et al. Green tea and cocoa enhance cognition in Lymnaea. Commun Integr Biol. 2018;11(1):e1434390.
144. Zhang J, de Freitas E, Lukowiak K. Black tea differs from green tea: it suppresses long-term memory formation in Lymnaea. Commun Integr Biol. 2018;11(3):1–4. https://doi.org/10.1080/19420889.2018.1491245.
145. Chow HH, Hakim I. Pharmacokinetic and chemo-prevention studies on tea in humans. Pharmacol Res. 2011;64:105–12.
146. Shen W, Xiao Y, Ying X, Li S, Zhai Y, Shang X, et al. Tea consumption and cognitive impairment: a cross-sectional study among Chinese elderly. PLoS One. 2015;10:e0137781. https://doi.org/10.1371/journal.pone.0140739.
147. Borota D, Murray E, Keceli G, et al. Post-study caffeine administration enhances memory consolidation in humans. Nat Neurosci. 2014;17:201–3.
148. McLellan T, Caldwell J, Lieberman HA. Review of caffeine's effects on cognitive, physical and occupational performance. Neurosci Biobehav Rev. 2016;71:294–312.
149. Wright GA, Baker DD, Palmer MJ, Stevenson PC, et al. Caffeine in floral nectar enhances a pollinator's memory of reward. Science. 2013;339:1202–4.

150. Xu H, Wang Y, Yuan Y, Zhang X, Zuo X, Cui L, et al. Gender differences in the protective effects of green tea against amnestic mild cognitive impairment in the elderly Han population. Neuropsychiatr Dis Treat. 2018;14:1795–801.
151. Lindsay J, Laurin D, Verreault R, et al. Risk factors for Alzheimer's disease: a prospective analysis from the Canadian Study of Health and Aging. Am J Epidemiol. 2002;156(5):445–53.
152. Panza F, Solfrizzi V, Barulli MR, et al. Coffee, tea, and caffeine consumption and prevention of late-life cognitive decline and dementia: a systematic review. J Nutr Health Aging. 2015;19(3):313–28.
153. Mashal RH. Hyperhomocysteinemia, lifestyle factors and cognitive impairment in heathy older subjects in Jordan. Pak J Nutr. 2013;12:71–9. https://doi.org/10.3923/pjn.2013.71.79.
154. Flores MF, Martins A, Schimidt HL, Santos FW, Izquierdo I, Mello-Carpes PB, et al. Effects of green tea and physical exercise on memory impairments associated with aging. Neurochem Int. 2014;78:53–60.
155. Lee LS, Kim SH, Kim YB, Kim YC. Quantitative analysis of major constituents in green tea with different plucking periods and their antioxidant activity. Molecules. 2014;19:9173–86.
156. Bieschke J, Russ J, Friedrich RP, Ehrnhoefer DE, Wobst H, Neugebauer K, Wanker EE. EGCG remodels mature alpha-synuclein and amyloid-beta fibrils and reduces cellular toxicity. Proc Natl Acad Sci U S A. 2010;107:7710–5.
157. Pastoriza S, Mesías M, Cabrera C, Rufián-Henares JA. Healthy properties of green and white teas: an update. Food Funct. 2017;8(8):2650–62. https://doi.org/10.1039/c7fo00611j.
158. Mancini E, Beglinger C, Drewe J, Zanchi D, Lang UE, Borgwardt S. Green tea effects on cognition, mood and human brain function: a systematic review. Phytomedicine. 2017;34:26–37. https://doi.org/10.1016/j.phymed.2017.07.008.
159. Zhang Y, He F, Hua T, Sun Q. Green tea polyphenols ameliorate ethanol-induced spatial learning and memory impairments by enhancing hippocampus NMDAR1 expression and CREB activity in rats. Neuroreport. 2018;29(18):1564–70. https://doi.org/10.1097/WNR.0000000000001152.
160. Ali B, Jamal QM, Shams S, et al. In silico analysis of green tea polyphenols as inhibitors of AChE and BChE enzymes in Alzheimer's disease treatment. CNS Neurol Disord Drug Targets. 2016;15:624–8. https://doi.org/10.2174/1871527315666160321110607.
161. Halliwell B. Are polyphenols antioxidants or pro-oxidants? What do we learn from cell culture and in vivo studies? Arch Biochem Biophys. 2008;476:107–12.
162. Bonkovsky HL. Hepatotoxicity associated with supplements containing Chinese green tea (Camellia sinensis). Ann Intern Med. 2006;144:68–71.
163. Werba JP, Misaka S, Giroli MG, Shimomura K, Amato M, Simonelli M, et al. Update of green tea interactions with cardiovascular drugs and putative mechanisms. J Food Drug Anal. 2018;26(2):S72–7. https://doi.org/10.1016/j.jfda.2018.01.008.
164. Albassam AA, Markowitz JS. An appraisal of drug-drug interactions with green tea (Camellia sinensis). Planta Med. 2017;83:496–508.
165. Li F, Wang Y, Li D, Chen Y, Qiao X, Fardous R, et al. Perspectives on the recent developments with green tea polyphenols in drug discovery. Expert Opin Drug Discovery. 2018;24:1–18.
166. Chu C, Deng J, Man Y, Qu Y. Green tea extracts epigallocatechin-3-gallate for different treatments. Biomed Res Int. 2017;2017:5615647.
167. Chakrawarti L, Agrawal R, Dang S, Gupta S, Gabrani R. Therapeutic effects of EGCG: a patent review. Expert Opin Ther Pat. 2016;26(8):907–16. https://doi.org/10.1080/13543776.2016.1203419.
168. Mandel S, Amit T, Reznichenko L, Weinreb O, Youdim MB. Green tea catechins as brain-permeable, natural iron chelators-antioxidants for the treatment of neurodegenerative disorders. Mol Nutr Food Res. 2006;50:229–34.
169. Serban C, Sahebkar A, Antal D, Ursoniu S, Banach M. Effects of supplementation with green tea catechins on plasma C-reactive protein concentrations: a systematic review and meta-analysis of randomized controlled trials. Nutrition. 2015;31(9):1061–71. https://doi.org/10.1016/j.nut.2015.02.004.

170. Singh NA, Mandal AK, Khan ZA. Potential neuroprotective properties of epigallocatechin-3-gallate (EGCG). Nutr J. 2016;15(1):60. https://doi.org/10.1186/s12937-016-0179-4.
171. Ehrnhoefer DE, Bieschke J, Boeddrich A, Herbst M, Masino L, Lurz R, Engemann S, Pastore A, Wanker EE. EGCG redirects amyloidogenic polypeptides into unstructured, off pathway oligomers. Nat Struct Mol Biol. 2008;15:558–66.
172. Lin CL, Chen TF, Chiu MJ, et al. Epigallocatechin gallate (EGCG) suppresses beta-amyloid-induced neurotoxicity through inhibiting c-Abl/FE65 nuclear translocation and GSK3 beta activation. Neurobiol Aging. 2009;30:81–92. https://doi.org/10.1016/j.neurobiolaging.2007.05.012.
173. Cheng-Chung Wei J, Huang HC, Chen WJ, et al. Epigallocatechin gallate attenuates amyloid β-induced inflammation and neurotoxicity in EOC 13.31 microglia. Eur J Pharmacol. 2016;770:16–24. https://doi.org/10.1016/j.ejphar.2015.11.048.
174. Cascella M, Bimonte S, Muzio MR, Schiavone V, Cuomo A. The efficacy of Epigallocatechin-3-gallate (green tea) in the treatment of Alzheimer's disease: an overview of pre-clinical studies and translational perspectives in clinical practice. Infect Agent Cancer. 2017;12:36.
175. He M, Liu MY, Wang S, Tang QS, Yao WF, Zhao HS, Wei MJ. Research on EGCG improving the degenerative changes of the brain in AD model mice induced with chemical drugs. Zhong Yao Cai. 2012;35:1641–4.
176. Walker JM, Klakotskaia D, Ajit D, Weisman GA, Wood WG, Sun GY, et al. Beneficial effects of dietary EGCG and voluntary exercise on behavior in an Alzheimer's disease mouse model. J Alzheimers Dis. 2015;44:561–72. https://doi.org/10.3233/JAD-140981.
177. Li Q, Gordon M, Tan J, et al. Oral administration of green tea epigallocatechin-3-gallate (EGCG) reduces amyloid beta deposition in transgenic mouse model of Alzheimer's disease. Exp Neurol. 2006;198:576. https://doi.org/10.1016/j.expneurol.2006.02.062.
178. Lee YJ, Choi DY, Yun YP, et al. Epigallocatechin-3-gallate prevents systemic inflammation-induced memory deficiency and amyloidogenesis via its anti-neuroinflammatory properties. J Nutr Biochem. 2013;24:298–310. https://doi.org/10.1016/j.jnutbio.2012.06.011.
179. Biasibetti R, Tramontina AC, Costa AP, Dutra MF, Quincozes-Santos A, Nardin P, et al. Green tea (−)epigallocatechin-3-gallate reverses oxidative stress and reduces acetylcholinesterase activity in a streptozotocin-induced model of dementia. Behav Brain Res. 2013;236:186–93. https://doi.org/10.1016/j.bbr.2012.08.039.
180. Aguiar S, Borowski T. Neuropharmacological review of the nootropic herb Bacopa monnieri. Rejuvenation Res. 2013;16(4):313–26. https://doi.org/10.1089/rej.2013.1431.
181. Türközü D, Şanlier N. L-theanin, unique aminoacid of tea, and its metabolism, health effects, safety. Crit Rev Food Sci Nutr. 2017;57(8):1681–7. https://doi.org/10.1080/10408398.2015.1016141.
182. Gomez-Ramirez M, Kelly SP, Montesi JL, Foxe JJ. The effects of L-theanine on alpha-band oscillatory brain activity during a visuo-spatial attention task. Brain Topogr. 2009;22(1):44–51. https://doi.org/10.1007/s10548-008-0068-z.
183. Nathan PJ, Lu K, Gray M, Oliver C. The neuropharmacology of L-theanine(N-ethyl-L-glutamine): a possible neuroprotective and cognitive enhancing agent. J Herb Pharmacother. 2006;6(2):21–30.
184. Juneja LR, Chu DC, Okubo T, Nagato Y, Yokogoshi H. L-theanine – a unique amino acid of green tea and its relaxation effect in humans. Trends Food Sci Technol. 1999;10:199–204.
185. Dufresne CJ, Farnworth ER. A review of latest research findings on the health promotion properties of tea. J Nutr Biochem. 2001;12:404–21.
186. Maia L, de Mendonca A. Does caffeine intake protect from Alzheimer's disease? Eur J Neurol. 2002;9:377–82.
187. Xu K, Xu Y, Brown-Jermyn D, Chen JF, Ascherio A, Dluzen DE, et al. Estrogen prevents neuroprotection by caffeine in the mouse 1-methyl-4-phenyl-1,2,3,6-tetrahydropyridine model of Parkinson's disease. J Neurosci. 2006;26:535–41.
188. Eskelinen MH, Kivipelto M. Caffeine as a protective factor in dementia and Alzheimer's disease. J Alzheimers Dis. 2010;20:167–74.

189. Chen X, Ghribi O, Geiger JD. Caffeine protects against disruptions of the blood-brain barrier in animal models of Alzheimer's and Parkinson's diseases. J Alzheimers Dis. 2010;20(Suppl 1):S127–41.
190. Pelligrino DA, Xu HL, Vetri F. Caffeine and the control of cerebral hemodynamics. J Alzheimers Dis. 2010;20:S51–62.
191. Klaassen EB, de Groot RH, Evers EA, Snel J, Veerman EC, Ligtenberg AJ, Jolles J, Veltman DJ. The effect of caffeine on working memory load-related brain activation in middle-aged males. Neuropharmacology. 2013;64:160–7.
192. Koppelstaetter F, Poeppel TD, Siedentopf CM, Ischebeck A, Verius M, Haala I, et al. Does caffeine modulate verbal working memory processes? An fMRI study. NeuroImage. 2007;39:492–9.
193. Haller S, Rodriguez C, Moser D, Toma S, Hofmeister J, Sinanaj I, et al. Acute caffeine administration impact on working memory-related brain activation and functional connectivity in the elderly: a BOLD and perfusion MRI study. Neuroscience. 2013;250:364–71.
194. Santos C, Costa J, Santos J, Vaz-Carneiro A, Lunet N. Caffeine intake and dementia: systematic review and meta-analysis. J Alzheimers Dis. 2010;20(Suppl 1):S187–204. https://doi.org/10.3233/JAD-2010-091387.
195. Wierzejska R. Can coffee consumption lower the risk of Alzheimer's disease and Parkinson's disease? A literature review. Arch Med Sci. 2017;13(3):507–14. https://doi.org/10.5114/aoms.2016.63599.
196. Kim YS, Kwak SM, Myung SK. Caffeine intake from coffee or tea and cognitive disorders: a meta-analysis of observational studies. Neuroepidemiology. 2015;44:51–63. https://doi.org/10.1159/000371710.
197. Tyas SL, Manfreda J, Strain LA, Montgomery P. Risk factors for Alzheimer's disease: a population-based., longitudinal study in Manitoba, Canada. Int J Epidemiol. 2001;30:590–7.
198. Arab L, Biggs ML, O'Meara ES, Longstreth WT, Crane PK, Fitzpatrick AL. Gender differences in tea, coffee, and cognitive decline in the elderly: the cardiovascular health study. J Alzheimers Dis. 2011;27:553–66. https://doi.org/10.3233/JAD-2011-110431.
199. Feng L, Gwee X, Kua EH, Ng TP. Cognitive function and tea consumption in community dwelling older Chinese in Singapore. J Nutr Health Aging. 2010;14:433–8. https://doi.org/10.1007/s12603-010-0095-9.
200. Lane J, Steege J, Rupp S, Kuhn C. Menstrual cycle effects on caffeine elimination in the human female. Eur J Clin Pharmacol. 1992;43:543–6. https://doi.org/10.1007/BF02285099.
201. Camandola S, Plick N, Mattson MP. Impact of coffee and cacao purine metabolites on neuroplasticity and neurodegenerative disease. Neurochem Res. 2019;44(1):214–27. https://doi.org/10.1007/s11064-018-2492-0.
202. Moreira A, Diogenes MJ, de Mendonca A, Lunet N, Barros H. Chocolate consumption is associated with a lower risk of cognitive decline. J Alzheimers Dis. 2016;53:85–93. https://doi.org/10.3233/JAD-160142.
203. Desideri G, Kwik-Uribe C, Grassi D, Necozione S, Ghiadoni L, Mastroiacovo D, et al. Benefits in cognitive function, blood pressure, and insulin resistance through cocoa flavanol consumption in elderly subjects with mild cognitive impairment: the cocoa, cognition, and aging (CoCoA) study. Hypertension. 2012;60(3):794–801.
204. Mastroiacovo D, Kwik-Uribe C, Grassi D, Necozione S, Raffaele A, Pistacchio L, et al. Cocoa flavanol consumption improves cognitive function, blood pressure control, and metabolic profile in elderly subjects: the cocoa, cognition, and aging (CoCoA) study – a randomized controlled trial. Am J Clin Nutr. 2015;101:538–48.
205. Wang J, Varghese M, Ono K, Yamada M, Levine S, Tzavaras N, et al. Cocoa extracts reduce oligomerization of amyloid-β:implications for cognitive improvement in Alzheimer's disease. J Alzheimers Dis. 2014;41(2):643–50. https://doi.org/10.3233/JAD-132231.
206. Rozan P, Hidalgo S, Nejdi A, Bisson JF, Lalonde R, Messaoudi M. Preventive antioxidant effects of cocoa polyphenolic extract on free radical production and cognitive performances after heat exposure in Wistar rats. J Food Sci. 2007;72:2–5.

207. Bisson JF, Nejdi A, Rozan P, Hidalgo S, Lalonde R, Messaoudi M. Effects of long-term administration of a cocoa polyphenolic extract (Acticoa powder) on cognitive performances in aged rats. Br J Nutr. 2008;100:94–101.
208. Massee LA, Ried K, Pase M, Travica N, Yoganathan J, Scholey A, et al. The acute and sub-chronic effects of cocoa flavanols on mood, cognitive and cardiovascular health in young healthy adults: a randomized, controlled trial. Front Pharmacol. 2015;6:93.
209. Grassi D, Ferri C, Desideri G. Brain protection and cognitive function: cocoa flavonoids as nutraceuticals. Curr Pharm Des. 2016;22(2):145–51.
210. Brickman AM, Khan UA, Provenzano FA, Yeung LK, Suzuki W, Schroeter H, et al. Enhancing dentate gyrus function with dietary flavanols improves cognition in older adults. Nat Neurosci. 2014;17(12):1798–803. https://doi.org/10.1038/nn.3850.
211. Nehlig A. The neuroprotective effects of cocoa flavanol and its influence on cognitive performance. Br J Clin Pharmacol. 2013;75(3):716–27. https://doi.org/10.1111/j.1365-2125.2012.04378.x.
212. Blanchard J, Sawers SJ. The absolute bioavailability of caffeine in man. Eur J Clin Pharmacol. 1983;24:93–8.
213. Chvasta TE, Cooke AR. Emptying and absorption of caffeine from the human stomach. Gastroenterology. 1971;61:838–43.
214. Oñatibia-Astibia A, Franco R, Martínez-Pinilla E. Health benefits of methylxanthines in neurodegenerative diseases. Mol Nutr Food Res. 2017;61:1600670.
215. Franco R, Oñatibia-Astibia A, Martínez-Pinilla E. Health benefits of methylxanthines in cacao and chocolate. Nutrients. 2013;5:4159–73.
216. Oñatibia-Astibia A, Martínez-Pinilla E, Franco R. The potential of methylxanthine-based therapies in pediatric respiratory tract diseases. Respir Med. 2016;112:1–9.
217. Smit HJ, Gaffan EA, Rogers PJ. Psychopharmacology. 2004;176:412. https://doi.org/10.1007/s00213-004-1898-3.
218. Judelson DA, Preston AG, Miller DL, Munoz CX, Kellogg MD, Lieberman HR. Effects of theobromine and caffeine on mood and vigilance. J Clin Psychopharmacol. 2013;33:499–506.
219. Baggott MJ, Childs E, Hart AB, et al. Psychopharmacology. 2013;228:109. https://doi.org/10.1007/s00213-013-3021-0.
220. Fernandez-Fernandez L, Esteban G, Giralt M, Valente T, Bolea I, Sole M, et al. Catecholaminergic and cholinergic systems of mouse brain are modulated by LMN diet, rich in theobromine, polyphenols and polyunsaturated fatty acids. Food Funct. 2015;6:1251–60.
221. Travassos M, Santana I, Baldeiras I, Tsolaki M, Gkatzima O, Sermin G, et al. Does caffeine consumption modify cerebrospinal fluid amyloid-β levels in patients with Alzheimer's disease? J Alzheimers Dis. 2015;47:1069–78. https://doi.org/10.3233/JAD-150374.
222. Cova I, Leta V, Mariani C, et al. Psychopharmacology. 2019;236:561. https://doi.org/10.1007/s00213-019-5172-0.
223. Sweitzer S, De Leo J. Propentofylline: glial modulation, neuroprotection, and alleviation of chronic pain. In: Methylxanthines. Berlin: Springer Berlin Heidelberg; 2011. p. 235–50.
224. Stough C, Downey LA, Lloyd J. Examining the nootropic effects of a special extract of *Bacopa monniera* on human cognitive functioning: 90 day double-blind placebo-controlled randomized trial. Phytother Res. 2008;22:1629–34. https://doi.org/10.1002/ptr.2537.
225. Sharma PC, Yelne MB, Dennis TJ. Database on medicinal plants used in ayurveda, vol. I. New Delhi: Central Council for Research in Ayurveda and Siddha Department of ISM & H, Ministry of Health and Family Welfare, Government of India; 2000. p. 93–101.
226. Rastogi S, Kulshreshtha DK. Bacoside A2 – a triterpenoid saponin from *Bacopa monnieri*. Indian J Chem. 1998;38:353–6.
227. Basu N, Rastogi RP, Dhar ML. Chemical examination of *Bacopa monnieri* Wettst: part III, bacoside B. Indian J Chem. 1967;5:84–6.
228. Sivaramakrishna C, Rao CV, Trimurtulu G, Vanisree M, Subbaraju GV. Triterpenoid glycosides from Bacopamonnieri. Phytochemistry. 2005;66(23):2719–28.

229. Chandel RS, Kulshreshtha DK, Rastogi RP. Bacogenin A3: a new sapogenin from *Bacopa monnieri*. Phytochemistry. 1977;16:141–3.
230. Stough C, Singh H, Zangara A. Mechanisms, efficacy, and safety of Bacopa monnieri (Brahmi) for cognitive and brain enhancement. Evid Based Complement Alternat Med. 2015;2015:717605. https://doi.org/10.1155/2015/717605.
231. Agrawal A. A comparative study of psychotropic drugs and bio-feedback therapy in the prevention and management of psychosomatic disorder. Thesis. Varanasi: Banaras Hindu University; 1993.
232. Bhattacharya SK, Kumar A, Ghosal S. Effect of Bacopa monniera on animal models of Alzheimer's disease and perturbed central cholinergic markers of cognition in rats. Res Commun Pharmacol Toxicol. 1999;4(3&4):1–12.
233. Jain SK. Ethnobotany and research on medicinal plants in India. CIBA Found Symp. 1994;185:153–64.
234. Dethe S, Deepak M, Agarwal A. Elucidation of molecular mechanism(s) of cognition enhancing activity of Bacomind(®): a standardized extract of Bacopa monnieri. Pharmacogn Mag. 2016;12(Suppl 4):S482–7.
235. Rastogi M, Ojha R, Prabu PC, Devi DP, Agrawal A, Dubey GP. Amelioration of age associated neuroinflammation on long term bacosides treatment. Neurochem Res. 2012;37:869–74. https://doi.org/10.1007/s11064-011-0681-1.
236. Promsuban C, Limsuvan S, Akaraseereenont P, Tilokskulchai K, Tapechum S, Pakaprot N. Bacopa monnieri extract enhances learning-dependent hippocampal long-term synaptic potentiation. Neuroreport. 2017;28(16):1031–5. https://doi.org/10.1097/WNR.0000000000000862.
237. Vohora D, Pal SN, Pillai KK. Protection from phenytoin-induced cognitive deficit by Bacopa monniera, a reputed Indian nootropic plant. J Ethnopharmacol. 2000;71:383–90.
238. Saraf MK, Prabhakar S, Pandhi P, Anand A. Bacopa monniera ameliorates amnesic effects of diazepam qualifying behavioral-molecular partitioning. Neuroscience. 2008;155:476–84.
239. Saini N, Singh D, Sandhir R. Neuroprotective effects of Bacopa monnieri in experimental model of dementia. Neurochem Res. 2012;37:1928–37.
240. Kishore K, Singh M. Effect of bacosides, alcoholic extract of Bacopa monniera Linn. (Brahmi), on experimental amnesia in mice. Indian J Exp Biol. 2005;43:640–5.
241. Kamkaew N, Norman Scholfield C, Ingkaninan K, Taepavarapruk N, Chootip K. Bacopa monnieri increases cerebral blood flow in rat independent of blood pressure. Phytother Res. 2013;27:135–8.
242. Singh HK, Dharwan BN. Neuropsychopharmacological effects of the Ayurvedic nootropic Bacopa monniera linn (brahmi). Indian J Pharm. 1997;29:S359–65.
243. Mathew M, Subramanian S. Evaluation of the anti-amyloidogenic potential of nootropic herbal extracts in vitro. Int J Pharm Sci Res. 2012;3:4276–80.
244. Saini N, Singh D, Sandhir R. Bacopa monnieri prevents colchicine-induced dementia by anti-inflammatory action. Metab Brain Dis. 2019;34(2):505–18. https://doi.org/10.1007/s11011-018-0332-1.
245. Pandareesh MD, Anand T, Khanum F. Cognition enhancing and neuromodulatory propensity of Bacopa monniera extract against scopolamine induced cognitive impairments in rat hippocampus. Neurochem Res. 2016;41(5):985–99. https://doi.org/10.1007/s11064-015-1780-1.
246. Kwon HJ, Jung HY, Hahn KR, Kim W, Kim JW, Yoo DY, et al. Bacopa monnieri extract improves novel object recognition, cell proliferation, neuroblast differentiation, brain-derived neurotrophic factor, and phosphorylation of cAMP response element-binding protein in the dentate gyrus. Lab Anim Res. 2018;34(4):239–47.
247. Pandey SP, Singh HK, Prasad S. Alterations in hippocampal oxidative stress, expression of AMPA receptor GluR2 subunit and associated spatial memory loss by Bacopa monnieri extract (CDRI-08) in streptozotocin-induced diabetes mellitus type 2 mice. PLoS One. 2015;10(7):e0131862.

248. Chaudhari KS, Tiwari NR, Tiwari RR, Sharma RS. Neurocognitive effect of nootropic drug brahmi (Bacopa monnieri) in Alzheimer's disease. Ann Neurosci. 2017;24(2):111–22.
249. Pase MP, Kean J, Sarris J, Neale C, Scholey AB, Stough C. The cognitive-enhancing effects of Bacopa monnieri: a systematic review of randomized, controlled human clinical trials. J Altern Complement Med. 2012;18(7):647–52.
250. Stough C, Lloyd J, Clarke J, Downey LA, Hutchison CW, Rodgers T, Nathan PJ. The chronic effects of an extract of *Bacopa monniera* (Brahmi) on cognitive function in healthy human subjects. Psychopharmacology. 2001;156(4):481–4.
251. Peth-Nui T, Wattanathorn J, Muchimapura S, Tong-Un T, Piyavhatkul N, Rangseekajee P, Ingkaninan K, Vittaya-Areekul S. Effects of 12-week *Bacopa monnieri* consumption on attention, cognitive processing, working memory, and functions of both cholinergic and monoaminergic systems in healthy elderly volunteers. Evid Based Complement Alternat Med. 2012;2012:606424.
252. Kean JD, Downey LA, Stough C. A systematic review of the ayurvedic medicinal herb *Bacopa monnieri* in child and adolescent populations. Complement Ther Med. 2016;29:56–62. https://doi.org/10.1016/j.ctim.2016.09.002.
253. Negi K, Singh Y, Kushwaha K, Rastogi C, Rathi A, Srivastava J, et al. Clinical evaluation of memory enhancing properties of memory plus in children with attention deficit hyperactivity disorder. Indian J Psychiatry. 2000;42:2.
254. Mitra-Ganguli T, Kalita S, Bhushan S, Stough C, Kean J, Wang N, et al. A randomized, double-blind study assessing changes in cognitive function in Indian school children receiving a combination of Bacopa monnieri and Micronutrient supplementation vs placebo. Front Pharmacol. 2017;8:678.
255. Kongkeaw C, Dilokthornsakul P, Thanarangsarit P, Limpeanchob N, Norman Scholfield C. Meta-analysis of randomized controlled trials on cognitive effects of Bacopa monnieri extract. J Ethnopharmacol. 2014;151(1):528–35. https://doi.org/10.1016/j.jep.2013.11.008.
256. Singh HK, Rastogi RP, Srimal RC, Dhawan BN. Effect of Bacosides A and B on avoidance responses in rats. Phytother Res. 1988;2:70–5. https://doi.org/10.1002/ptr.2650020205.
257. Uabundit N, Wattanathorn J, Mucimapura S, Ingkaninan K. Cognitive enhancement and neuroprotective effects of *Bacopa monnieri* in Alzheimer's disease model. J Ethnopharmacol. 2010;127:26–31. https://doi.org/10.1016/j.jep.2009.09.056.
258. Holcomb LA, Dhanasekaran M, Hitt AR. *Bacopa monniera* extract reduces amyloid levels in psapp mice. J Alzheimers Dis. 2006;9:243–51. https://doi.org/10.3233/JAD-2006-9303.
259. Schmidt M, Betti G, Hensel A. Saffron in phytotherapy: pharmacology and clinical uses. Wien Med Wochenschr. 2007;157(13–14):315–9.
260. Finley JW, Gao S. A perspective on Crocus sativus L. (saffron) constituent crocin: a potent water-soluble antioxidant and potential therapy for Alzheimer's disease. J Agric Food Chem. 2017;65(5):1005–20. https://doi.org/10.1021/acs.jafc.6b04398.
261. Khazdair MR, Boskabady MH, Hosseini M, Rezaee R, Tsatsakis AM. The effects of Crocus sativus (saffron) and its constituents on nervous system: a review. Avicenna J Phytomed. 2015;5:376–91.
262. Rios J, Recio M, Giner R, Manez S. An update review of saffron and its active constituents. Phytother Res. 1996;10:189–93.
263. Pitsikas N. The effect of Crocus sativus L. and its constituents on memory: basic studies and clinical applications. Evid Based Complement Alternat Med. 2015;2015:926284. https://doi.org/10.1155/2015/926284.
264. Naghizadeh B, Mansouri MT, Ghorbanzadeh B, Farbood Y, Sarkaki A. Protective effects of oral crocin against intracerebroventricular streptozotocin-induced spatial memory deficit and oxidative stress in rats. Phytomedicine. 2013;20(6):537–42. https://doi.org/10.1016/j.phymed.2012.12.019.
265. Linardaki ZI, Lamari FN, Margarity M. Saffron (Crocus sativus L.) tea intake prevents learning/memory defects and neurobiochemical alterations induced by Aflatoxin B_1

exposure in adult mice. Neurochem Res. 2017;42(10):2743–54. https://doi.org/10.1007/s11064-017-2283-z.

266. Akhondzadeh S, Sabet MS, Harirchian MH, Togha M, Cheraghmakani H, Razeghi S, et al. Saffron in the treatment of patients with mild to moderate Alzheimer's disease: a 16-week, randomized and placebo-controlled trial. J Clin Pharm Ther. 2010;35(5):581–8. https://doi.org/10.1111/j.1365-2710.2009.01133.x.

267. Farokhnia M, Shafiee Sabet M, Iranpour N, Gougol A, Yekehtaz H, Alimardani R, et al. Comparing the efficacy and safety of Crocus sativus L. with memantine in patients with moderate to severe Alzheimer's disease: a double-blind randomized clinical trial. Hum Psychopharmacol. 2014;29(4):351–9. https://doi.org/10.1002/hup.2412.

268. Tsolaki M, Karathanasi E, Lazarou I, Dovas K, Verykouki E, Karacostas A, et al. Efficacy and safety of Crocus sativus L. in patients with mild cognitive impairment: one year single-blind randomized, with parallel groups, clinical trial. J Alzheimers Dis. 2016;54(1):129–33. https://doi.org/10.3233/JAD-160304.

269. Pitsikas N, Tarantilis PA. Effects of the active constituents of Crocus sativus L. crocins and their combination with memantine on recognition memory in rats. Behav Pharmacol. 2018;29(5):400–12. https://doi.org/10.1097/FBP.0000000000000380.

270. Kim HJ, Kim P, Shin CY. A comprehensive review of the therapeutic and pharmacological effects of ginseng and ginsenosides in central nervous system. J Ginseng Res. 2013;37:8–29.

271. Sticher O. Getting to the root of ginseng. ChemTech. 1998;28:26–32.

272. Im DS, Nah SY. Yin and Yang of ginseng pharmacology: ginsenosides vs gintonin. Acta Pharmacol Sin. 2013;34:1367–73.

273. Tachikawa E, Kudo K, Harada K, Kashimoto T, Miyate Y, Kakizaki A, Takahashi E. Effects of ginseng saponins on responses induced by varoius receptor stimuli. Eur J Pharmacol. 1999;369:23–32. https://doi.org/10.1016/S0014-2999(99)00043-6.

274. Zhu JD, Wang JJ, Zhang XH, Yu Y, Kang ZS. Panax ginseng extract attenuates neuronal injury and cognitive deficits in rats with vascular dementia induced by chronic cerebral hypoperfusion. Neural Regen Res. 2018;13(4):664–72.

275. Al-Hazmi MA, Rawi SM, Arafa NM, Wagas A, Montasser AO. The potent effects of ginseng root extract and memantine on cognitive dysfunction in male albino rats. Toxicol Ind Health. 2015;31(6):494–509.

276. Kennedy DO, Scholey AB, Wesnes KA. Modulation of cognition and mood following administration of single doses of *Ginkgo biloba*, ginseng, and a ginkgo/ginseng combination to healthy young adults. Physiol Behav. 2002;75:739–51. https://doi.org/10.1016/S0031-9384(02)00665-0.

277. Wesnes KA, Ward T, McGinty A, Petrini O. The memory enhancing effects of a *Ginkgo biloba/Panax ginseng* combination in healthy middle-aged volunteers. Psychopharmacology. 2000;152:353–61. https://doi.org/10.1007/s002130000533.

278. Heo JH, Park MH, Lee JH. Effect of Korean red ginseng on cognitive function and quantitative EEG in patients with Alzheimer's disease: a preliminary study. J Altern Complement Med. 2016;22:280–5.

279. Kim HJ, Jung SW, Kim SY, Cho IH, Kim HC, Rhim H, et al. *Panax* ginseng as an adjuvant treatment for Alzheimer's disease. J Ginseng Res. 2018;42(4):401–11. https://doi.org/10.1016/j.jgr.2017.12.008.

280. Lee HW, Lim HJ, Jun JH, Choi J, Lee MS. Ginseng for treating hypertension: a systematic review and meta-analysis of double blind, randomized, placebo-controlled trials. Curr Vasc Pharmacol. 2017;15:549–56. https://doi.org/10.2174/1570161115666170713092701.

281. Wang Y, Yang G, Gong J, Lu F, Diao Q, Sun J, et al. Ginseng for Alzheimer's disease: a systematic review and meta-analysis of randomized controlled trials. Curr Top Med Chem. 2016;16:529–36. https://doi.org/10.2174/1568026615666150813143753.

282. Rajabian A, Rameshrad M, Hosseinzadeh H. Therapeutic potential of Panax ginseng and its constituents, ginsenosides and gintonin, in neurological and neurodegenerative disorders:

a patent review. Expert Opin Ther Pat. 2019;29(1):55–72. https://doi.org/10.1080/1354377 6.2019.1556258.

283. Tu TT, Sharma N, Shin EJ, Tran HQ, Lee YJ, Nah SY, et al. Treatment with mountain-cultivated ginseng alleviates trimethyltin-induced cognitive impairments in mice via IL-6-dependent JAK2/STAT3/ERK Signaling. Planta Med. 2017;83(17):1342–50. https://doi.org/10.1055/s-0043-111896.

284. Chen C, Zhang H, Xu H, Zheng Y, Wu T, Lian Y. Ginsenoside Rb1 ameliorates cisplatin-induced learning and memory impairments. J Ginseng Res. 2019;43:409–507. https://doi.org/10.1016/j.jgr.2017.07.009.

285. Miao HH, Zhang Y, Ding GN, Hong FX, Dong P, Tian M. Ginsenoside Rb1 attenuates isoflu-rane/surgery-induced cognitive dysfunction via inhibiting neuroinflammation and oxidative stress. Biomed Environ Sci. 2017;30:363–72.

286. Zhao Y, Liu J, Lu D, Zhao Y, Li P. Improvement effect of ginsenoside Re on learning and memory abilities of natural apolexis eats and its mechanisms. Tradit Chin Drug Res Clin Pharm. 2007;18:20–2.

287. Liu YW, Zhu X, Li W, Lu Q, Wang JY, Wei YQ, Yin XX. Ginsenoside Re attenuates diabetes-associated cognitive deficits in rats. Pharmacol Biochem Behav. 2012;101:93–8.

288. Kim JM, Park CH, Park SK, Seung TW, Kang JY, Ha JS, et al. Ginsenoside Re ameliorates brain insulin resistance and cognitive dysfunction in high fat diet-induced C57BL/6 mice. J Agric Food Chem. 2017;65:2719–29.

289. Qi D, Zhu Y, Wen L, Liu Q, Qiao H. Ginsenoside Rg1 restores the impairment of learning induced by chronic morphine administration in rats. J Psychopharmacol. 2009;23:74–83.

290. Wang Q, Sun LH, Jia W, Liu XM, Dang HX, Mai WL, Wang N, Steinmetz A, Wang YQ, Xu CJ. Comparison of ginsenosides Rg1 and Rb1 for their effects on improving scopolamine-induced learning and memory impairment in mice. Phytother Res. 2010;24:1748–54.

291. Zhu J, Mu X, Zeng J, Xu C, Liu J, Zhang M, et al. Ginsenoside Rg1 prevents cognitive impairment and hippocampus senescence in a rat model of D-galactose-induced aging. PLoS One. 2014;9:e101291.

292. Kezhu W, Pan X, Cong L, Liming D, Beiyue Z, Jingwei L, et al. Effects of ginsenoside Rg1 on learning and memory in a reward-directed instrumental conditioning task in chronic restraint stressed rats. Phytother Res. 2017;31:81–9.

293. Zhang Y, Zhang Z, Wang H, Cai N, Zhou S, Zhao Y, et al. Neuroprotective effect of gin-senoside Rg1 prevents cognitive impairment induced by isoflurane anesthesia in aged rats via antioxidant, anti-inflammatory and anti-apoptotic effects mediated by the PI3K/AKT/GSK-3β pathway. Mol Med Rep. 2016;14:2778–84.

294. Jin Y, Peng J, Wang X, Zhang D, Wang T. Ameliorative effect of ginsenoside Rg1 on lipopolysaccharide-induced cognitive impairment: role of cholinergic system. Neurochem Res. 2017;42:1299–307.

295. Zhang Y, Hu W, Zhang B, Yin Y, Zhang J, Huang D, et al. Ginsenoside Rg1 protects against neuronal degeneration induced by chronic dexamethasone treatment by inhibiting NLRP-1 inflammasomes in mice. Int J Mol Med. 2017;40:1134–42.

296. Zhang G, Liu A, Zhou Y, San X, Jin T, Jin Y. Panax ginseng ginsenoside-Rg2 protects mem-ory impairment via anti-apoptosis in a rat model with vascular dementia. J Ethnopharmacol. 2008;115:441–8.

297. Lee B, Sur B, Park J, Kim SH, Kwon S, Yeom M, et al. Ginsenoside rg3 alleviates lipopolysaccharide-induced learning and memory impairments by anti-inflammatory activity in rats. Biomol Ther (Seoul). 2013;21:381–90.

298. Kim J, Shim J, Lee S, Cho WH, Hong E, Lee JH, et al. Rg3-enriched ginseng extract ame-liorates scopolamine-induced learning deficits in mice. BMC Complement Altern Med. 2016;16:66.

299. Peña ID, Yoon SY, Kim HJ, Park S, Hong EY, Ryu JH, et al. Effects of ginseol k-g3, an Rg3-enriched fraction, on scopolamine-induced memory impairment and learning deficit in mice. J Ginseng Res. 2014;38:1–7.

300. Wang YZ, Chen J, Chu SF, Wang YS, Wang XY, Chen NH, Zhang JT. Improvement of memory in mice and increase of hippocampal excitability in rats by ginsenoside Rg1's metabolites ginsenoside Rh1 and protopanaxatriol. J Pharmacol Sci. 2009;109:504–10.
301. Kim EJ, Jung IH, Van Le TK, Jeong JJ, Kim NJ, Kim DH. Ginsenosides Rg5 and Rh3 protect scopolamine-induced memory deficits in mice. J Ethnopharmacol. 2013;146:294–9.
302. Lu C, Shi Z, Dong L, Lv J, Xu P, Li Y, Qu L, Liu X. Exploring the effect of ginsenoside Rh1 in a sleep deprivation-induced mouse memory impairment model. Phytother Res. 2017;31:763–70.
303. Jakaria M, Haque E, Kim J, Cho DY, Kim IS, Choi K. Active ginseng components in cognitive impairment: therapeutic potential and prospects for delivery and clinical study. Oncotarget. 2018;9(71):33601–20.
304. Hwang SH, Shin EJ, Shin TJ, Lee BH, Choi SH, Kang J, et al. Gintonin, a ginseng-derived lysophosphatidic acid receptor ligand, attenuates Alzheimer's disease-related neuropathies: involvement of non-amyloidogenic processing. J Alzheimers Dis. 2012;31:207–23.
305. Lee ST, Chu K, Sim JY, Heo JH, Kim M. Panax ginseng enhances cognitive performance in Alzheimer disease. Alzheimer Dis Assoc Disord. 2008;22:222–6.
306. Yeo HB, Yoon HK, Lee HJ, Kang SG, Jung KY, Kim L. Effects of Korean red ginseng on cognitive and motor function: a double-blind, randomized, placebo-controlled trial. J Ginseng Res. 2012;36:190–7.
307. Park K, Jin H, Rhee HY, Kim S, Lee SE, Kim YO, et al. A randomized, double-blind, placebo-controlled clinical trial of Korean ginseng as a functional food in mild cognitive impairment. Alzheimers Dement. 2013;9:804.
308. Scholey A, Ossoukhova A, Owen L, Ibarra A, Pipingas A, He K, et al. Effects of American ginseng (Panax quinquefolius) on neurocognitive function: an acute, randomised, double-blind, placebo-controlled, crossover study. Psychopharmacology. 2010;212:345–56.
309. Sutherland SK, Purdon SE, Lai C, Wang LJ, Liu GZ, Shan JJ. Memory enhancement from two weeks' exposure to North American ginseng extract HT1001 in young and middle aged healthy adults. Open Nutraceuticals J. 2010;3:20–4.
310. Lho SK, Kim TH, Kwak KP, Kim K, Kim BJ, Kim SG, et al. Effects of lifetime cumulative ginseng intake on cognitive function in late life. Alzheimers Res Ther. 2018;10:50.
311. Kim H, Lee JH, Kim JE, Kim YS, Ryu CH, Lee HJ, et al. Micro-/nano-sized delivery systems of ginsenosides for improved systemic bioavailability. J Ginseng Res. 2018;42:361–9.
312. Hasegawa H. Proof of the mysterious efficacy of ginseng: basic and clinical trials: metabolic activation of ginsenoside: deglycosylation by intestinal bacteria and esterification with fatty acid. J Pharmacol Sci. 2004;95:153–7. https://doi.org/10.1254/jphs.FMJ04001X4.
313. Sahebkar A, Saboni N, Pirro M, Banach M. Curcumin: an effective adjunct in patients with statin-associated muscle symptoms? J Cachexia Sarcopenia Muscle. 2017;8(1):19–24. https://doi.org/10.1002/jcsm.12140.
314. Sarker MR, Franks SF. Efficacy of curcumin for age-associated cognitive decline: a narrative review of preclinical and clinical studies. GeroScience. 2018;40(2):73–95.
315. Nelson KM, Dahlin JL, Bisson J, Graham J, Pauli GF, Walters MA. The essential medicinal chemistry of curcumin. J Med Chem. 2017;60:1620–37. https://doi.org/10.1021/acs.jmedchem.6b00975.
316. Lee WH, Loo CY, Bebawy M, Luk F, Mason RS, Rohanizadeh R. Curcumin and its derivatives: their application in neuropharmacology and neuroscience in the 21st century. Curr Neuropharmacol. 2013;11(4):338–78. https://doi.org/10.2174/1570159X11311040002.
317. Ullah F, Liang A, Rangel A, Gyengesi E, Niedermayer G, Münch G. High bioavailability curcumin: an anti-inflammatory and neurosupportive bioactive nutrient for neurodegenerative diseases characterized by chronic neuroinflammation. Arch Toxicol. 2017;91(4):1623–34. https://doi.org/10.1007/s00204-017-1939-4.
318. Ganjali S, Blesso CN, Banach M, Pirro M, Majeed M, Sahebkar A. Effects of curcumin on HDL functionality. Pharmacol Res. 2017;119:208–18. https://doi.org/10.1016/j.phrs.2017.02.008.

319. Lim GP, Chu T, Yang F, Beech W, Frautschy SA, Cole GM. The curry spice curcumin reduces oxidative damage and amyloid pathology in an Alzheimer transgenic mouse. J Neurosci. 2001;21:8370–7.
320. Yang F, Lim GP, Begum AN, Ubeda OJ, Simmons MR, Ambegaokar SS, et al. Curcumin inhibits formation of amyloid beta oligomers and fibrils, binds plaques, and reduces amyloid invivo. J Biol Chem. 2005;280:5892–901.
321. Sreejayan Rao MN. Nitric oxide scavenging by curcuminoids. J Pharm Pharmacol. 1997;49:105–7.
322. Sreejayan N, Rao MN. Free radical scavenging activity of curcuminoids. Arzneimittelforschung. 1996;46:169–71.
323. Fu XY, Yang MF, Cao MZ, Li DW, Yang XY, Sun JY, et al. Strategy to suppress oxidative damage-induced neurotoxicity in PC12 cells by curcumin: the role of ROS-mediated DNA damage and the MAPK and Akt pathways. Mol Neurobiol. 2016;53:369–78. https://doi.org/10.1007/s12035-014-9021-1.
324. Jin ML, Park SY, Shen Q, Lai YH, Ou XM, Mao Z, et al. Anti-neuroinflammatory effect of curcumin on Pam3CSK4-stimulated microglial cells. Int J Mol Med. 2018;41:521–30. https://doi.org/10.3892/ijmm.2017.3217.
325. Kodali M, Hattiangady B, Shetty GA, Bates A, Shuai B, Shetty AK. Curcumin treatment leads to better cognitive and mood function in a model of Gulf War illness with enhanced neurogenesis, and alleviation of inflammation and mitochondrial dysfunction in the hippocampus. Brain Behav Immun. 2018;69:499–514. https://doi.org/10.1016/j.bbi.2018.01.009.
326. Liu ZJ, Li ZH, Liu L, Tang WX, Wang Y, Dong MR, Xiao C. Curcumin attenuates beta-amyloid-induced neuroinflammation via activation of peroxisome proliferator-activated receptor-gamma function in a rat model of Alzheimer's disease. Front Pharmacol. 2016;7:261. https://doi.org/10.3389/fphar.2016.00261.
327. Wang YL, Li JF, Wang YT, Xu CY, Hua LL, Yang XP, et al. Curcumin reduces hippocampal neuron apoptosis and JNK-3 phosphorylation in rats with Aβ-induced Alzheimer's disease: protecting spatial learning and memory. J Neuro-Oncol. 2017;5:117–23. https://doi.org/10.2147/JN.S125567.
328. Rinwa P, Kumar A. Piperine potentiates the protective effects of curcumin against chronic unpredictable stress-induced cognitive impairment and oxidative damage in mice. Brain Res. 2012;1488:38–50. https://doi.org/10.1016/j.brainres.2012.10.002.
329. Wang P, Su C, Li R, Wang H, Ren Y, Sun H, et al. Mechanisms and effects of curcumin on spatial learning and memory improvement in APPswe/PS1dE9 mice. J Neurosci Res. 2014;92:218–31. https://doi.org/10.1002/jnr.23322.
330. Wullschleger S, Loewith R, Hall MN. Tor signaling in growth and metabolism. Cell. 2006;124:471–84. https://doi.org/10.1016/j.cell.2006.01.016.
331. He Y, Wang P, Wei P, Feng H, Ren Y, Yang J, et al. Effects of curcumin on synapses in APPswe/PS1dE9 mice. Int J Immunopathol Pharmacol. 2016;29:217–25. https://doi.org/10.1177/0394632016638099.
332. Franco-Robles E, Campos-Cervantes A, Murillo-Ortiz BO, Segovia J, Lopez-Briones S, Vergara P, et al. Effects of curcumin on brain-derived neurotrophic factor levels and oxidative damage in obesity and diabetes. Appl Physiol Nutr Metab. 2014;39:211–8. https://doi.org/10.1139/apnm-2013-0133.
333. Nam SM, Choi JH, Yoo DY, Kim W, Jung HY, Kim JW, et al. Effects of curcumin (Curcuma longa) on learning and spatial memory as well as cell proliferation and neuroblast differentiation in adult and aged mice by upregulating brain-derived neurotrophic factor and CREB signaling. J Med Food. 2014;17(6):641–9. https://doi.org/10.1089/jmf.2013.2965.
334. Kang G, Kong PJ, Yuh YJ, Lim SY, Yim SV, Chun W, Kim SS. Curcumin suppresses lipopolysaccharide-induced cyclooxygenase-2 expression by inhibiting activator protein 1 and nuclear factor kappaB bindings in BV2 microglial cells. J Pharmacol Sci. 2004;94:325–8. https://doi.org/10.1254/jphs.94.325.

335. Jin CY, Lee JD, Park C, Choi YH, Kim GY. Curcumin attenuates the release of pro-inflammatory cytokines in lipopolysaccharide-stimulated BV2 microglia. Acta Pharmacol Sin. 2007;28:1645–51. https://doi.org/10.1111/j.1745-7254.2007.00651.x.
336. Dong S, Zeng Q, Mitchell ES, Xiu J, Duan Y, Li C, Zhao Z. Curcumin enhances neurogenesis and cognition in aged rats: implications for transcriptional interactions related to growth and synaptic plasticity. PLoS One. 2012;7(2):e31211. https://doi.org/10.1371/journal.pone.0031211.
337. Sun CY, Qi SS, Zhou P, Cui HR, Chen SX, Dai KY, Tang ML. Neurobiological and pharmacological validity of curcumin in ameliorating memory performance of senescence-accelerated mice. Pharmacol Biochem Behav. 2013;105:76–82. https://doi.org/10.1016/j.pbb.2013.02.002.
338. Shailaja M, Damodara Gowda KM, Vishakh K, Suchetha Kumari N. Anti-aging role of curcumin by modulating the inflammatory markers in albino Wistar rats. J Natl Med Assoc. 2017;109(1):9–13. https://doi.org/10.1016/j.jnma.2017.01.005.
339. Vidal B, Vázquez-Roque RA, Gnecco D, Enríquez RG, Floran B, Díaz A, Flores G. Curcuma treatment prevents cognitive deficit and alteration of neuronal morphology in the limbic system of aging rats. Synapse. 2017;71:e21952.
340. Ishrat T, Hoda MN, Khan MB, Yousuf S, Ahmad M, Khan MM, et al. Amelioration of cognitive deficits and neurodegeneration by curcumin in rat model of sporadic dementia of Alzheimer's type (SDAT). Eur Neuropsychopharmacol. 2009;19(9):636–47. https://doi.org/10.1016/j.euroneuro.2009.02.002.
341. Ataie A, Sabetkasaei M, Haghparast A, Moghaddam AH, Kazeminejad B. Neuroprotective effects of the polyphenolic antioxidant agent, curcumin, against homocysteine-induced cognitive impairment and oxidative stress in the rat. Pharmacol Biochem Behav. 2010;96(4):378–85. https://doi.org/10.1016/j.pbb.2010.06.009.
342. Kawamoto EM, Scavone C, Mattson MP, Camandola S. Curcumin requires tumor necrosis factor alpha signaling to alleviate cognitive impairment elicited by lipopolysaccharide. Neurosignals. 2013;21(1–2):75–88. https://doi.org/10.1159/000336074.
343. Muthuraman A, Thilagavathi L, Jabeen S, Ravishankar SB, Ahmed SS, George T, et al. Curcumin prevents cigarette smoke extract induced cognitive impairment. Front Biosci (Elite Ed). 2019;11:109–20.
344. Bassani TB, Bonato JM, Machado MMF, Coppola-Segovia V, Moura ELR, Zanata SM, et al. Decrease in adult neurogenesis and neuroinflammation are involved in spatial memory impairment in the streptozotocin-induced model of sporadic Alzheimer's disease in rats. Mol Neurobiol. 2018;55(5):4280–96. https://doi.org/10.1007/s12035-017-0645-9.
345. Mazzanti G, Di Giacomo S. Curcumin and resveratrol in the management of cognitive disorders: what is the clinical evidence? Molecules. 2016;21(9):pii: E1243. https://doi.org/10.3390/molecules21091243.
346. Cicero AFG, Fogacci F, Banach M. Botanicals and phytochemicals active on cognitive decline: the clinical evidence. Pharmacol Res. 2018;130:204–12. https://doi.org/10.1016/j.phrs.2017.12.029.
347. Small GW, Siddarth P, Li Z, Miller KJ, Ercoli L, Emerson ND, et al. Memory and brain amyloid and tau effects of a bioavailable form of curcumin in non-demented adults: a double-blind, placebo-controlled 18-month trial. Am J Geriatr Psychiatry. 2018;26:266–77. https://doi.org/10.1016/j.jagp.2017.10.010.
348. Rainey-Smith SR, Brown BM, Sohrabi HR, Shah T, Goozee KG, Gupta VB, Martins RN. Curcumin and cognition: a randomised, placebo-controlled, double-blind study of community-dwelling older adults. Br J Nutr. 2016;115(12):2106–13. https://doi.org/10.1017/S0007114516001203.
349. Baum L, Lam CW, Cheung SK, Kwok T, Lui V, Tsoh J, et al. Six-month randomized, placebo-controlled, double-blind, pilot clinical trial of curcumin in patients with Alzheimer disease. J Clin Psychopharmacol. 2008;28(1):110–3. https://doi.org/10.1097/jcp.0b013e318160862c.

350. Ringman JM, Frautschy SA, Teng E, Begum AN, Bardens J, Beigi M, et al. Oral curcumin for Alzheimer's disease: tolerability and efficacy in a 24-week randomized, double blind, placebo-controlled study. Alzheimers Res Ther. 2012;4(5):43. https://doi.org/10.1186/alzrt146.

351. Haskell CF, Kennedy DO, Wesnes KA, Milne AL, Scholey AB. A double-blind, placebo-controlled, multi-dose evaluation of the acute behavioural effects of guarana in humans. J Psychopharmacol. 2007;21:65–70.

352. Scholey A, Haskell C. Neurocognitive effects of guaraná plant extract. Drugs Future. 2008;33:869–74. https://doi.org/10.1358/dof.2008.33.10.1250977.

353. Espinola EB, Dias RF, Mattei R, Carlini EA. Pharmacological activity of guarana (*Paullinia cupana* Mart.) in laboratory animals. J Ethnopharmacol. 1997;55:223–9. https://doi.org/10.1016/S0378-8741(96)01506-1.

354. Mattei R, Dias RF, Espínola EB, Carlini EA, Barros SB. Guarana (*Paullinia cupana*): toxic behavioral effects in laboratory animals and antioxidants activity in vitro. J Ethnopharmacol. 1998;60:111–6. https://doi.org/10.1016/S0378-8741(97)00141-4.

355. Pomportes L, Davranche K, Brisswalter I, Hays A, Brisswalter J. Heart rate variability and cognitive function following a multi-vitamin and mineral supplementation with added Guarana (*Paullinia cupana*). Nutrients. 2014;7:196–208. https://doi.org/10.3390/nu7010196.

356. Kennedy DO, Haskell CF, Wesnes KA, Scholey AB. Improved cognitive performance in human volunteers following administration of guarana (*Paullinia cupana*) extract: comparison and interaction with Panax ginseng. Pharmacol Biochem Behav. 2004;79:401–11. https://doi.org/10.1016/j.pbb.2004.07.014.

357. Veasey RC, Haskell-Ramsay CF, Kennedy DO, Wishart K, Maggini S, Fuchs CJ, Stevenson EJ. The effects of supplementation with a vitamin and mineral complex with guaraná prior to fasted exercise on affect, exertion, cognitive performance, and substrate metabolism: a randomized controlled trial. Nutrients. 2015;7:6109–27. https://doi.org/10.3390/nu7085272.

358. Ruchel JB, Braun JBS, Adefegha SA, Guedes Manzoni A, Abdalla FH, de Oliveira JS, et al. Guarana (Paullinia cupana) ameliorates memory impairment and modulates acetylcholinesterase activity in Poloxamer-407-induced hyperlipidemia in rat brain. Physiol Behav. 2017;168:11–9. https://doi.org/10.1016/j.physbeh.2016.10.003.

359. Pomportes L, Brisswalter J, Casini L, Hays A, Davranche K. Cognitive performance enhancement induced by caffeine, carbohydrate and guarana mouth rinsing during submaximal exercise. Nutrients. 2017;9(6):589.

360. Pomportes L, Brisswalter J, Hays A, Davranche K. Effects of carbohydrate, caffeine and guarana on cognitive performance, perceived exertion and shooting performance in high level athletes. Int J Sports Physiol Perform. 2018;9:1–26. https://doi.org/10.1123/ijspp.2017-0865.

361. Scholey A, Bauer I, Neale C, Savage K, Camfield D, White D, et al. Acute effects of different multivitamin mineral preparations with and without Guaraná on mood, cognitive performance and functional brain activation. Nutrients. 2013;5:3589–604. https://doi.org/10.3390/nu5093589.

362. Liang W, Lee AH, Binns CW, Huang R, Hu D, Shao H. Soy consumption reduces risk of ischemic stroke: a case-control study in southern China. Neuroepidemiology. 2009;33:111–6. https://doi.org/10.1159/000222093.

363. Katayama S, Imai R, Sugiyama H, Nakamura S. Oral administration of soy peptides suppresses cognitive decline by induction of neurotrophic factors in SAMP8 mice. J Agric Food Chem. 2014;62(16):3563–9. https://doi.org/10.1021/jf405416s.

364. Lu C, Wang Y, Wang D, Zhang L, Lv J, Jiang N, et al. Neuroprotective effects of soy isoflavones on scopolamine-induced amnesia in mice. Nutrients. 2018;10(7):853.

365. Bagheri M, Joghataei MT, Mohseni S, Roghani M. Genistein ameliorates learning and memory deficits in amyloid beta(1–40) rat model of Alzheimer's disease. Neurobiol Learn Mem. 2011;95:270–6. https://doi.org/10.1016/j.nlm.2010.12.001.

366. Ma WW, Xiang L, Yu HL, Yuan LH, Guo AM, Xiao YX, Li L, Xiao R. Neuroprotection of soybean isoflavone co-administration with folic acid against beta-amyloid 1–40-induced neurotoxicity in rats. Br J Nutr. 2009;102:502–5. https://doi.org/10.1017/S0007114509274757.
367. Russell AL, Grimes JM, Larco DO, Cruthirds DF, Joanna W, Wooten L, et al. The interaction of dietary isoflavones and estradiol replacement on behavior and brain-derived neurotrophic factor in the ovariectomized rat. Neurosci Lett. 2017;640:53–9. https://doi.org/10.1016/j.neulet.2017.01.011.
368. MacLusky NJ, Thomas G, Leranth C. Low dietary soy isoflavonoids increase hippocampal spine synapse density in ovariectomized rats. Brain Res. 1657;2017:361–7. https://doi.org/10.1016/j.brainres.2017.01.002.
369. Gleason CE, Carlsson CM, Barnet JH, Meade SA, Setchell KD, Atwood CS, Johnson SC, Ries ML, Asthana S. A preliminary study of the safety, feasibility and cognitive efficacy of soy isoflavone supplements in older men and women. Age Ageing. 2009;38:86–93.
370. John JAS, Henderson VW, Hodis HN, Kono N, McCleary CA, Franke AA, Mack WJ. Associations of urine excretion of isoflavonoids with cognition in postmenopausal women in the Women's Isoflavone Soy Health clinical trial. J Am Geriatr Soc. 2014;62(4):629–35.
371. Woo J, Lynn H, Lau WY, Leung J, Lau E, Wong SY, Kwok T. Nutrient intake and psychological health in an elderly Chinese population. Int J Geriatr Psychiatry. 2006;21:1036–43.
372. Hogervorst E, Mursjid F, Priandini D, Setyawan H, Ismael RI, Bandelow S, Rahardjo TB. Borobudur revisited: soy consumption may be associated with better recall in younger, but not in older, rural Indonesian elderly. Brain Res. 2011;1379:206–12.
373. Gleason CE, Fischer BL, Dowling NM, Setchell KDR, Atwood CS, Carlsson CM, Asthana S. Cognitive effects of soy isoflavones in patients with Alzheimer's disease. J Alzheimers Dis. 2015;47(4):1009–19.
374. Henderson VW, St John JA, Hodis HN, Kono N, McCleary CA, Franke AA, Mack WJ, Group WR. Long-term soy isoflavone supplementation and cognition in women: a randomized, controlled trial. Neurology. 2012;78:1841–8.
375. Kreijkamp-Kaspers S, Kok L, Grobbee DE, de Haan EH, Aleman A, van der Schouw YT. Dietary phytoestrogen intake and cognitive function in older women. J Gerontol A Biol Sci Med Sci. 2007;62:556–62.
376. Huang MH, Luetters C, Buckwalter GJ, Seeman TE, Gold EB, Sternfeld B, Greendale GA. Dietary genistein intake and cognitive performance in a multiethnic cohort of midlife women. Menopause. 2006;13:621–30.
377. Franco OH, Burger H, Lebrun CE, Peeters PH, Lamberts SW, Grobbee DE, Van Der Schouw YT. Higher dietary intake of lignans is associated with better cognitive performance in postmenopausal women. J Nutr. 2005;135:1190–5.
378. Kreijkamp-Kaspers S, Kok L, Grobbee DE, et al. Effect of soy protein containing isoflavones on cognitive function, bone mineral density, and plasma lipids in postmenopausal women: a randomized controlled trial. JAMA. 2004;292:65–74.
379. Ho SC, Chan AS, Ho YP, et al. Effects of soy isoflavone supplementation on cognitive function in Chinese postmenopausal women: a double-blind, randomized, controlled trial. Menopause. 2007;14(Pt 1):489–99.
380. White LR, Petrovitch H, Ross GW, Masaki K, Hardman J, Nelson J, Davis D, Markesbery W. Brain aging and midlife tofu consumption. J Am Coll Nutr. 2000;19:242–55.
381. Setchell KD, Brown NM, Lydeking-Olsen E. The clinical importance of the metabolite equol – a clue to the effectiveness of soy and its isoflavones. J Nutr. 2002;132:3577–84.
382. Setchell KDR, Brown NM, Desai P, et al. Bioavailability of pure isoflavones in healthy humans and analysis of commercial soy isoflavone supplements. J Nutr. 2001;131:1362S–75S.
383. Setchell KD, Cole SJ. Method of defining equol-producer status and its frequency among vegetarians. J Nutr. 2006;136:2188–93.
384. Frankenfeld CL, Atkinson C, Thomas WK, et al. Familial correlations, segregation analysis, and nongenetic correlates of soy isoflavone-metabolizing phenotypes. Exp Biol Med (Maywood). 2004;229:902–13.

385. Zajac IT, Herreen D, Bastiaans K, Dhillon VS, Fenech M. The effect of whey and soy protein isolates on cognitive function in older Australians with low vitamin B12: a randomised controlled crossover trial. Nutrients. 2019;11(1):19.
386. Kritz-Silverstein D, Von Muhlen D, Barrett-Connor E, Mathias B. Isoflavones and cognitive function in older women: the SOy and postmenopausal health in aging (SOPHIA) Study. Menopause. 2003;10:196–202. https://doi.org/10.1097/00042192-200310030-00004.
387. Nakamoto M, Otsuka R, Nishita Y, Tange C, Tomida M, Kato Y, et al. Soy food and isoflavone intake reduces the risk of cognitive impairment in elderly Japanese women. Eur J Clin Nutr. 2018;72(10):1458–62. https://doi.org/10.1038/s41430-017-0061-2.
388. Cheng PF, Chen JJ, Zhou XY, Ren YF, Huang W, Zhou JJ, Xie P. Do soy isoflavones improve cognitive function in postmenopausal women? A meta-analysis. Menopause. 2015;22(2):198–206. https://doi.org/10.1097/GME.0000000000000290.
389. Soni M, Rahardjo TB, Soekardi R, Sulistyowati Y, Lestariningsih CL, Yesufu-Udechuku A, et al. Phytoestrogens and cognitive function: a review. Maturitas. 2014;77(3):209–20. https://doi.org/10.1016/j.maturitas.2013.12.010.
390. Islam F, Sparkes C, Roodenrys S, Astheimer L. Short-term changes in endogenous estrogen levels and consumption of soy isoflavones affect working and verbal memory in young adult females. Nutr Neurosci. 2008;11(6):251–62. https://doi.org/10.1179/147683008X301612.
391. Lee YB, Lee HJ, Sohn HS. Soy isoflavones and cognitive function. J Nutr Biochem. 2005;16(11):641–9.
392. Kajta M, Rzemieniec J, Litwa E, Lason W, Lenartowicz M, Krzeptowski W, Wojtowicz AK. The key involvement of estrogen receptor beta and G-protein-coupled receptor 30 in the neuroprotective action of daidzein. Neuroscience. 2013;238:345–60.
393. Pike AC, Brzozowoski AM, Hubbard RE, et al. Structure of the ligand-binding domain of oestrogen receptor beta in the presence of a partial agonist and a full antagonist. EMBO J. 1999;18:4608–18.
394. Nadal-Serrano M, Pons DG, Sastre-Serra J, Blanquer-Rossello MD, Roca P, Oliver J. Genistein modulates oxidative stress in breast cancer cell lines according to ER alpha/ER beta ratio: effects on mitochondrial functionality, sirtuins, uncoupling protein 2 and antioxidant enzymes. Int J Biochem Cell Biol. 2013;45:2045–51.
395. Chung MJ, Kang AY, Lee KM, Oh E, Jun HJ, Kim SY, et al. Water-soluble genistin glycoside isoflavones up-regulate antioxidant metallothionein expression and scavenge free radicals. J Agric Food Chem. 2006;54:3819–26.
396. Butterfield DA, Reed T, Newman SF, Sultana R. Roles of amyloid beta-peptide-associated oxidative stress and brain protein modifications in the pathogenesis of Alzheimer's disease and mild cognitive impairment. Free Radic Biol Med. 2007;43:658–77.
397. Henry-Vitrac C, Berbille H, Merillon JM, Vitrac X. Soy isoflavones as potential inhibitors of Alzheimer beta-amyloid fibril aggregation in vitro. Food Res Int. 2010;43:2176–8.
398. Setchell KDR. Soy isoflavones--benefits and risks from nature's selective estrogen receptor modulators (SERMs). J Am Coll Nutr. 2001;20:354S–63S.
399. Mirahmadi SM, Shahmohammadi A, Rousta AM, Azadi MR, Fahanik-Babaei J, Baluchnejadmojarad T, Roghani M. Soy isoflavone genistein attenuates lipopolysaccharide-induced cognitive impairments in the rat via exerting antioxidative and anti-inflammatory effects. Cytokine. 2018;104:151–9. https://doi.org/10.1016/j.cyto.2017.10.008.
400. Seo JY, Kim BR, Oh J, Kim JS. Soybean-derived phytoalexins improve cognitive function through activation of Nrf2/HO-1 signaling pathway. Int J Mol Sci. 2018;19(1):268.
401. Wu L, Tong T, Wan S, Yan T, Ren F, Bi K, Jia Y. Protective effects of puerarin against Aβ 1-42-induced learning and memory impairments in mice. Planta Med. 2017;83(3–04):224–31. https://doi.org/10.1055/s-0042-111521.
402. Seo YM, Choi SJ, Park CK, Gim MC, Shin DH. Synergistic effect of Korean red ginseng and Pueraria montana var. lobata against trimethyltin-induced cognitive impairment. Food Sci Biotechnol. 2018;27(4):1193–200. https://doi.org/10.1007/s10068-018-0362-9.

403. Anukulthanakorn K, Parhar IS, Jaroenporn S, Kitahashi T, Watanbe G, Malaivijitnond S. Neurotherapeutic effects of Pueraria mirifica extract in early- and late-stage cognitive impaired rats. Phytother Res. 2016;30(6):929–39. https://doi.org/10.1002/ptr.5595.
404. Xu XH, Zhao TQ. Effects of puerarin on D-galactose-induced memory deficits in mice. Acta Pharmacol Sin. 2002;23(7):587–90.
405. Li J, Wang G, Liu J, Zhou L, Dong M, Wang R, et al. Puerarin attenuates amyloid-beta-induced cognitive impairment through suppression of apoptosis in rat hippocampus in vivo. Eur J Pharmacol. 2010;649(1–3):195–201. https://doi.org/10.1016/j.ejphar.2010.09.045.
406. Hosoi M, Belcaro G, Saggino A, Luzzi R, Dugall M, Feragalli B. Pycnogenol® supplementation in minimal cognitive dysfunction. J Neurosurg Sci. 2018;62(3):279–84. https://doi.org/10.23736/S0390-5616.18.04382-5.
407. Belcaro G, Dugall M, Ippolito E, Hu S, Saggino A, Feragalli B. The COFU3 Study. Improvement in cognitive function, attention, mental performance with Pycnogenol® in healthy subjects (55–70) with high oxidative stress. J Neurosurg Sci. 2015;59(4):437–46.
408. Ryan J, Croft K, Mori T, Wesnes K, Spong J, Downey L, Kure C, Lloyd J, Stough C. An examination of the effects of the antioxidant Pycnogenol on cognitive performance, serum lipid profile, endocrinological and oxidative stress biomarkers in an elderly population. J Psychopharmacol. 2008;22(5):553–62. https://doi.org/10.1177/0269881108091584.
409. Paarmann K, Prakash SR, Krohn M, Möhle L, Brackhan M, Brüning T, et al. French maritime pine bark treatment decelerates plaque development and improves spatial memory in Alzheimer's disease mice. Phytomedicine. 2019;57:39–48. https://doi.org/10.1016/j.phymed.2018.11.033.
410. Fan B, Dun SH, Gu JQ, Guo Y, Ikuyama S. Pycnogenol attenuates the release of proinflammatory cytokines and expression of Perilipin 2 in lipopolysaccharide-stimulated microglia in part via inhibition of NF-kappaB and AP-1 activation. PLoS One. 2015;10:e0137837.
411. Gu JQ, Ikuyama S, Wei P, Fan B, Oyama J, Inoguchi T, Nishimura J. Pycnogenol, an extract from French maritime pine, suppresses toll-like receptor 4-mediated expression of adipose differentiation-related protein in macrophages. Am J Physiol Endocrinol Metab. 2008;295:E1390–400.
412. Kobayashi MS, Han D, Packer L. Antioxidants and herbal extracts protect HT-4 neuronal cells against glutamate-induced cytotoxicity. Free Radic Res. 2000;32(2):115–24. https://doi.org/10.1080/10715760000300121.
413. Liu F, Lau BHS, Peng Q, Shah V. Pycnogenol protects vascular endothelial cells from α-amyloid-induced injury. Biol Pharm Bull. 2000;23(6):735–7. https://doi.org/10.1248/bpb.23.735.
414. Peng QL, Buzzard AR, Lau BHS. Pycnogenol® protects neurons from amyloid-β peptide-induced apoptosis. Mol Brain Res. 2002;104(1–2):55–65.
415. Ansari MA, Roberts KN, Scheff SW. Dose- and time-dependent neuroprotective effects of Pycnogenol following traumatic brain injury. J Neurotrauma. 2013;30:1542–9.
416. Norris CM, Sompol P, Roberts KN, Ansari M, Scheff SW. Pycnogenol protects CA3-CA1 synaptic function in a rat model of traumatic brain injury. Exp Neurol. 2016;276:5–12.
417. Scheff SW, Ansari MA, Roberts KN. Neuroprotective effect of Pycnogenol(R) following traumatic brain injury. Exp Neurol. 2013;239:183–91.
418. Wattanathorn J, Mator L, Muchimapura S. Positive modulation of cognition and mood in the healthy elderly volunteer following the administration of Centella asiatica. J Enthnopharmacol. 2008;116:325–32. https://doi.org/10.1016/j.jep.2007.11.038.
419. Chengappa KNR, Bowie CR, Schlicht PJ, Fleet D, Brar JS, Jindal R. Randomized placebo-controlled adjunctive study of an extract of withania somnifera for cognitive dysfunction in bipolar disorder. J Clin Psychiatry. 2013;74:1076–83. https://doi.org/10.4088/JCP.13m08413.
420. Joshi H, Parle M. Nardostachys jatamansi improves learning and memory in mice. J Med Food. 2006;9:113–8. https://doi.org/10.1089/jmf.2006.9.113.

421. Vinutha B, Prashanth D, Salma K, Sreeja SL, Pratiti D, Padmaja R, et al. Screening of selected Indian medicinal plants for acetylcholinesterase inhibitory activity. J Ethnopharmacol. 2007;109:359–63. https://doi.org/10.1016/j.jep.2006.06.014.
422. Bhanumathy M, Harish MS, Shivaprasad HN, Sushma G. Nootropic activity of celastrus paniculatus seed. Pharm Biol. 2010;48:324–7. https://doi.org/10.3109/13880200903127391.
423. Rahimi R, Ardekani MRS. Medicinal properties of *Foeniculum vulgare* Mill. in traditional Iranian medicine and modern phytotherapy. Chin J Integr Med. 2013;19:73–9. https://doi.org/10.1007/s11655-013-1327-0.
424. Sethiya NK, Nahata A, Dixit VK, Mishra SH. Cognition boosting effect of *Canscora decussata* (a south Indian shankhpushpi). Eur J Int Med. 2012;4:e113–21. https://doi.org/10.1016/j.eujim.2011.11.003.
425. Kothiyal P, Rawat MSM. Comparative nootropic effect of *Evolvulus alsinoides* and convolvulus pluricaulis. Int J Pharm Bio Sci. 2011;2:616–21.
426. Geller SE, Studee L. Soy and red clover for midlife and aging. Climacteric. 2006;9(4):245–63.
427. Kennedy DO, Wake G, Savelev S. Modulation of mood and cognitive performance following acute administration of single doses of *Melissa officinalis* (lemon balm) with human CNS nicotinic and muscarinic receptor-binding properties. Neuropsychopharmacology. 2003;28:1871–81. https://doi.org/10.1038/sj.npp.1300230.
428. McNamara RK, Kalt W, Shidler MD, McDonald J, Summer S, Stein AL, et al. Cognitive response to fish oil, blueberry, and combined supplementation in older adults with subjective cognitive impairment. Neurobiol Aging. 2018;64:147–56.
429. Katagiri M, Satoh A, Tsuji S, Shirasawa T. Effects of astaxanthin-rich Haematococcus pluvialis extract on cognitive function: a randomised, double-blind, placebo-controlled study. J Clin Biochem Nutr. 2012;51:102–7.
430. Wu H, Niu H, Shao A, Wu C, Dixon BJ, Zhang J, Yang S, Wang Y. Astaxanthin as a potential neuroprotective agent for neurological diseases. Mar Drugs. 2015;13:5750–66.
431. Grimmig B, Kim SH, Nash K, Bickford PC, Douglas SR. Neuroprotective mechanisms of astaxanthin: aotential therapeutic role in preserving cognitive function in age and neurodegeneration. GeroScience. 2017;39:19–32.
432. Cheng FC, Jinn TR, Hou RC, Tzen JT. Neuroprotective effects of sesamin and sesamolin on gerbil brain in cerebral ischemia. Int J Biomed Sci. 2006;2:284–8.
433. Guo H, Tian J, Wang X, Tian Z, Li X, Yang L, Zhao M, Liu S. Neuroprotection of sesamin against cerebral ischemia in-vivo and N-Methyl-D-Aspartate-induced apoptosis in-vitro. Biochem Pharmacol (Los Angeles). 2015;4:185.
434. Liu Y, Xu Z, Yang G, Yang D, Ding J, Chen H, Yuan F, Tian H. Sesamin alleviates blood-brain barrier disruption in mice with experimental traumatic brain injury. Acta Pharmacol Sin. 2017;38:1445–55.
435. Dimpfel W, Schombert L, Biller A. Psychophysiological effects of *Sideritis* and *Bacopa* extract and three combinations thereof – a quantitative EEG study in subjects suffering from mild cognitive impairment (MCI). Adv Alzheimer's Dis. 2016;5(1):1–22. https://doi.org/10.4236/aad.2016.51001.
436. Kotsirilos V. Complementary and alternative medicine. Part 2–evidence and implications for GPs. Aust Fam Physician. 2005;34:689–91.

Chapter 11
Nutraceuticals Supporting Heart Function in Heart Failure

Arrigo F.G. Cicero and Alessandro Colletti

Introduction

Heart failure (HF) is defined by the American Heart Association /American College of Cardiology guidelines as "a complex clinical syndrome that can result from any structural or functional cardiac disorder that impairs the ability of the ventricle to fill or eject blood" [1, 2]. In USA the prevalence of HF is about of 5 million people [3], while it affects 23 million people worldwide [4]. In Europe the prevalence and incidence of HF are quite similar [5, 6]. This condition is the main responsible for hospitalization and disability in the elderly and it is the cause of one in nine death in the USA [3]. The estimated economic burden of HF to the health-care system amounts more than $39 billion annually in the USA [7]. The main HF risk factors are coronary artery disease, ageing, cardiomyopathy, hypertension and valvular heart disease [1, 2]. Even though there have been relevant improvements in the HF prevention and treatment, quality of life is often impaired and mortality rates are greater than 10% per year, reaching 20–50% in more serious patients [8]. An improvement in life-style is suggested when HF is already diagnosed, and at the same time HF could be prevented in part by improving lifestyle [9, 10]. Lifestyle changes include first of all adherence to a Mediterranean diet as well as a reduced-sodium diet or Dietary Approaches to Stop Hypertension (DASH) [11, 12], that are able to reduce the risk of developing HF and improve endothelial function, exercise

A. F.G. Cicero
Medicine and Surgery Sciences Department, Alma Mater Studiorum University of Bologna, Bologna, Italy

Italian Nutraceutical Society (SINut), Bologna, Italy
e-mail: arrigo.cicero@unibo.it

A. Colletti (✉)
Italian Nutraceutical Society (SINut), Bologna, Italy

Department of Drug Science and Technology, University of Turin, Turin, Italy

© Springer Nature Switzerland AG 2021
A. F.G. Cicero, M. Rizzo (eds.), *Nutraceuticals and Cardiovascular Disease*,
Contemporary Cardiology, https://doi.org/10.1007/978-3-030-62632-7_11

capacity and quality of life in HF patients [13]. In particular, DASH-diet can protect against HF risk by 29% [14]. Moreover, increased aerobic exercise, weight loss, and moderation of alcohol consumption are recommended, as well [15]. In the recent years, epidemiological studies and clinical trials have investigated the possibility that some dietary supplements and phytochemicals can contribute to the prevention of incident HF and or to the improvement of related symptoms and/or instrumental parameters (Table 11.1). The aim of this chapter is to describe the nutraceuticals potentially active on HF based on data of scientific literature.

Table 11.1 Nutraceuticals supporting heart function: active daily doses, effects on symptoms, effects on lab or instrumental parameters and on hard outcomes

Nutraceutical	Active daily doses	Effects on symptoms	Effects on lab or instrumental parameters	Effects on hard outcomes
Beetroot	10–15 mmol of NO3-	↑ self-perceived quality of life	↑ Exercise capacity, CO, VO2 max, submaximal aerobic endurance, ↓ blood pressure,	Not investigated
Cocoa and dark chocolate	25–100 g of dark chocolate or 400-1000 mg of cocoa polyphenols	↑ self- perceived quality of life	↑ vascular function (FMD, PWV), LKB1, AMPK, NO bioavailability, ↓ NT-proBNP, total cholesterol, LDL-cholesterol, insulin resistance, HOMA-index, SBP, DBP, and vascular inflammation (hsCRP, ET-1)	↓ of HF hospitalization, cardiovascular disease (epidemiological data)
Coenzyme Q10	100–300 mg	↑ self-perceived quality of life, improvement in NYHA class	↑ EF (if >30%), ↑ LVEF, ↑ CO and CI, ↑ SV, ↑ EDV, ↑ Exercise capacity, ↓ ventricular arrhythmias after surgery and need of inotropic drugs (after cardiac surgery), ↓ lipid peroxidation, Lp(a), triglycerides and low-grade inflammation (TNF-alpha, IL-6, hsCRP), ↑ insulin sensitivity	↓ MACE, total mortality and incidence of hospital stays for HF
D-ribose	5 g/day	↑ self-perceived quality of life and physical activity performance	↑ vascular stiffness, ATP bioavailability, diastolic function, ventilatory efficiency	Not investigated

Table 11.1 (continued)

Nutraceutical	Active daily doses	Effects on symptoms	Effects on lab or instrumental parameters	Effects on hard outcomes
Hawthorn	160–1800 mg	↑ self-perceived quality of life, symptom burden, ability to enjoy and relax, positive and negative mood, socialness, and allegiance	↑ EF, ↑ LVEF, ↑ Exercise capacity, maximal workload and exercise tolerance, ↑ maximal workload, ↑ endothelium stiffness, ↓ lipid peroxidation, pressure-heart rate product	↓ sudden death (patients with less compromised LV function)
Iron	30–150 mg/day (?)	↓ asthenia (?)	↑serum iron and transferrin	No data available
L-carnitine	1500–6000 mg	↓ angina symptoms (?)	↑ LVEF, ↑ CO and CI, ↑ SV, ↑ EDV, ↓ NP, NT-proBNP, LVESD, LVEDD and LVESV, ↓ hs-CRP, ↓ Lp(a), ↓ body weight	↓ ventricular arrhythmias and total mortality ? (conflicting data)
L-carnosine	500 mg (L-carnosine) 3–6 g (magnesium orotate)	↑ self-perceived quality of life and physical activity performance	↑ peak VO2, VO2 at anaerobic threshold and peak exercise workload	↓ mortality ? (few data available)
Magnesium	200–400 mg	Low serum magnesium seems to be associated to poor QoL	↓ LVEF, DBP, SBP, ↑ glucose homeostasis and insulin action	Low serum magnesium appear to be associated to the increase risk of all cause of mortality, CVD, HF, atrial fibrillation and number of hospitalization
Omega-3	1 4 g	Not investigated	↓ TG, hsCRP, TNF-alpha, BNP, Adhesion molecules, ↑ LVEF and LAEF, ↓ Blood pressure, ↑ FMD, ↓ PWV	↓ cardiovascular mortality (epidemiological data), cardiac death and sudden death post myocardial infarction
Vitamin B1	25–300 mg/day	Improvement of fatigue and asthenia	↑ LVEF	Not investigated
Vitamin C	1–2 g	Not investigated	↓ hsCRP, ↓ lipid peroxidation, ↑ FMD, ↓ PWV	Unavailable data

(continued)

Table 11.1 (continued)

Nutraceutical	Active daily doses	Effects on symptoms	Effects on lab or instrumental parameters	Effects on hard outcomes
Vitamin D	1000–100000 UI	Improvement of quality of life (6MWT)	Improvement of serum 25-(OH)-D, LVEF, LVEDD, LVESD, myocardial performance index, interleukin-10 and reduction of TNF-alpha	No clear data available
Vitamin E	160–1800 mg	Not investigated	↓ ApoB, ↓ LDL-C, ↑ HDL-C ↑ FMD, ↓ PWV	↑ risk of HF, ↓ risk of myocardial infarction

AMPK AMP-activated Protein Kinase, *ApoB* Apolipoprotein B, *ATP* Adenosine Triphosphate, *CI* Cardiac Input, *CO* Cardiac Output, *CVD* Cardiovascular Disease, *DBP* Diastolic Blood Pressure, *EDV* End-Diastolic Volume, *EF* Ejection Fraction, *ET-1* Endothelin 1, *FMD* Flow Mediated Dilatation, *HDL-C* HDL Cholesterol, *HF* Heart Failure, *hsCRP* high sensible C-Reactive Protein, *IL-6* Interleukin 6, *LDL-C* LDL Cholesterol, *LKB1* Liver Kinase B1, *Lp(a)* Lipoprotein a, *LVEDD* left ventricular end diastolic diameter, *LVEF* Left Ventricular Ejection Fraction, *LVESD* left ventricular end systolic diameter, *MACE* Major Adverse Cardiac Events, *NO* Nitric Oxide, *NYHA* New York Heart Association, *LVESV* Left Ventricular End Systolic Volume, *PWV* Pulse Wave Velocity, *QoL* Quality of Life, *SBP* Systolic Blood Pressure, *SV* Stroke Volume, *TG* Triglycerides, *TNF-alpha* Tumor Necrosis Factor-alpha, *VO2 max* Maximal Oxygen Consumption, *6MWT* six-minute walking test

Nutraceuticals

Beetroot and Inorganic Nitrates

Nitric oxide (NO) is both endothelium-derived relaxing factor and a key cellular signaling molecule with pleiotropic effects in many tissues [16]. In failing cardiac muscle, the increased production of ROS leads to more rapid destruction of NO which in turn is thought to contribute to reduced contractility in HF [17]. Emerging evidence suggests that supplementation of dietary inorganic nitrate (NO3−) has beneficial effects on vascular health, blood pressure, exercise capacity, and oxygen metabolism though targeted NO production [18]. NO3− is reduced to bioactive NO2− by bacteria found in the oral cavity, and can be converted to nitric oxide (NO) after absorption [19]. Inorganic nitrates slowly produce NO and determine more mild but sustained vasodilation while organic nitrates rapidly release relatively large amounts of NO [20, 21], with potentially adverse effect on myocardial functionality in HF patients [22]. As underline by the study of *Miller et al.* a single, acute dose or one week of daily dosing of beetroot juice significantly increased plasma NO2− similarly, by 138% and 129% respect to placebo, respectively [23]. Today, no epidemiological evidences exist on the association between beetroot juice or dietary nitrates use and HF incidence or prognosis. However, i some RCTs, (randomized clinical trials) beetroot has been shown to increase time to exhaustion during high-intensity exercise and to reduce oxygen consumption (VO2) during submaximal exercise (i.e. reduce oxygen cost at a given submaximal work rate) [24–26]. These results were obtained in healthy people [27], elite adults [28] and also in HF patients [29]. Daily supplementation with beetroot juice containing 11.2 mmol of NO3- increase NO production and muscle function with an improvement of physical exercise in HF patients [30]. In another RCT including elderly people with HF, the consumption of 6.1 mmol of inorganic nitrate (beetroot juice), significantly improves submaximal aerobic endurance (p = 0.02 compared with placebo) and blood pressure (p < 0.001) [31]. Acute dietary NO3- intake was also related to increase of VO2 peak, improved physical performances [32] and may have positive effects also combined with aerobic exercise training regimen in patients with HF [33]. Finally, a meta-analysis of RCTs including 1248 patients showed that beetroot juice is associated to significant reduction in blood pressure (SBP: −3.55 mm Hg; 95% CI: −4.5, −2.5 mm Hg; DBP: −1.3 mm Hg; 95%CI: −1.9 to −0.7 mm Hg) compared to controls, thus reducing the afterload [34]. In general, beetroot supplementation seems to be tolerable and safe after short-term administration. Long-term effects on EF (ejection fraction) and hard outcomes are still lacking.

Cocoa and Dark Chocolate

Cocoa (*Theobroma cacao*) is a rich source of polyphenols, generally varying from 12% to 18% of dry weight depending on variety, growing region and processing operations of the bean [35]. Among polyphenols, cocoa is particularly rich in flavonoids, in particular flavanols that are present as aglycones both in the monomeric and polymerized form: among the monomeric flavanols the flavan-3-ols (37% of total monomeric flavanols form), with (−)-epicatechin occurring in largest quantities, represent 35% of the total content of phenolic compounds in cocoa beans. Cocoa contains also procyanidins that represent about the 58% of the total polyphenol, anthocyanins which constitute the 4% of total polyphenols, and finally flavonols (quercetin), flavones (apigenin, luteolin) and flavanones (naringenin) that are present in small quantities with other non-flavanoids polyphenols as derivatives of hydroxy-benzoic acids and hydroxy-cinnamic acids [36]. Dark chocolate is particularly rich in polyphenols, even if the treatment of cocoa beans through fermentation, roasting, drying and alkalization processes is the cause of a significant loss of polyphenol content and of the antioxidant, metabolic and vascular effects [37]. The possible mechanisms of action through which cocoa polyphenols could act on HF concern the improvement of the endothelium-dependent vasodilator responses, mediated by increase of nitric oxide synthesis, the suppression of endothelin-1 (ET-1) synthesis, and the reduction of N-terminal pro-B-type natriuretic peptide [38, 39]. A recent meta-analysis of prospective studies showed that light-to-moderate, but not high, consumption of dark chocolate was associated with a reduced risk of HF. Compared to no chocolate consumption, a moderate consumption was associated with a risk reduction in HF incidence of 16% [40]. A similar result was further obtained in a prospective cohort study: in this case, the moderate chocolate consumption was associated with a lower rate of HF hospitalization or death [41]. However, a higher than moderate intake was not associated with a decreased risk, probably to the high calorie content of commercially available chocolate even if in the large Physician's Health Study, the association between chocolate consumption and incident HF was stronger in lean than in overweight/obese subjects [42], making the interpretation of this relationship more complex. In RCT, 32 patients with chronic HF were randomized to consume 50 g/day of high-flavanol dark chocolate (HFDC; 1064 mg of flavanols/day) or low-flavanol dark chocolate (LFDC; 88 mg of flavanols/day) for 4 weeks and then crossed over to consume the alternative dark chocolate for a further 4 weeks. At the end of treatment of HFDC, NT-proBNP was significantly reduced compared with baseline ($-44 \pm 69\%$), LFDC ($-33 \pm 72\%$), and follow-up ($-41 \pm 77\%$) values. HFDC also reduced diastolic blood pressure compared with values after LFDC (-6.7 ± 10.1 mmHg) [43]. In addition, flavanol-rich chocolate acutely improves also vascular function in patients with CHF [44]. Dark chocolate consumption in patients with HF it was also related to an improvement of VO2 max ($p = 0.056$) and maximum work (watts) ($p = 0.026$), with no changes with placebo. It was observed also a significant increase in protein levels for LKB1, AMPK and PGC1α and in their active forms (phosphorylated AMPK and LKB1) as well as in citrate synthase [45]. At dosages of 25–100 g of dark chocolate or 400-1000 mg of cocoa polyphenols, it has been demonstrated a significant reduction of LDL-C, HDL-C, hs-CRP levels, blood pressure and platelet aggregation, with small but controversial improvements of the HDL-C [46–48]. In addition, two meta-analyses of RCTs observed also an improvement of insulin resistance and flow-mediated dilation [49, 50]. Cocoa is usually very well-tolerated, both as functional food and as dietary supplement (cocoa flavanols). However, larger and longer studies with a designed treatment and a specific population sample are needed to have clearer and more consistent results.

Hawthorn Flavonoid Fraction

Hawthorn extract from *Crataegus monogyna* and *oxyacantha* is a flavonoid-rich herbal remedy with known anti-inflammatory, antioxidant, inotropic and coronary vasodilator effects. The most studied extract (WS 1442) is a dry extract from hawthorn leaves that contains about 17.3–20.1% oligomeric procyanidins (OPCs) and several flavonoids, including hyperoside, vitexin-rhamnoside, rutin, and vitexin as well as triterpenoids and phenol carboxylic acids. *In vitro* experiments with human myocardial tissue demonstrated a positive inotropic effect of hawthorn with a concentration-dependent increase of myocardial contractility accompanied by a transient rise in intracellular calcium [51, 52]. In addition, in contrast to cardiac glycosides, hawthorn possess pronounced anti-arrhythmic properties especially evaluated in animal models and it increases the release of NO from the endothelium [53, 54]. Hawthorn has also shown to raise endothelial calcium levels by inhibition of SERCA and activation of the IP3 pathway [55].

The SPICE study has investigated the effect of 900 mg/day of WS 1442 on mortality and hospitalization rate in NYHA class II–III patients, in a 24-month, randomized, placebo-controlled trial: the trend for cardiac mortality reduction with WS 1442 was not statistically significant (p = 0.269) even if, in the subgroup with LVEF ≥25%, WS 1442 reduced sudden cardiac death by 39.7% (HR 0.59; 95%CI: 0.37–0.94) at month 24; p = 0.025) [56, 57]. Hawthorn supplementation has shown to improve maximum workload (p = 0.024) and general capability, lassitude, early fatigability, and effort dyspnoea at dosages of 900 mg/day (p = 0.04) and 1800 mg/day (p = 0.004) [58]. A Cochrane meta-analysis of RCTs concluded that the treatment with hawthorn compared to placebo was more beneficial for the physiologic outcome of maximal workload (p < 0.02, n = 380), exercise tolerance and the pressure-heart rate product, an index of cardiac oxygen consumption. Furthermore, shortness of breath and fatigue were also improved [59]. These results were confirmed by a more recent meta-analysis of RCTs [60]. Hawthorn also seems to be able to improve lipid metabolism [61] and could improve endothelial dysfunction and atherosclerosis related diseases [62].

The recommended daily dose of hawthorn extract is 160–900 mg (equivalent to 30–169 mg of epicatechin or 3.5–19.8 mg of flavonoids), which must be taken in two or three doses to reach a therapeutic effect. Side effects reported were mild, transient and infrequent and in general compared to placebo; they included a mild rash, headache, sweating, dizziness, and gastrointestinal symptoms [63]. In conclusion, according to clinical evidence, *Crataegus* extracts have proven benefits regarding functional capacity, symptom control and health-related QoL in HF people.

Nutritional Supplements

Coenzyme Q10

Coenzyme Q10 (CoQ10) is an organic molecule which is composed of a lipophilic core (benzoquinone) and an isoprenoid side chain; it was identified in 1940 and isolated for the first time from beef heart mitochondria by Frederick Crane of Wisconsis (USA), in 1957 [64]. CoQ10 is universally present in the cells of the body, particularly concentrated in the mitochondria, in both reduced form (ubiquinol) and oxidized form (ubiquinone) [65]. The overall body content of CoQ10 is only about 500–1500 mg (highest in organs with high rates of metabolism such as the heart, kidney, and liver) and decreases with age. It is naturally contained in oily fish, organ meats and whole grains, but it can be assumed also as dietary supplement [66]. CoQ10 has two important roles as an essential cofactor of the mitochondrial respiratory chain used for production of adenosine triphosphate (ATP) [67] and the only lipid-soluble antioxidant that slows lipid peroxidation in the circulation [68]. Other functions of CoQ10 in cell membrane include stabilization of calcium-dependent channels, metabolic regulation, cell signalling and cell growth [69]. Being the CoQ10 an essential cofactor for the synthesis of ATP, it is not surprising that the highest concentration compared to other tissues, is focused in myocardium mitochondria [70]. There are not studies investigating the association between serum CoQ10 level and incidence of HF even if some evidence suggest that decreased myocardial function is associated with decreased CoQ10 myocardial tissue concentrations [71–73], and greater is the depletion of CoQ10 more serious is the development of the disease [74, 75]. One of the most important study in the field of nutraceuticals is the Q-SYMBIO multicenter clinical trials that assessed the impact of the daily intake of CoQ10 on total mortality and not just on the surrogate endpoints. 420 patients with moderate or severe HF for a period of two years, were treated with 300 mg of CoQ10 (n = 202) or placebo (n = 218): at the end of treatments they have benefited from a significant reduction in MACE (15% of the patients in the CoQ10 group versus 26% in the placebo group, hazard ratio: 0.50; 95%CI: 0.32 to 0.80; p = 0.003), cardiovascular mortality (9% vs. 16%, p = 0.026), all-cause mortality (10% vs. 18%, p = 0.018) and incidence of hospital stays for HF (p = 0.033) [76]. A meta-analysis of 14 RCTs including 2149 patients has shown that administration of CoQ10 reduces mortality (RR = 0.69; 95%CI: 0.50–0.95; p = 0.02; I2 = 0%) and improves exercise capacity (SMD = 0.62; 95%CI: 0.02–0.30; p = 0.04; I2 = 54%) compared with placebo. No significant difference was observed in the endpoints of LVEF between "active group" and placebo (SMD = 0.62; 95% CI: 0.02–1.12; p = 0.04; I2 = 75%) [77]. The effect on LVEF could be more relevant patients with preserved EF [78] and patients untreated with statins and/or ACE inhibitors (ACEi) compared to the subgroup of patients treated with these drugs [79]. The heterogeneity of results obtained on EF may therefore be partly explained by many factors such as the diversity of CoQ10 supplemented through different pharmaceutical forms and dosages [80–82], diversity of HF grade of patients enrolled (NYHA I-II-III-IV), duration of treatments and co-treatment with conventional therapies [83]. CoQ10 supplementation could exert pleiotropic activities such as the reduction of serum triglycerides levels and the improvement of lipid profiles in patients with metabolic disorders [84]. CoQ10 also exert a mild but significant reduction in plasma lipoprotein(a) levels [85]. In elderly healthy people who received CoQ10 supplementation for over 4 years, an increase in insulin-like growth factor 1 (IGF-1) and postprandial insulin-like growth factor-binding protein 1 (IGFBP-1) levels, and greater age-corrected IGF-1 score based on the standard deviation of the mean value were observed compared with placebo [86]. A recent meta-analysis of RCT show that CoQ10 is responsible for the significant reduction of the plasma levels of tumor necrosis factor alpha (TNF-α), C-reactive protein and interleukin 6 (IL-6) in patients afflicted by inflammatory diseases [87]. Similar results were obtained by the meta-analysis of RCTs of *Zhai et al.* [88]. Finally, CoQ10 lowers the need of inotropic drugs and reduces the appearance of ventricular arrhythmias after surgery in the prevention of complications in patients undergoing cardiac surgery: the results showed that this molecule [89]. CoQ10 has high safety profile and at dosages ranging from 60 to 600 mg/day it does not cause clinically relevant adverse events. In conclusion, meta-analyses suggest that supplementation with CoQ10 (≥200 mg/day) can be of benefit in patients with chronic HF, in particular in early stage of HF, and potentially responsible of a reduction in MACE and total mortality.

D-ribose

D-ribose is a pentose carbohydrate that has a key role in the interaction between calcium and the sarcoplasmic reticulum (important for ventricular relaxation) and thus to maintain the cell's integrity and function [90]. Supplementation of D-ribose enhances the regeneration of ATP levels by bypassing rate-limiting, slow enzymatic steps in glycolysis through the pentose phosphate pathway [91, 92]. The supplementation with D-ribose in an experimental model of ischemic injury quickly increase the levels of ATP, improving diastolic dysfunction and substantially shortens the lengthy time recovery that normally occurs following ischemia [93]. However, no epidemiological evidence exist on the association between D-ribose use and HF incidence or prognosis. In a prospective feasibility study D-ribose improved diastolic dysfunction, self-perceived QoL, and physical function [94], while in a pilot trial D-ribose improved ventilatory efficiency [95]. In RCT, 5 g daily of D-ribose for 6 weeks in patients with NYHA II-IV showed an improvement of tissue doppler velocity (E') (3/4 of the patients), also maintained in the follow-up visit at nine weeks. In addition, half of the patients achieved an improvement in their ratio of early diastolic filling velocity € to early annulus relaxation velocity (E') [96]. Part of these effects might be related to the anti-ischemic properties of this molecule that enabled patients with stable coronary artery disease to exercise longer without developing angina or electrocardiographic changes [97]. In addition, improvement in heamodynamic parameters have been also recorded perioperatively, in patients undergoing off-pump coronary artery bypass [98] and in people following aortic valve replacement [99]. In conclusion, D-ribose might offer an energetic benefit in patients with ischemic cardiovascular diseases, including HF with a good safety profile. Even if the preliminary data are encouraging, clinical studies conducted to date are still few, small and short. For this reason, new long-term RCTs are needed.

Iron

Iron deficiency is defined in the general population as serum ferritin <30 ng/ml and transferrin (TfS) saturation below 20%: however, in the presence of inflammatory comorbidities such as chronic kidney disease or inflammatory bowel disease different cutoff values of ferritin and TfS are used to diagnose iron deficiency [100]. The burdening prevalence of this comorbid condition is illustrated by the findings of such deficit in 30–50% in chronic stable disease [101, 102] and 70–80% in acute HF [103, 104]. Iron deficiency independently predicts more severe symptomatic burden, higher morbidity, as noted by markedly increased hospitalizations and readmission rates, and mortality [105], which underscores its importance in HF. Iron deficiency in HF patients (as in general population) may be due to either reduced iron intake, increased iron body and/or losses impaired iron absorption [106]. No epidemiological evidences exist on the association between iron intake and HF incidence or prognosis. The study of *Noghes et al.* noted that iron intake was markedly decreased in HF patients, aggravating with increased disease severity [107]. Nervetheless, the multicentre double-blinded IRONOUT HF study (255 patients with symptomatic iron deficiency and reduced ejection fraction treated for 16 weeks with oral intake of 150 mg twice/daily of iron polysaccharide or placebo), it found no significant differences between groups regarding natriuretic peptides levels, symptomatic score, 6MWT or pVO2 [108]. Today, no trial has formally tested the role of oral iron in patients with HF and mid-range ejection fraction or HF with preserved ejection fraction. While intravenous iron administration in stable symptomatic (NYHA II-III) chronic HF (LVEF <40–45%) is supported by several clinical trial, no convincing evidence is available as it regards oral iron supplementation. Moreover, oral iron supplementation is often associated with multiple unwanted events, particularly gastrointestinal adverse effects [109] which clearly outweighs the null benefit of such dietary supplement in reduced ejection fraction.

L-carnitine

Levo-carnitine is a hydrophilic quaternary amine, chemically analogue of choline, that is involved in several physiological activities such as mitochondrial defence and lipid metabolism (it acts as an obligatory cofactor for oxidation of fatty acids and the transport of long-chain fatty acids from the cytosol to the mitochondrial matrix for β-oxidation) [110]. It seems possible that L-carnitine improves energy metabolism in cardiomyocytes and contribute to the improvement of clinical symptoms and cardiac function: this ability, is in agreement with the "energy starvation" hypothesis, suggesting that insufficient ATP supply underlies the contractile dysfunction presenting in HF [111]. L-carnitine exerts cardioprotective effects through the reduction of arterial hypertension, cardiac inflammation and fibrosis [112, 113], oxidative stress [114], and interstitial remodelling [115], as well as by improving endothelial function and nitric oxide bioavailability [116, 117]. No epidemiological evidences exist on the association between L-carnitine use and HF incidence or improvement. In a first meta-analysis of RCTs not specifically including HF patients, L-carnitine use was associated with a 27% reduction in all-cause mortality, a 65% reduction in ventricular arrhythmias, and a 40% reduction in angina in patients experiencing an acute myocardial infarction [118]. A more recent meta-analysis of 17 RCTs enrolling 1625 HF subjects showed a considerable improvement in overall efficacy (p < 0.01), LVEF (p = 0.01), stroke volume (SV) (p = 0.01), cardiac output (CO) (p < 0.01), and E/A (p<0.01) compared to control. In addition, treatment with L-carnitine also resulted in significant decrease in serum levels of BNP (p = 0.01), serum levels of NT-proBNP (p<0.01), LV end systolic diameter (LVESD) (p<0.01), LV end diastolic diameter (LVEDD) (p<0.01), and LV end systolic volume (LVESV) (p<0.01). No significant differences were reported in all-cause mortality, 6-minute walk, and adverse events between L-carnitine and control groups [119]. The partially contrasting data reported in the above cited meta-analyses, is probably related to the higher heterogeneity in the studies included in the more recent one as it regards severity of patients, background therapy, L-carnitine tested doses (ranging from 1.5 to 6 g/day) and follow-up length (ranging from 7 days to 3 years). In a further meta-analysis of RCTs, the L-carnitine assumption was associated to a significant reduction of serum CRP and TNF-α concentrations [120]. Then, L-carnitine supplementation could have mild but significant impact on body weight [121] and plasma level of Lipoprotein (a) [122]. The clinical relevance of these effects has to be clarified. In general, L-carnitine is usually well tolerated even if dry mouth, rash and mild gastrointestinal problems could unfrequently occur. In conclusion, L-carnitine treatment is effective for chronic HF patients in improving clinical symptoms and cardiac functions, decreasing serum levels of BNP and NT-proBNP. Further research is required to more accurately assess the results of L-carnitine for supporting HF care.

L-carnosine

L-carnosine, chemically β-alanyl-L-histidine, is a dipeptide produced from β-alanine, through carnosine synthase (in the liver) and stored especially in the skeletal muscle and in the heart [123]. The oral administration of β-alanine has shown to increase the levels of L-carnosine in the heart probably because the rate limiting step in the synthesis of L-carnosine is represented by the tissue concentration of β-alanine (produced as a result of uracil hepatic metabolism) [124]. It exerts a positive effect on HF patients through different mechanisms of action: the inhibition of the fragmentation and inactivation of Cu, Zn-superoxide dismutase (SOD) by peroxyl radicals, the prevention of hydroxyl radicals production via chemical Fenton catalysis by iron and copper chelation antioxidant and through its peroxyl radical-trapping ability at physiological concentrations due to its imidazole ring [125–127]. In addition, L-carnosine plays a sensitizing action of calcium in cardiac contraction, probably related to an upregulation of calcium release from the sarcoplasmic reticulum [128]. This effect could led to a procontractile action [129], potentially useful in HF patients. No epidemiological evidence exist on the association between L-carnosine use and HF incidence or improvement (L-carnosine is not a nutrient or food but a supplement). In RCT the oral administration of 500 mg of orodisperible

L-carnosine for six months has been tested in 50 patients with stable HF and severe LVEF: at the end of the study, patients who received this supplement experienced an improvement in 6-minute walking test (6MWT) distance (p = 0.014) and an improvement in self-perceived quality of life (assessed with a Visual Analogue Scale – VAS score, p = 0.039) between baseline and follow-up. In addition, L-carnosine group compared to controls, at the end of six months of treatment showed an improvement in peak VO2 (p < 0.0001), VO2 at anaerobic threshold, 6MWT, peak exercise workload and self-perceived quality of life assessed by the EuroQoL five dimensions questionnaire (EQ-5D test) and the VAS score [130]. A potential precursor of uridine, a nucleoside used from cardiac tissue as a source of β-alanine and subsequently of L-carnosine is magnesium orotate, that seems also to be clinically useful in HF [131]. In patients with severe HF, treated with magnesium orotate (6 g per day for 1 month, 3 g per day for 11 months) the survival rate was of 75.7% compared to 51.5% to those treated with placebo (p < 0.05) [132]. Orotate can be considered as a "delayed release" form of β-alanine, better tolerated than β-alanine itself because the evolution of β-alanine proceeds gradually [133]. Magnesium orotate is in generally safe and well tolerated. However, the intake of β-alanine active doses at one time can give "pins and needles" paraesthesia that can last one hour, during the peak of plasma β-alanine [134]. Timed-release β-alanine preparations may also be employed to prevent the above cited paresthesias [135], but this formulation has not yet tested in HF patients.

Magnesium

Magnesium plays a role in electrophysiologic and hemodynamics functioning through many enzymatic processes: first of all, it is an important component in the mitochondrial function, modulating cellular potassium permeability and affecting calcium uptake and its distribution [136, 137]. Even if is not infrequently observed in HF patients respect to other electrolyte alterations, the pathophysiology of hypo-magnesemia (serum magnesium <1.5 mg/dL) remains less studied: the prevalence is 7% of well-compensated ambulatory subjects to 52 % in more advanced HF patients who are aggressively treated with diuretics [138]. The effective correction of magnesium disturbances is favourable in HF subjects, in particular preventive potentially life-threatening arhytmias [139]. Magnesium depletion in HF people appears to be due to several factors that include the reduced dietary intake, altered distribution of the ion, renal losses, edematous states of intestinal mucosa that might interfere with the absorption of microelements, respiratory alkalosis and excessive catecholamine release [140]. In addition, diuretics produce most of renal magnesium loss, especially in the volume-expanded setting of HF and in associated hyper-aldosteronism and it has been demonstrated that potassium depletion inhibits the renal reabsorption of magnesium, leading to hypermagnesiuria and hypomagnese-mia [141]. In HF people, the presence of adequate total-body magnesium stores has been associated with a reduction in the risk of arrhythmias, digitalis toxicity, and hemodynamic abnormalities [142]. The most part of evidence supporting magnesium supplementation in HF patients comes from observational data, even if small RCTs carried out on HF people have underlined that magnesium supplementation improves LVEF [143] and heart rate variability [144]. Observational studies have linked low serum magnesium to more adverse cardiovascular disease (CVD) risk factor profiles [145–147] and greater risk of CVD events [148]. Many studies have underlined an inverse correlation was noted between mortality and plasma magnesium and in some cases, magnesium supplementation determines the reversal of HF [149, 150]. In particular in the ARIC study, participants in the lowest quintile of magnesium were at 2.5 times greater risk of incident HF (and after adjustment for demographic factors and for behaviors and CVD risk factors, individuals in the lowest quintile of magnesium were at 66% greater risk of developing incident HF than those in the highest quintile) [151]. Evidences to date suggested that patients with HF are more likely to have low serum magnesium than are other older individuals [152], and among patients with HF, low serum magnesium has been associated with increased all-cause mortality [153]. The prospective British Heart Regional Study showed that serum magnesium was inversely related to risk of incident HF and the benefit of high serum magnesium on HF risk was most evident in men with ECG evidence of ischaemia (HR 0.29; 95%CI: 0.13–0.68, p < 0.05) [154]. In the Jackson Heart Study cohort, magnesium intake <2.3 mg/kg was related to increased risk of subsequent HF hospitalizations [155], and in a more recent study, the magnesium deficiency independently predicted poor HRQoL and earlier cardiac event-free survival in HF patients [156]. However, a meta-analysis of 7 eligible prospective studies did not observed a clear correlation between hypomagnesemia and HF, if not in elderly HF patients with reduced LVEF [157]. Nevertheless, low serum magnesium seems to be associated with an increased risk of incident atrial fibrillation [158, 159] that is closely related with HF [160, 161]. In addition, magnesium is believed to be linked to CVD risk through a broad range of physiologic roles; low serum concentrations have been associated with impaired glucose homeostasis and insulin action, elevated blood pressure, chronic inflammation, impaired vasomotor tone and peripheral blood flow, and electrocardiogram abnormalities [162]. A recent meta-analysis of forty prospective cohort studies (more than 1 million participants) has shown that increasing dietary magnesium intake is associated with a reduced risk of stroke, HF, diabetes, and all-cause mortality, but not CHD or total CVD [163]. The prognostic significance of serum magnesium concentration in HF patients is currently under investigation. Additional work is needed to elucidate whether the association between HF and magnesium deficiency is causal and to clarify the specific mechanisms that underlie the association. Whether this biomarker will be useful candidates for HF risk prediction or targets for prevention remains to be confirmed. Stomach upset, mild diarrhea, nausea and heartbeat are the most common dose-dependent side effects after the use of magnesium. Magnesium toxicity rarely occurs except in patients with renal dysfunction: severe kidney failure and heart block are the two relative contraindications [164].

Omega-3 Polyunsaturated Fatty Acids (PUFAs)

Supplementation with omega-3 PUFAs could exert some positive effects in HF patients: it is possible that eicosapentaenoic (EPA) and docosahexaenoic (DHA) fatty acids have a direct action on mitochondrial membrane, modifying its structure and function [165–167]. DHA could in fact decreases viscosity of the membrane and a greater ease of movement of membrane proteins [168, 169]. PUFAs exhibit wide-ranging biological actions that include regulating both vasomotor tone and renal sodium excretion, they also reduce angiotensin-converting enzyme activity, angiotensin II formation, tumor growth factor-beta expression, enhance endothelial nitric oxide generation and activate the parasympathetic nervous system [170]. PUFAs inhibit natriuretic peptide production and alters the diacylglycerol composition in the heart and prevents activation of protein kinase C [171, 172]. In a meta-analysis of 7 prospective epidemiological studies involving 176441 subjects with 5480 incident cases of HF, the pooled relative risk for HF comparing the highest to lowest category of fish intake was 0.85 (95%CI: 0.73–0.99; p = 0.04); corresponding value for marine omega-3 PUFAs was 0.86 (95%CI: 0.74–1.00; p = 0.05) [173]. In the large GISSI-HF trial patients with chronic HF of NYHA class II-IV, were randomly assigned to omega-3 PUFA 1 g daily (n = 3494) or placebo (n = 3481). 955 (27%) patients died from any cause in the n-3 PUFA group and 1014 (29%) in the placebo group (HR 0.91; 95%CI: 0.833-0.998; p = 0.041). 57% patients in the omega-3 PUFA group and 59% in the placebo group died or were admitted to hospital for cardiovascular reasons (HR 0.92; 99%CI: 0.849–0.999; p = 0.009). In absolute terms, 56 patients needed to be treated for a median duration of 3.9 years to avoid one death or 44 to avoid one event like death or admission to hospital for cardiovascular reasons [174]. In the same trial, baseline LVEF increased with n-3 PUFA by 8.1% at 1 year, 11.1% at 2 years, and 11.5% at 3 years vs. 6.3% at 1 year, 8.2% at 2 years, and 9.9% at 3 years in the placebo group (p = 0.005) [175]. A meta-analysis of RCTs highlighted also a significant reduction in cardiac death in active group compared with control, in particular in subgroup analysis with EPA+DHA dosages >1 g/day [176]. Similar results were obtained by the study of *Dabkowsky et al.* in more than two hundred patients with ischemic HF or dilated cardiomyopathy [177]. The effect of omega-3 PUFA on HF seems to be dose-related [178]. In a double-blind, placebo controlled, cross-over trial the treatment with 2 g/daily of omega-3 PUFAs for 8 weeks in 31 patients with ischemic HF has shown to improve LVEF, global longitudinal strain, E/e' ratio (early ventricular filling to early mitral annulus velocities), ST2 levels, FMD and hsCRP levels (p < 0.05 for all) compared to placebo [179]. These results confirm those from previous investigations suggesting beneficial effects of EPA/DHA on LV indices, hemodynamics and inflammation [180, 181]. As parallel effects, omega-3 PUFAs exert a significant dose-related reduction in triglycerides level, systemic inflammation, arterial stiffness and a mild improving effect on blood pressure [182]. Omega-3 PUFAs are well tolerated beyond some mild gastrointestinal adverse events [183]. the available evidences support the supplementation of EPA and DHA to improve HF prognosis, especially after a myocardial infarction.

Probiotics

Recent clinical and preclinical studies underline the key role of intestinal microbiota in cardiovascular health and in particular in HF prognosis [184]. Intestinal eubiosis is important in regulation of the function of the intestinal barrier, together with mucosal immunity, sodium and water homeostasis and the functionality of tight junctions. Subjects with HF manifest gastrointestinal disorders of absorption, motility, tissue perfusion and edema, which determine alterations of the intestinal bacterial flora that are responsible of an increase in translocation of endotoxins in the blood, an increase in preload and afterload and an aggravation of the clinical picture [185, 186]. An altered intestinal microbiota is associated with a modification in permeability and an increase in trimethylamine N-oxide (TMAO) levels, which is also indirectly responsible for an exacerbation of HF and renal dysfunction. At the same time, the translocation in the bloodstream of microbes and endotoxins increase in pro-inflammatory cytokine levels and this "phenomenon" is called leaky gut syndrome. It appears to exist a strong correlation between the HF severity and the severity of intestinal dysbiosis, measured through the serum levels of trimethylamine-N-oxide (TMAO), an amine produced by the metabolism of choline and phosphatidylcholine from opportunistic/pathogenic microorganisms [187, 188]. The etiopathogenetic mechanism is not clear yet but it is evident that there is a direct proportionality between the blood levels of TMAO and the increase in intestinal oedema, inflammatory metabolites and cardiac and vascular remodelling. In a prospective trial, it was studied the role of TMAO in HF, measured through fasting blood samples in 720 subjects and for a duration of 5 years of follow-up -up. The study found that the highest TMAO levels were reported in patients with HF (mean TMAO levels: 5.0 μM) compared to healthy subjects (mean TMAO levels: 3.5 μM, $p < 0.001$), with a risk of mortality increased by 3.4 times [189]. It has been shown also that elevated TMAO levels modify lipid metabolism through changes in the functionality of reverse cholesterol transport, sterol metabolism and modification of the quality and quantity of bile acids [190, 191]. The potential role of probiotics supplementation was confirmed in RCT conducted in patients with HF: at the end of the study (3 months) the group treated with probiotics (1000 mg/day of *S. boulardii*) benefited from a significant reduction in uric acid levels (-1.08 mg/dL, $p = 0.014$ vs. placebo: -0.01 mg/dL, $p = 0.930$), total cholesterol ($-7,63$ mg/dL, $p = 0.010$ vs placebo: -2.02 mg/dL, $p = 0.603$), hsCRP (-0.23 mg/dL, $p = 0.116$ vs placebo: $+0.44$ mg/dL, $p = 0.011$), an improvement in LVEF ($+6.6\%$, $p = 0.005$ vs. placebo: $+4.2\%$, $p = 0.173$) and of the left atrial diameter (-0.29 cm, $p = 0.044$ vs. placebo: $+0.2$ cm, $p = 0.079$) [192]. Preclinical data have shown results comparable to *L. rhamnosus* [193]. Probiotics have different pleiotropic activities in cardiovascular prevention confirmed by several meta-analysis, such as blood pressure lowering effect [194], lipid-lowering activities [195] and also they can modulate some glyco-metabolic parameters (in particular fasting plasma glucose (FPG), insulin levels and glycated hemoglobin (HbA1c)) [196, 197] and vascular inflammation (reduction of plasmatic hsCRP, IL-6, fibrinogen, F2-isoprostane and TNF-alpha, improvement of NO plasmatic levels) [198, 199]. However, in agreement with the results of literature, duration of treatment should be ≥8 weeks and the daily dose ≥1011 CFU. In general, supplementation with probiotics in HF proved to be safe and free of any relevant side effects. Further long-term clinical trials are needed to investigate the effects of probiotic supplementation on hard outcomes.

Vitamins

Vitamin B1 (thiamine)

Thiamine is an essential vitamin required for cellular energy production and humans neither synthesize thiamine nor store it in large quantities [200]. In particular thiamine pyrophosphate (TPP) is the key coenzyme in the pentose phosphate pathway for transketolation of glucose-6-phosphate to ribose-5-phosphate, it is essential for the ATP metabolism and specifically for the functioning of the pyruvate dehydrogenase complex and alpha-ketoglutarate dehydrogenase in the Kreb's cycle [201]. Thiamine deficiency is related to a several non-specific signs, that including anorexia, fatigue, weight loss, sleep disorders, depression [202]. Many studies have shown that thiamine deficiency is more prevalent in HF patients than in general population: the meta-analysis of *Jane et al.* including nine observational studies, it showed that the incidence of thiamine deficiency in patients with HF was higher compared to that of control subjects without HF (OR 2.53 [95% CI 1.65–3.87]) [203]. The reduction of thiamine intake and/or its poor absorption due to cardiac cachexia and splanchnic congestion, associated to the increased urinary excretion determined by the treatment with high-dose loop diuretics are the possible mechanisms for thiamine deficiency in HF [204]. Decreased activity of pyruvate dehydrogenase due to thiamine deficiency results in build-up of pyruvate, which is then shunted towards anaerobic conversion into lactate [205]. This accumulation of lactate causes a decrease in peripheral resistance, thereby increasing the preload, that, coupled with myocardial dysfunction, has been proposed to be a basis of congestive HF in thiamine deficiency [206]. In a cross-sectional prospective observational analysis on 32 male NYHA II HF patients on prolonged diuretic therapy, 16 patients received 300 mg/day of thiamine for 28 days: a 13.5% increase in EF was observed in thiamine recipients (p = 0.021) when compared to control [207]. *Shimon et al.* randomized 30 hospitalized HF patients secondary to myocardial ischemia and administered intravenous thiamine for 7 days or placebo in a double-blind manner followed by 6 weeks of oral thiamine 200 mg/day in all patients. At the end of complete treatment patients experienced a 22% increase in EF as compared to the baseline value (p < 0.01) [208]. Similar results were obtained in a RCT carried out of nine symptomatic patients with HF with an increase in LVEF from 29.5% to 32.8% (p = 0.024) after supplementation with oral thiamine 300 mg/day for 28 days [209]. A meta-analysis of the available RCTs showed a small increase in LVEF (3.28%, 95%CI 0.64–5.93%) with thiamine therapy in HF patients compared to control [210]. However, a recent RCT (52 patients with HF and LVEF <40% treated with

300 mg/day of thiamine or placebo for a period of 1 month) showed no significant difference in either systolic or diastolic echocardiographic parameters and dyspnea between the two groups, even if patients in the thiamine group showed a significant improvement in peripheral edema (34.6 vs 3.8%, p = 0.005) [211]. In this study, however, the proportion of patients who were on furosemide in this study was incredibly low (10 out of 52). Second, spironolactone was prescribed to most (22 out of 26) patients in the thiamine group which may have caused a decrease in the incidence of thiamine deficiency in this small cohort of patients [212]. In general, at dosages between 25 and 300 mg/day thiamine confirms to have an excellent profile of safety. Given the small sample size and inherent limitations of the individual studies, long-term RCTs with large samples are needed to confirm or not the positive effects of thiamine on heart [213].

Vitamin C

Ascorbic acid (Vitamin C) is contained mostly in fruits and vegetables and is well known to protect against oxidative stress by reducing levels of free oxygen radicals and inhibiting low density lipoprotein oxidation and oxidative cell damage [214]. It also improves arterial stiffness and immune function, and it reduces inflammatory markers responsible of systemic inflammation [215]. Some [216, 217], but not all the studies [218] have underlined that high diet in fruit and vegetable rich in antioxidants is associated with reduced risk of HF. Few studies have examined the association between plasma vitamin C levels and incidence of HF, suggesting a positive correlation between elevated vitamin C levels and reduction of the risk of HF [219]. However, as reported also by the European Investigation into Cancer and Nutrition (EPIC) Norfolk study the association between vitamin C and HF seems to involve plasma vitamin C rather than dietary vitamin C, [220]. A possible mechanism of correlation between plasma vitamin C levels and its beneficial effects may be relate to the arterial dilation mediated by the modulation of nitric oxide release [221]. In a prospective study (3919 men aged 60–79 years with no HF at the baseline and followed up for a mean period of 11 years), higher plasma vitamin C level was associated with significantly lower risk of incident HF in both men with and without previous myocardial infarction after adjustment for lifestyle characteristics, diabetes mellitus, blood lipids, blood pressure, and heart rate (hazards ratio 95% CI 0.81 [0.70, 0.93] and 0.75 [0.59, 0.97] for 1 SD increase in log vitamin C, respectively) [222]. In another study, 200 HF patients completed a 3-day food diary to determine vitamin C intake: 39% of patients had vitamin C deficiency that was associated with an hsCRP level higher than 3 mg/L in the hierarchical logistic regression (odds ratio, 2.40; 95% confidence interval, [1.13–5.10]; p = 0.023). In addition, both vitamin C deficiency and hsCRP level higher than 3 mg/L predicted shorter cardiac event-free survival in hierarchical Cox regression and produced a 2.3-fold higher risk for cardiac events (p = 0.002) in moderation analysis. Higher level of hsCRP predicted shorter cardiac event-free survival only in patients with vitamin C deficiency (p = 0.027), but not in those with vitamin C adequacy [223]. In addition, a meta-analysis of 44 RCTs showed a significant positive effect of vitamin C on endothelial function (SMD: 0.50, 95%CI: 0.34, 0.66, p < 0.001), in particular in the HF subgroup (SMD: 0.48, 95% CI: 0.08, 0.88, p < 0.02) [224]. In general, supplementation with vitamin C at dosages between 500 mg and 3 g/day is considered safe and well tolerated [225], even if to date no study direct investigated the impact of chronic vitamin C supplementation on HF incidence nor prognosis.

Vitamin D

Vitamin D is a collection of fat-soluble steroids, obtained via endogenous production or from dietary intake, with the latter accounting for nearly 10–20% of our total supply [226]. Vitamin D, is commonly referred to D2 and D3, respectively ergocalciferol and cholecalciferol [227]. In the last years, the biological influence of Vitamin D has been significantly expanded beyond just calcium regulation: vitamin D receptor has been isolated from a number of different tissues not traditionally involved in calcium homeostasis, such as the myocardium [228] and fibroblasts [229]. Many observational studies have suggested a possible relationship between vitamin D status and prevalence, incidence and severity of HF [230–232]]. Despite emerging evidence supporting a pathophysiological relationship between Vitamin D and HF, the exact mechanism by which vitamin D deficiency leads to poor clinical outcome has not been clearly established. Vitamin D deficiency in HF patients could be linked to an over activation of the RAAS and the sympathetic nervous system and thus to an increased risk in clinical entity called cardiorenal syndrome [233, 234]. In general, mean serum 25(OH)D concentration is usually lower in patients with HF compared with controls [235–237] and vitamin D status may be related to physical functioning and prognosis in HF [238–241]. In RCT, 123 patients with HF treated for 9 months with vitamin D, 2000 IU/day + 500 mg/day of calcium, experienced a significantly increased of serum 25-(OH)-D and interleukin-10 and reduction of TNF-alpha compared with placebo (only calcium 500 mg/day) [242]. Similar results were obtained in pediatric HF patients with daily vitamin D supplementation of 1000 IU [243]. Vitamin D supplementation (between 800 and 1000 IU per day) in HF patients with low 25(OH)D levels was associated with a significant reduction in mortality, independent of the baseline 25(OH)D levels [244]. However, the supplementation with high dosage is not associated with improvement of 6MWT distance after 20 weeks of treatment, despite a significant reduction in BNP levels [245].To date, vitamin D should be supplemented in vitamin D deficient subjects: however, large-scale RCTs are needed before routine vitamin D supplementation can be recommended as part of clinical care of HF patients. Vitamin D is believed to be safe and well tolerated even if use of thiazide diuretics in combination with calcium and this supplement may cause hypercalcemia in the elderly or those with compromised renal function or hyperparathyroidism. [246].

Vitamin E

Vitamin E includes eight distinct chemical entities: α-, β-, g-, and δ-tocopherol and α-, β-, g-, and δ-tocotrienol even if the most studied is α-tocopherol. *In vitro* and animal studies suggest that oxidative stress characterized by the excessive production of ROS and reduction of antioxidant defence capacity, may play an important role in the pathophysiology of HF [247]. In this sense, vitamin E can protect against oxidative stress and also it inhibits low density lipoprotein oxidation and oxidative cell damage and it has a small but significant and documented lipid-lowering activity through the peroxisome proliferator-activated receptor (PPAR-α, PPAR-β, and PPAR-g) activation and the HMG-CoA reductase inhibition [248]. Finally, vitamin E showed an improvement of endothelial function and arterial stiffness at doses between 50 and 200 mg [249, 250]. Studies conducted to date, regarding the role of vitamin E in HF, are still inconclusive and conflicting. In the meta-analysis of RCTs by *Loffredo et al.* the supplementation of vitamin E given alone (33–800 IU) significantly decreased myocardial infarction (3.0% vs 3.4%) (random effects RR: 0.82; 95%CI 0.70–0.96; p = 0.01). This effect was driven by reduction of fatal myocardial infarction (RR: 0.84; 95%CI 0.73–0.96; p = 0.01) [251]. At the same time the Physician's Health Study II and the Women's Health Study reported no association between vitamin E supplements and HF in a primary prevention population [252, 253] while other studies reported increased risk of HF with vitamin E supplements in those with CVD [254, 255] raising concern about the use of vitamin E supplements. Moreover, in a prospective study of 3919 men aged 60–79 years with no HF followed up for a mean period of 11 years, the high intake of dietary vitamin E was associated with increased HF risk [256]. The reason for an increased risk of HF in particular in older men [257] is still unclear, but it may relate to the suggestion that α–tocopherol may become a pro-oxidant in a pre-existing environment with increased oxidative stress, suppress other fat-soluble antioxidants such as γ-tocopherol (more powerful antioxidant than α-tocopherol), disrupting the natural balance of antioxidant systems and increasing vulnerability to oxidative damage [258]. In contrast to dietary vitamin E, it was observed no association between plasma vitamin E and risk of HF [259]. In conclusion, epidemiological data and results from RCTs do not suggest supplementation of vitamin E in prevention or as adjuvant to conventional therapy in HF.

Conclusion

It's well known that HF is highly prevalent in Western countries and the prevention of this condition is necessary not only to improve the quality of life, but also because of the great economic burden that imposes to both healthcare systems and society, through hospitalizations, pharmacological therapy, lost productivity, morbidity and premature mortality [260–262]. The overall economic cost of HF was estimated at $108 billion/year worldwide: specifically, direct costs for healthcare system accounted for ~60%, while indirect costs for society accounted for ~40% of the overall expenditure [263]. The therapeutic goal for the HF is to increase the cardiac efficiency to improve the quality of life, exercise performance and in particular increase the duration of life. Therefore, drugs as digitalis and phosphodiesterase inhibitors (that increase the force of heart muscle contraction), ACE inhibitors or B-blockers (vasodilators) and natriuretics (drugs that cause a reduction in the volume of extracellular fluid) are commonly used in clinical practice [264]. Parallel to the drug therapy used, a potential support is given by the nutraceuticals or dietary supplements recommended as adjuvants of conventional treatments in HF. Nutraceuticals (Fig. 11.1) would seem to have an ameliorative action as well as the symptoms (QoL and 6MWT), in some cardiac parameters (LVEF, SV, CO). However, it is important to evaluate the impact of the nutraceutical approach in terms of reduction of cardiovascular events and mortality; until now, the GISSI HF trial (about w-3) and the Q-SYMBIO study (about coenzyme q10) are the most convincing ones [76, 265]. It is really important to stress the observation that the positive results obtained with some nutraceuticals in the above cited trials have been achieved with the use of highly standardized and full dosed products, not always similar to what is available in the market and sometime expensive for everyday use. In conclusion, a growing clinical evidence suggests that the intake of adequate dosages of some nutraceuticals (Hawthorn extract, Coenzyme Q10, L-carnitine, D-ribose, Carnosine, Vitamin D, Probiotics, Omega-3 PUFAs, Beet nitrates) is associated with improvements in self-perceived quality of life and/or functional

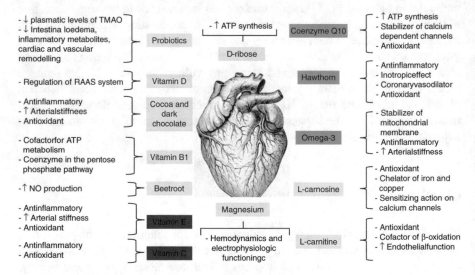

Fig. 11.1 Nutraceuticals with clinical effects on heart failure: main mechanisms of action. Green colour: evidence A (very good) – Yellow colour: evidence B (good) – Red colour: evidence C (poor)

parameters such as ejection fraction, stroke volume and cardiac output in HF patients, with the advantage of excellent safety profile. Those benefits tended to be greater in earlier HF stage. In no case, the use of nutraceuticals can replace the consolidated pharmacological treatment of HF. Finally, it is necessary to evaluate the cost/benefit ratio in the long term with clinical trials on larger and heterogeneous sample of HF patients.

References

1. Bozkurt B. What is new in heart failure management in 2017? Update on ACC/AHA heart failure guidelines. Curr Cardiol Rep. 2018;20(6):39. https://doi.org/10.1007/s11886-018-0978-7.
2. Jessup M, Marwick TH, Ponikowski P, Voors AA, Yancy CW. 2016 ESC and ACC/AHA/HFSA heart failure guideline update – what is new and why is it important? Nat Rev Cardiol. 2016;13(10):623–8. https://doi.org/10.1038/nrcardio.2016.134.
3. Writing Group Members, Mozaffarian D, Benjamin EJ, Go AS, Arnett DK, Blaha MJ, Cushman M, Das SR, de Ferranti S, Després JP, Fullerton HJ, Howard VJ, Huffman MD, Isasi CR, Jiménez MC, Judd SE, Kissela BM, Lichtman JH, Lisabeth LD, Liu S, Mackey RH, Magid DJ, McGuire DK, Mohler ER, Moy CS, Muntner P, Mussolino ME, Nasir K, Neumar RW, Nichol G, Palaniappan L, Pandey DK, Reeves MJ, Rodriguez CJ, Rosamond W, Sorlie PD, Stein J, Towfighi A, Turan TN, Virani SS, Woo D, Yeh RW, Turner MB, American Heart Association Statistics Committee; Stroke Statistics Subcommittee. Heart disease and stroke statistics-2016 Update: A report from the American Heart Association. Circulation. 2016;133:e38–e360.
4. Liu L, Eisen HJ. Epidemiology of heart failure and scope of the problem. Cardiol Clin. 2014;32(1):1–8.
5. Maggioni AP. Epidemiology of heart failure in Europe. Heart Fail Clin. 2015;11(4):625–35.
6. Meyer S, Brouwers FP, Voors AA, Hillege HL, de Boer RA, Gansevoort RT, van der Harst P, Rienstra M, van Gelder IC, van Veldhuisen DJ, van Gilst WH, van der Meer P. Sex differences in new-onset heart failure. Clin Res Cardiol. 2015;104(4):342–50.
7. Bui AL, Horwich TB, Fonarow GC. Epidemiology and risk profile of heart failure. Nat Rev Cardiol. 2011;8:30–41.
8. Kannel WB. Incidence and epidemiology of heart failure. Heart Fail Rev. 2000;5(2):167–73.
9. ACCF/AHA. Guideline for the management of heart failure 2013. J Am Coll Cardiol. 2013;62(16):e147–239.
10. Ponikowski P, Voors A, D Anker S, Bueno H, Cleland JGF, Coats AJS, Falk V, Ramón González-Juanatey J, Harjola VP, Jankowska EA, Jessup M, Linde C, Nihoyannopoulos P, Parissis JT, Pieske B, Riley JP, Rosano GMC, Ruilope LM, Ruschitzka F, Rutten FH, van der Meer P, ESC Scientific Document Group. 2016 ESC Guidelines for the diagnosis and treatment of acute and chronic heart failure: The Task Force for the diagnosis and treatment of acute and chronic heart failure of the European Society of Cardiology (ESC) Developed with the special contribution of the Heart Failure Association (HFA) of the ESC. Europ Heart J. 2016;37–27, 2129–2200.
11. Rifai L, Silver MA. A review of the DASH diet as an optimal dietary plan for symptomatic heart failure. Prog Cardiovasc Dis. 2016;58(5):548–54. https://doi.org/10.1016/j.pcad.2015.11.001.
12. Rifai L, Pisano C, Hayden J, Sulo S, Silver MA. Impact of the DASH diet on endothelial function, exercise capacity, and quality of life in patients with heart failure. Proc. 2015;28(2):151–6.

13. Tektonidis TG, Åkesson A, Gigante B, Wolk A, Larsson SC. Adherence to a Mediterranean diet is associated with reduced risk of heart failure in men. Eur J Heart Fail. 2016;18(3):253–9. https://doi.org/10.1002/ejhf.481.
14. Salehi-Abargouei A, Maghsoudi Z, Shirani F, Azadbakht L. Effects of Dietary Approaches to Stop Hypertension (DASH)-style diet on fatal or nonfatal cardiovascular diseases – incidence: a systematic review and meta-analysis on observational prospective studies. Nutrition. 2013;29(4):611–8.
15. Wexler R, Pleister A, Raman SV, Borchers JR. Therapeutic lifestyle changes for cardiovascular disease. Phys Sports Med. 2012;40:109–15.
16. Coggan AR, Peterson LR. Dietary nitrate and skeletal muscle contractile function in heart failure. Curr Heart Fail Rep. 2016;13(4):158–65.
17. Hare JM, Stamler JS. NO/redox disequilibrium in the failing heart and cardiovascular system. J Clin Invest. 2005;115:509–17.
18. Kapil V, Weitzberg E, Lundberg JO. Clinical evidence demonstrating the utility of inorganic nitrate in cardiovascular health. Nitric Oxide. 2014;38:45–57.
19. Cosby K, Partovi KS, Crawford JH, Patel RP, Reiter CD, Martyr S, Yang BK, Waclawiw MA, Zalos G, Xu X, Huang KT, Shields H, Kim-Shapiro DB, Schechter AN, Cannon RO 3rd, Gladwin MT. Nitrite reduction to nitric oxide by deoxyhemoglobin vasodilates the human circulation. Nat Med. 2003;9:1498–505.
20. Lundberg JO, Carlstrom M, Larsen FJ, Weitzberg E. Roles of dietary inorganic nitrate in cardiovascular health and disease. Cardiovasc Res. 2011;89:525–32.
21. Omar SA, Artime E, Webb AJ. A comparison of organic and inorganic nitrates/nitrites. Nitric Oxide-Biol Chem. 2012;26:229–40.
22. Redfield MM, Anstrom KJ, Levine JA, Koepp GA, Borlaug BA, Chen HH, LeWinter MM, Joseph SM, Shah SJ, Semigran MJ, Felker GM, Cole RT, Reeves GR, Tedford RJ, Tang WH, McNulty SE, Velazquez EJ, Shah MR, Braunwald E, Heart Failure Clinical Research Network NHLBI. Isosorbide mononitrate in heart failure with preserved ejection fraction. N Engl J Med. 2015;373(24):2314–24.
23. Miller GD, Marsh AP, Dove RW, Beavers D, Presley T, Helms C, Bechtold E, King SB, Kim-Shapiro D. Plasma nitrate and nitrite are increased by a high-nitrate supplement but not by high-nitrate foods in older adults. Nutr Res. 2012;32:160–8.
24. Lansley K, Winyard P, Fulford J, Vanhatalo A, Bailey SJ, Blackwell JR, DiMenna FJ, Gilchrist M, Benjamin N, Jones AM. Dietary nitrate supplementation reduces the O2 cost of walking and running: a placebo-controlled study. J Appl Physiol. 2011;110:591–600.
25. Bailey SJ, Winyard P, Vanhatalo A, Blackwell JR, Dimenna FJ, Wilkerson DP, Tarr J, Benjamin N, Jones AM. Dietary nitrate supplementation reduces the O2 cost of low-intensity exercise and enhances tolerance to high-intensity exercise in humans. J Appl Physiol. 2009;107:1144–55.
26. Hoon MW, Johnson NA, Chapman PG, Burke LM. The effect of nitrate supplementation on exercise performance in healthy individuals: a systematic review and meta-analysis. Int J Sport Nutr Exerc Metab. 2014;23:522–32.
27. Kelly J, Fulford J, Vanhatalo A, Blackwell JR, French O, Bailey SJ, Gilchrist M, Winyard PG, Jones AM. Effects of short-term dietary nitrate supplementation on blood pressure, O2 uptake kinetics, and muscle and cognitive function in older adults. Am J Physiol Regul Integr Comp Physiol. 2013;304:R73–83.
28. Balsalobre-Fernández C, Romero-Moraleda B, Cupeiro R, et al. The effects of beetroot juice supplementation on exercise economy, rating of perceived exertion and running mechanics in elite distance runners: a double-blinded, randomized study. PLoS One. 2018;13(7):e0200517. https://doi.org/10.1371/journal.pone.0200517. eCollection 2018
29. Zamani P, Rawat D, Shiva-Kumar P, Geraci S, Bhuva R, Konda P, Doulias PT, Ischiropoulos H, Townsend RR, Margulies KB, Cappola TP, Poole DC, Chirinos JA. Effect of inorganic nitrate on exercise capacity in heart failure with preserved ejection fraction. Circulation. 2015;131:371–80.

30. Coggan AR, Leibowitz JL, Spearie CA, Kadkhodayan A, Thomas DP, Ramamurthy S, Mahmood K, Park S, Waller S, Farmer M, Peterson LR. Acute dietary nitrate intake improves muscle contractile function in patients with heart failure: a double-blind, placebo-controlled, Randomized Trial. Circ Heart Fail. 2015;85:914–20.
31. Eggebeen J, Kim-Shapiro DB, Haykowsky M, Morgan TM, Basu S, Brubaker P, Rejeski J, Kitzman DW. One week of daily dosing with beetroot juice improves submaximal endurance and blood pressure in older patients with heart failure and preserved ejection fraction. JACC Heart Fail. 2016;4(6):428–37.
32. Coggan AR, Broadstreet SR, Mahmood K. Dietary nitrate increases VO$_2$peak and performance but does not alter ventilation or efficiency in patients with heart failure with reduced ejection fraction. J Card Fail. 2018;24(2):65–73.
33. Shaltout HA, Eggebeen J, Marsh AP, Miguel-Carrasco JL, Arias JL, Arévalo M, Mate A, Aramburu O, Vázquez CM. Effects of supervised exercise and dietary nitrate in older adults with controlled hypertension and/or heart failure with preserved ejection fraction. Nitric Oxide. 2017;69:78–90.
34. Bahadoran Z, Mirmiran P, Kabir A, Azizi F, Ghasemi A. The Nitrate-independent blood pressure-lowering effect of beetroot juice: a systematic review and meta-analysis. Adv Nutr. 2017 Nov 15;8(6):830–8. https://doi.org/10.3945/an.117.016717.
35. Fernández-Murga L, Tarín JJ, García-Perez MA, Cano A. The impact of chocolate on cardiovascular health. Maturitas. 2011;69(4):312–21.
36. Oracz J, Zyzelewicz D, Nebesny E. The content of polyphenolic compounds in cocoa beans (Theobroma cacao L.), depending on variety, growing region, and processing operations: a review. Crit Rev Food Sci Nutr. 2015;55:1176–92.
37. Ortega N, Romero MP, Macià A, Reguant J, Anglès N, Morelló JR, Motilva MJ. Obtention and characterization of phenolic extracts from different cocoa sources. J Agric Food Chem. 2008;56(20):9621–7.
38. Schroeter H, Heiss C, Balzer J, Kleinbongard P, Keen CL, Hollenberg NK, Sies H, Kwik-Uribe C, Schmitz HH, Kelm M. (-)-Epicatechin mediates beneficial effects of flavanol-rich cocoa on vascular function in humans. Proc Natl Acad Sci U S A. 2006;103:1024–9.
39. Heiss C, Jahn S, Taylor M, Real WM, Angeli FS, Wong ML, Amabile N, Prasad M, Rassaf T, Ottaviani JI, Mihardja S, Keen CL, Springer ML, Boyle A, Grossman W, Glantz SA, Schroeter H, Yeghiazarians Y. Improvement of endothelial function with dietary flavanols is associated with mobilization of circulating angiogenic cells in patients with coronary artery disease. J Am Coll Cardiol. 2010;56:218–24.
40. Gong F, Yao S, Wan J, Chocolate Consumption GX. Risk of heart failure: a meta-analysis of prospective studies. Nutrients. 2017;9(4):402.
41. Steinhaus DA, Mostofsky E, Levitan EB, Dorans KS, Håkansson N, Wolk A, Mittleman MA. Chocolate intake and incidence of heart failure: findings from the cohort of Swedish men. Am Heart J. 2017;183:18–23.
42. Petrone AB, Gaziano JM, Djousse L. Chocolate consumption and risk of heart failure in the Physicians' Health Study. Eur J Heart Fail. 2014;16:1372–6.
43. De Palma R, Sotto I, Wood EG, Khan NQ, Butler J, Johnston A, Rothman MT, Corder R. Cocoa flavanols reduce N-terminal pro-B-type natriuretic peptide in patients with chronic heart failure. ESC Heart Fail. 2016;3(2):97–106.
44. Flammer AJ, Sudano I, Wolfrum M, Thomas R, Enseleit F, Périat D, Kaiser P, Hirt A, Hermann M, Serafini M, Lévêques A, Lüscher TF, Ruschitzka F, Noll G, Corti R. Cardiovascular effects of flavanol-rich chocolate in patients with heart failure. Eur Heart J. 2012;33(17):2172–80.
45. Taub PR, Ramirez-Sanchez I, Patel M, Higginbotham E, Moreno-Ulloa A, Román-Pintos LM, Phillips P, Perkins G, Ceballos G, Villarreal F. Beneficial effects of dark chocolate on exercise capacity in sedentary subjects: underlying mechanisms. A double blind, randomized, placebo controlled trial. Food Funct. 2016;7(9):3686–93.

46. Hamed MS, Gambert S, Bliden KP, Bailon O, Singla A, Antonino MJ, Hamed F, Tantry US, Gurbel PA. Dark chocolate effect on platelet activity, C-reactive protein and lipid profile: a pilot study. South Med J. 2008;101(12):1203–8.
47. Mursu J, Voutilainen S, Nurmi T, Rissanen TH, Virtanen JK, Kaikkonen J, Nyyssönen K, Salonen JT. Dark chocolate consumption increases HDL cholesterol concentration and chocolate fatty acids may inhibit lipid peroxidation in healthy humans. Free Radic Biol Med. 2004;37(9):1351–9.
48. Ludovici V, Barthelmes J, Nägele MP, Enseleit F, Ferri C, Flammer AJ, Ruschitzka F, Sudano I. Cocoa, blood pressure, and vascular function. Front Nutr. 2017;4:36.
49. Hooper L, Kay C, Abdelhamid A, Kroon PA, Cohn JS, Rimm EB, Cassidy A. Effects of chocolate, cocoa, and flavan-3-ols on cardiovascular health: a systematic review and meta-analysis of randomized trials. Am J Clin Nutr. 2012;95(3):740–51.
50. Shrime MG, Bauer SR, McDonald AC, Chowdhury NH, Coltart CE, Ding EL. Flavonoid-rich cocoa consumption affects multiple cardiovascular risk factors in a meta-analysis of short-term studies. J Nutr. 2011;141(11):1982–8.
51. Schwinger RH, Pietsch M, Frank K, Brixius K. Crataegus special extract WS 1442 increases force of contraction in human myocardium cAMP-independently. J Cardiovasc Pharmacol. 2000;35(5):700–7. https://doi.org/10.1097/00005344-200005000-00004.
52. Münch G, Brixius K, Frank K, Erdmann EWS. 1442 (extract of Crataegus species) increases force of contraction in human failing myocardium by inhibition of the Na+/K+-ATPase. Circulation. 1997;96(S):I–729. Abstract No. 4090
53. Brixius K, Willms S, Napp A, Tossios P, Ladage D, Bloch W, Mehlhorn U, Schwinger RH. Crataegus special extract WS 1442 induces an endothelium-dependent, NO-mediated vasorelaxation via eNOS-phosphorylation at serine 1177. Cardiovasc Drugs Ther. 2006;20(3):177–84. https://doi.org/10.1007/s10557-006-8723-7.
54. Anselm E, Socorro VF, Dal-Ros S, Schott C, Bronner C, Schini-Kerth VB. Crataegus special extract WS 1442 causes endothelium-dependent relaxation via a redox-sensitive Src- and Akt-dependent activation of endothelial NO synthase but not via activation of estrogen receptors. J Cardiovasc Pharmacol. 2009;53(3):253–60. https://doi.org/10.1097/FJC.0b013e31819ccfc9.
55. Willer EA, Malli R, Bondarenko AI, Zahler S, Vollmar AM, Graier WF, Fürst R. The vascular barrier protecting hawthorn extract WS® 1442 raises endothelial calcium levels by inhibition of SERCA and activation of the IP3 pathway. J Mol Cell Cardiol. 2012;53(4):567–77.
56. Holubarsch CJ, Colucci WS, Meinertz T, Gaus W, Tendera M. Survival and Prognosis: Investigation of Crataegus Extract WS 1442 in congestive heart failure (SPICE)—rationale, study design and study protocol. Eur J Heart Fail. 2000;2(4):431–7.
57. Holubarsch CJ, Colucci WS, Meinertz T, Gaus W, Tendera M. The efficacy and safety of Crataegus extract WS 1442 in patients with heart failure: the SPICE trial. Eur J Heart Fail. 2008;10(12):1255–63.
58. Tauchert M. Efficacy and safety of Crataegus extract WS 1442 in comparison with placebo in patients with chronic stable New York Heart Association class-III heart failure. Am Heart J. 2002;143(5):910–5.
59. Pittler MH, Guo R, Ernst E. Hawthorn extract for treating chronic heart failure. Cochrane Database Syst Rev. 2008;1:CD005312.
60. Eggeling T, Regitz-Zagrosek V, Zimmermann A, Burkart M. Baseline severity but not gender modulates quantified Crataegus extract effects in early heart failure--a pooled analysis of clinical trials. Phytomedicine. 2011;18(14):1214–9.
61. Wang J, Xiong X, Feng B. Effect of crataegus usage in cardiovascular disease prevention: an evidence-based approach. Evid Based Complement Alternat Med. 2013;2013:149363.
62. Koch E, Malek FA. Standardized extracts from hawthorn leaves and flowers in the treatment of cardiovascular disorders--preclinical and clinical studies. Planta Med. 2011;77(11):1123–8.
63. Daniele C, Mazzanti G, Pittler MH, Ernst E. Adverse-event profile of Crataegus spp.: a systematic review. Drug Saf. 2006;29(6):523–35. https://doi.org/10.2165/00002018-200629060-00005.
64. Cicero AF, Colletti A. Nutraceuticals and dietary supplements to improve quality of life and outcomes in heart failure patients. Curr Pharm Des. 2017;23(8):1265–72.

65. Saini R. Coenzyme Q10: the essential nutrient. J Pharm Bioallied Sci. 2011;3(3):466–7.
66. Menke T, Niklowitz P, de Sousa G, Reinehr T, Andler W. Comparison of coenzyme Q10 plasma levels in obese and normal weight children. Clin Chim Acta. 2004;349(1-2):121–7.
67. Littarru GP, Tiano L. Clinical aspects of coenzyme Q10: an update. Nutrition. 2010;26:250–4.
68. Littarru GP, Tiano L. Bioenergetic and antioxidant properties of coenzyme Q10: recent developments. Mol Biotechnol. 2007;37:31–7.
69. Hernández-Camacho JD, Bernier M, López-Lluch G, Navas P. Coenzyme Q10 supplementation in aging and disease. Front Physiol. 2018;9:44.
70. Florkowski CM, Molyneux SL, Young JM. Coenzyme Q10 and congestive heart failure: an evolving evidence base. Kardiol Pol. 2015;73(2):73–9.
71. Folkers K, Vadhanavikit S, Mortensen SA. Biochemical rationale and myocardial tissue data on the effective therapy of cardiomyopathy with coenzyme Q10. Proc Natl Acad Sci U S A. 1985;82:901–4.
72. Kitamura N, Yamaguchi A, Otaki M, Sawatani O, Minoji T, Tamura H, Atobe M. Myocardial tissue level of coenzyme Q10 in patients with cardiac failure. Biomedical and Clinical Aspects of Coenzyme Q. 1984;4:221–9.
73. Judy WV, Stogsdill WW, Folkers K. Myocardial preservation by therapy with coenzyme Q10 during heart surgery. Clin Investig. 1993;71(S):155–61.
74. Weber C, Bysted A, Hǿlmer G. The coenzyme Q10 content of the average Danish diet. Int J Vitam Nutr Res. 1997;67(2):123–9.
75. Onur S, Niklowitz P, Jacobs G, et al. Association between serum level of ubiquinol and NT-proBNP, a marker for chronic heart failure, in healthy elderly subjects. Biofactors. 2015;41(1):35–43.
76. Mortensen SA, Rosenfeldt F, Kumar A, Dolliner P, Filipiak KJ, Pella D, Alehagen U, Steurer G, Littarru GP, Q-SYMBIO Study Investigators. The effect of coenzyme Q10 on morbidity and mortality in chronic heart failure: results from Q-SYMBIO: a randomized double-blind trial. JACC Heart Fail. 2014;2(6):641–9.
77. Lei L, Liu Y. Efficacy of coenzyme Q10 in patients with cardiac failure: a meta-analysis of clinical trials. BMC Cardiovasc Disord. 2017;17(1):196.
78. Fotino AD, Thompson-Paul AM, Bazzano LA. Effect of coenzyme Q10 supplementation on heart failure: a meta-analysis. Am J Clin Nutr. 2013;97(2):268–75.
79. Sander S, Coleman CI, Patel AA, Kluger J, White CM. The impact of coenzyme Q10 on systolic function in patients with chronic heart failure. J Card Fail. 2006;12(6):464–72.
80. Belardinelli R, Mucaj A, Lacalaprice F, Solenghi M, Principi F, Tiano L, Littarru GP. Coenzyme Q10 improves contractility of dysfunctional myocardium in chronic heart failure. Biofactors. 2005;25:137–45.
81. Munkholm H, Hansen HH, Rasmussen K. Coenzyme Q10 treatment in serious heart failure. Biofactors. 1999;9:285–9.
82. Keogh A, Fenton S, Leslie C, Aboyoun C, Macdonald P, Zhao YC, Bailey M, Rosenfeldt F. Randomised double-blind, placebo-controlled trial of coenzyme Q, therapy in class II and III systolic heart failure. Heart Lung Circ. 2003;12:135–41.
83. Langsjoen PH. Lack of effect of coenzyme Q on left ventricular function in patients with congestive heart failure. J Am Coll Cardiol. 2000;35:816–7.
84. Sharifi N, Tabrizi R, Moosazadeh M, Mirhosseini N, Lankarani KB, Akbari M, Chamani M, Kolahdooz F, Asemi Z. The effects of coenzyme Q10 supplementation on lipid profiles among patients with metabolic diseases: a systematic review and meta-analysis of randomized controlled trials. Curr Pharm Des. 2018; https://doi.org/10.2174/1381612824666180406104516.
85. Sahebkar A, Simental-Mendia LE, Stefanutti C, Pirro M. Supplementation with coenzyme Q10 reduces plasma lipoprotein(a) concentrations but not other lipid indices: a systematic review and meta-analysis. Pharmacol Res. 2016;105:198–209.
86. Alehagen U, Johansson P, Aaseth J, Alexander J, Brismar K. Increase in insulin-like growth factor 1 (IGF-1) and insulin-like growth factor binding protein 1 after supplementation with

selenium and coenzyme Q10. A prospective randomized double-blind placebo-controlled trial among elderly Swedish citizens. PLoS One. 2017;12:e0178614.

87. Fan L, Feng Y, Chen GC, Qin LQ, Fu CL, Chen LH. Effects of coenzyme Q10 supplementation on inflammatory markers: a systematic review and meta-analysis of randomized controlled trials. Pharmacol Res. 2017;119:128–36.

88. Zhai J, Bo Y, Lu Y, Liu C, Zhang L. Effects of coenzyme Q10 on markers of inflammation: a systematic review and meta-analysis. PLoS One. 2017;12:e0170172.

89. de Frutos F, Gea A, Hernandez-Estefania R, Rabago G. Prophylactic treatment with coenzyme Q10 in patients undergoing cardiac surgery: could an antioxidant reduce complications? a systematic review and meta-analysis. Interact Cardiovasc Thorac Surg. 2015;20:254–9.

90. Pauly DF, Pepine CJ. D-ribose as a supplement for cardiac energy metabolism. J Cardiovasc Pharmacol Therapeut. 2000;5(4):249–58. 11

91. JA SC, Bianco RW, Schneider JR, Mahoney JR Jr, Tveter K, Einzig S, Foker JE. Enhanced high energy phosphate recovery with ribose infusion after global myocardial ischemia in a canine model. J Surg Res. 1989;46(2):157–62.

92. Zimmer HG. Normalization of depressed heart function in rats by ribose. Science. 1983;220(4592):81–2.

93. Schneider J, St Cyr J, Mahoney J. Recovery of ATP and return of function after global ischemia. Circulation. 1985;72(Suppl III):298.

94. Omran H, Illien S, MacCarter D, St Cyr J, Lüderitz B. D-ribose improves diastolic function and quality of life in congestive heart failure patients: a prospective feasibility study. Eur J Heart Fail. 2003;5:615–9.

95. Vijay N, MacCarter D, Shecterle LM. D-ribose benefits heart failure patients. J Med Food. 2008;11(1):199–200.

96. Bayram M, St Cyr JA, Abraham WT. D-ribose aids heart failure patients with preserved ejection fraction and diastolic dysfunction: a pilot study. Ther Adv Cardiovasc Dis. 2015;9(3):56–65.

97. Pliml W, von Arnim T, Stablein A, Hofmann H, Zimmer HG, Erdmann E. Effects of ribose on exercise-induced ischaemia in stable coronary artery disease. Lancet. 1992;340:507–10.

98. Perkowski D, Wagner S, Marcus A. D-ribose improves cardiac indices in patients undergoing "off" pump coronary arterial revascularization. J Surg Res. 2007;137(2):295.

99. Vance R, Einzig S, Kreisler K. D-ribose maintains ejection fraction following aortic valve surgery. FASEB J. 2000;14(4):A419. (NIENTE LAVORO INTEGRALE?)

100. Jimenez K, Kulnigg-Dabsch S, Gasche C. Management of Iron Deficiency Anemia. Gastroenterol Hepatol. 2015;11(4):241–50.

101. Jankowska EA, Rozentryt P, Witkowska A, Nowak J, Hartmann O, Ponikowska B, Borodulin-Nadzieja L, von Haehling S, Doehner W, Banasiak W, Polonski L, Filippatos G, Anker SD, Ponikowski P. Iron deficiency predicts impaired exercise capacity in patients with systolic chronic heart failure. J Card Fail. 2011;17:899–906.

102. Tkaczyszyn M, Comín-Colet J, Voors AA, van Veldhuisen DJ, Enjuanes C, Moliner Borja P, Rozentryt P, Poloński L, Banasiak W, Ponikowski P, van der Meer P, Jankowska EA. Iron deficiency and red cell indices in patients with heart failure. Eur J Heart Fail. 2017;20:114–22.

103. Van Aelst LNL, Abraham M, Sadoune M, Lefebvre T, Manivet P, Logeart D. Iron status and inflammatory biomarkers in patients with acutely decompensated heart failure: Early in-hospital phase and 30-day follow-up. Eur J Heart Fail. 2017;19:1075–6.

104. Cohen-Solal A, Damy T, Hanon O, Terbah M, Laperche T, Kerebel S. High prevalence of iron deficiency in patients admitted for acute decompensated heart failure: A french study (CardioFer). J Am Coll Cardiol. 2014;63:A779. pp. Presentation Number: 1114-183. (mai pubblicato in extensor???)

105. Okonko DO, Mandal AK, Missouris CG, Poole-Wilson PA. Disordered iron homeostasis in chronic heart failure: prevalence, predictors, and relation to anemia, exercise capacity, and survival. J Am Coll Cardiol. 2011;58:1241–51.

106. Ganz T, Nemeth E. Iron imports. IV. Hepcidin and regulation of body iron metabolism. Am J Physiol Gastrointest Liver Physiol. 2006;290:G199–203.
107. Hughes CM, Woodside JV, McGartland C, Roberts MJ, Nicholls DP, McKeown PP. Nutritional intake and oxidative stress in chronic heart failure. Nutr Metab Cardiovasc Dis. 2012;22:376–82.
108. Lewis GD, Malhotra R, Hernandez AF, McNulty SE, Smith A, Felker GM, Tang WHW, LaRue SJ, Redfield MM, Semigran MJ, Givertz MM, Van Buren P, Whellan D, Anstrom KJ, Shah MR, Desvigne-Nickens P, Butler J, Braunwald E, NHLBI Heart Failure Clinical Research Network. Effect of oral iron repletion on exercise capacity in patients with heart failure with reduced ejection fraction and iron deficiency: The IRONOUT HF randomized clinical trial. JAMA. 2017;317:1958–66.
109. McDonagh T, Macdougall IC. Iron therapy for the treatment of iron deficiency in chronic heart failure: Intravenous or oral? Eur J Heart Fail. 2015;17:248–62.
110. El-Hattab AW, Scaglia F. Disorders of carnitine biosynthesis and transport. Mol Genet Metab. 2015;116:107–12.
111. Katz AM. Is the failing heart energy depleted? Cardiol Clin. 1998;16(4):633–44. https://doi.org/10.1016/S0733-8651(05)70040-0.
112. Blanca AJ, Ruiz-Armenta MV, Zambrano S, Miguel-Carrasco JL, Arias JL, Arévalo M, Mate A, Aramburu O, Vázquez CM. Inflammatory and fibrotic processes are involved in the cardiotoxic effect of sunitinib: protective role of L-carnitine. Toxicol Lett. 2016;241:9–18.
113. Omori Y, Ohtani T, Sakata Y, Mano T, Takeda Y, Tamaki S, Tsukamoto Y, Kamimura D, Aizawa Y, Miwa T, Komuro I, Soga T, Yamamoto K. L-Carnitine prevents the development of ventricular fibrosis and heart failure with preserved ejection fraction in hypertensive heart disease. J Hypertens. 2012;30(9):1834–44.
114. Flanagan JL, Simmons PA, Vehige J, Willcox MD, Garrett Q. Role of carnitine in disease. Nutr Metab. 2010;7:30. https://doi.org/10.1186/1743-7075-7-30.
115. Orlandi A, Francesconi A, Ferlosio A, Di Lascio A, Marcellini M, Pisano C, Spagnoli LG. Propionyl-L-carnitine prevents age-related myocardial remodeling in the rabbit. J Cardiovasc Pharmacol. 2007;50(2):168–75.
116. Dzugkoev SG, Mozhaeva IV, Otiev MA, Margieva OI, Dzugkoeva FS. Effect of L-carnitine, afobazole and their combination with L-arginine on biochemical and histological indices of endothelial dysfunctions in cobalt intoxication in rats. Patologicheskaia fiziologiia i eksperimental'naia terapiia. 2015;59(2):70–5.
117. Koc A, Ozkan T, Karabay AZ, Sunguroglu A, Aktan F. Effect of L-carnitine on the synthesis of nitric oxide in RAW 264·7 murine macrophage cell line. Cell Biochem Funct. 2011;29(8):679–85. https://doi.org/10.1002/cbf.1807.
118. DiNicolantonio JJ, Lavie CJ, Fares H, Menezes AR, O'Keefe JH. L-carnitine in the secondary prevention of cardiovascular disease: systematic review and meta-analysis. Mayo Clin Proc. 2013;88(6):544–51.
119. Song X, Qu H, Yang Z, Rong J, Cai W, Zhou H. Efficacy and safety of L-carnitine treatment for chronic heart failure: a meta-analysis of randomized controlled trials. Biomed Res Int. 2017;2017:6274854.
120. Mazidi M, Rezaie P, Banach M. Impact of L-carnitine on C-reactive protein: a systematic review and meta-analysis of 10 randomized control trials with 925 patients. Presentation at 2nd CPPEI Congress in Vienna, July 2017.
121. Pooyandjoo M, Nouhi M, Shab-Bidar S, Djafarian K, Olyaeemanesh A. The effect of (L-) carnitine on weight loss in adults: a systematic review and meta-analysis of randomized controlled trials. Obes Rev. 2016;17:970–6.
122. Serban MC, Sahebkar A, Mikhailidis DP, Toth PP, Jones SR, Muntner P, Blaha MJ, Andrica F, Martin SS, Borza C, Lip GY, Ray KK, Rysz J, Hazen SL, Banach M. Impact of L-carnitine on plasma lipoprotein(a) concentrations: a systematic review and meta-analysis of randomized controlled trials. Sci Rep. 2016;6:19188.

123. Boldyrev AA, Aldini G, Derave W. Physiology and pathophysiology of carnosine. Physiol Rev. 2013;93:1803–45.
124. Sale C, Saunders B, Harris RC. Effect of beta-alanine supplementation on muscle carnosine concentrations and exercise performance. Amino Acids. 2010;39:321–33.
125. Kohen R, Yamamoto Y, Cundy KC, Ames BN. Antioxidant activity of carnosine, homocarnosine, and anserine present in muscle and brain. Proc Natl Acad Sci U S A. 1988;85:3175–9.
126. Kang JH, Kim KS, Choi SY, Kwon HY, Won MH, Kang TC. Protective effects of carnosine, homocarnosine and anserine against peroxyl radical-mediated Cu,Zn-superoxide dismutase modification. Biochim Biophys Acta. 2002;1570(2):89–96.
127. Pavlov AR, Revina AA, Dupin AM, Boldyrev AA, Yaropolov AI. The mechanism of interaction of carnosine with superoxide radicals in water solutions. Biochim Biophys Acta. 1993;1157:304–12.
128. Zaloga GP, Roberts PR, Black KW, Lin M, Zapata-Sudo G, Sudo RT, Nelson TE. Carnosine is a novel peptide modulator of intracellular calcium and contractility in cardiac cells. Am J Physiol. 1997;272(1 Pt 2):H462–8.
129. Bokeriya LA, Boldyrev AA, Movsesyan RR, Alikhanov SA, Arzumanyan ES, Nisnevich ED, Artyukhina TV, Serov RA. Cardioprotective effect of histidine-containing dipeptides in pharmacological cold cardioplegia. Bull Exp Biol Med. 2008;145:323–7.
130. Lombardi C, Carubelli V, Lazzarini V, Vizzardi E, Quinzani F, Guidetti F, Rovetta R, Nodari S, Gheorghiade M, Metra M. Effects of oral amino acid supplements on functional capacity in patients with chronic heart failure. Clin Med Insights Cardiol. 2014;8:39–44.
131. Rosenfeldt FL. Metabolic supplementation with orotic acid and magnesium orotate. Cardiovasc Drugs Ther. 1998;12(Suppl 2):147–52.
132. Stepura OB, Martynow AI. Magnesium orotate in severe congestive heart failure (MACH). Int J Cardiol. 2009;134:145–7.
133. McCarty MF, Di Nicolantonio JJ. β-Alanine and orotate as supplements for cardiac protection. Open Heart. 2014;1(1):e000119.
134. Artioli GG, Gualano B, Smith A, Stout J, Lancha AH Jr. Role of beta-alanine supplementation on muscle carnosine and exercise performance. Med Sci Sports Exerc. 2010;42:1162–73.
135. Decombaz J, Beaumont M, Vuichoud J, Bouisset F, Stellingwerff T. Effect of slow-release beta-alanine tablets on absorption kinetics and paresthesia. AminoAcids. 2012;43:67–76.
136. Rude RK. Physiology of magnesium metabolism and the important role of magnesium in potassium deficiency. Am J Cardiol. 1989;63:31–4.
137. Gattlieb SS. Importance of magnesium in congestive heart failure. Am J Cardiol. 1989;63:39–42.
138. Ralston MA, Mumane MR, Unverferth DV, Leier CV. Serum and tissue magnesium concentrations in patients with heart failure and serious ventricular arrhythmias. Ann Intern Med. 1990;113:841–6.
139. Douban S, Brodsky MA, Whang DD, Whang R. Significance of magnesium congestive heart failure. Am Heart J. 1996;132:664–71.
140. Wester PO. Electrolyte balance in heart failure and the role of magnesium ions. Am J Cardiol. 1992;70:44–9.
141. Wu X, Ackermann U, Sonnenberg H. Potassium depletion and salt-sensitive hypertension in DAHL rats: effect on calcium, magnesium, and phosphate excretions. Clin Exp Hypertens. 1995;17:989–1008.
142. Douban S, Brodsky MA, Whang DD, Whang R. Significance of magnesium in congestive heart failure. Am Heart J. 1996;132(3):664–71.
143. Witte KKA, Nikitin NP, Parker AC, von Haehling S, Volk H-D, Anker SD, Clark AL, Cleland JGF. The effect of micronutrient supplementation on quality-of-life and left ventricular function in elderly patients with chronic heart failure. Eur Heart J. 2005;26:2238–44.
144. Almoznino-Sarafian D, Sarafian G, Berman S, Shteinshnaider M, Tzur I, Cohen N, Gorelik O. Magnesium administration may improve heart rate variability in patients with heart failure. Nutr Metab Cardiovasc Dis. 2009;19:641–5.

145. He K, Liu K, Daviglus ML, Morris SJ, Loria CM, Van Horn L, Jacobs DR, Savage PJ. Magnesium intake and incidence of metabolic syndrome among young adults. Circulation. 2006;113:1675–82.
146. Song Y, He K, Levitan EB, Manson JE, Liu S. Effects of oral magnesium supplementation on glycaemic control in type 2 diabetes: a meta-analysis of randomized double-blind controlled trials. Diabet Med. 2006;23:1050–6.
147. Lee SH, Miller ER, Guallar E, Singh VK, Appel LJ, Klag MJ. The effect of magnesium supplementation on blood pressure: a meta-analysis of randomized clinical trials. Am J Hypertens. 2002;15:691–6.
148. Misialek JR, Lopez FL, Lutsey PL, Huxley RR, Peacock JM, Chen LY, Soliman EZ, Agarwal SK, Alonso A. Serum and dietary magnesium and incidence of atrial fibrillation in whites and in African Americans; Atherosclerosis Risk in Communities (ARIC) Study. Circ J. 2013;77:323–9.
149. Gottlieb SS, Baruch L, Kukin ML, Bemstein JL, Fisher ML, Packer M. Prognostic importance of the serum magnesium concentration in patients with congestive heart failure. J Am Cardiol. 1990;6:827–83.
150. Altura BM, Altura BT. Biochemistry and pathophysiology of congestive heart failure: is there a role for magnesium. Magnesium. 1986;5:134–43.
151. Lutsey PL, Alonso A, Michos ED, Loehr LR, Astor BC, Coresh J, Folsom AR. Serum magnesium, phosphorus, and calcium are associated with risk of incident heart failure: the Atherosclerosis Risk in Communities (ARIC) Study. Am J Clin Nutr. 2014;100(3):756–64.
152. Arinzon Z, Peisakh A, Schrire S, Berner YN. Prevalence of hypomagnesemia (HM) in a geriatric long-term care (LTC) setting. Arch Gerontol Geriatr. 2010;51:36–40.
153. Adamopoulos C, Pitt B, Sui X, Love TE, Zannad F, Ahmed A. Low serum magnesium and cardiovascular mortality in chronic heart failure: a propensity-matched study. Int J Cardiol. 2009;136:270–7.
154. Wannamethee SG, Papacosta O, Lennon L, Whincup PH. Serum magnesium and risk of incident heart failure in older men: The British Regional Heart Study. Eur J Epidemiol. 2018;33(9):873–82. https://doi.org/10.1007/s10654-018-0388-6.
155. Taveira TH, Ouellette D, Gulum A, Choudhary G, Eaton CB, Liu S, Wu WC. Relation of magnesium intake with cardiac function and heart failure hospitalizations in Black adults: the Jackson heart study. Circ Heart Fail. 2016;9(4):e002698.
156. Song EK, Kang SM. Micronutrient deficiency independently predicts adverse health outcomes in patients with heart failure. J Cardiovasc Nurs. 2017;32(1):47–53.
157. Angkananard T, Anothaisintawee T, Eursiriwan S, Gorelik O, McEvoy M, Attia J, Thakkinstian A. The association of serum magnesium and mortality outcomes in heart failure patients: a systematic review and meta-analysis. Medicine. 2016;95(50):e5406.
158. Lopez FL, Agarwal SK, Grams ME, Loehr LR, Soliman EZ, Lutsey PL, Chen LY, Huxley RR, Alonso A. Relation of serum phosphorus levels to the incidence of atrial fibrillation (from the Atherosclerosis Risk in Communities [ARIC] Study). Am J Cardiol. 2013;111:857–62.
159. Khan AM, Lubitz SA, Sullivan LM, Sun JX, Levy D, Vasan RS, Magnani JW, Ellinor PT, Benjamin EJ, Wang TJ. Low serum magnesium and the development of atrial fibrillation in the community: the Framingham Heart Study. Circulation. 2013;127:33–8.
160. Wang TJ, Larson MG, Levy D, Vasan RS, Leip EP, Wolf PA, D'Agostino RB, Murabito JM, Kannel WB, Benjamin EJ. Temporal relations of atrial fibrillation and congestive heart failure and their joint influence on mortality: the Framingham Heart Study. Circulation. 2003;107:2920–5.
161. Chamberlain AM, Redfield MM, Alonso A, Weston SA, Roger VL. Atrial fibrillation and mortality in heart failure: a community study. Circ Heart Fail. 2011;4:740–6.
162. Rude RK. Magnesium. In: Coates PM, Betz JM, Blackman MR, Cragg GM, editors. Encyclopedia of dietary supplements. New York: Informa Healthcare; 2010. p. 527–37.
163. Fang X, Wang K, Han D, He X, Wei J, Zhao L, Imam MU, Ping Z, Li Y, Xu Y, Min J, Wang F. Dietary magnesium intake and the risk of cardiovascular disease, type 2 diabetes, and

all-cause mortality: a dose-response meta-analysis of prospective cohort studies. BMC Med. 2016;14(1):210.
164. Urso C, Brucculeri S, Caimi G. Acid-base and electrolyte abnormalities in heart failure: pathophysiology and implications. Heart Fail Rev. 2015;20(4):493–503.
165. Khairallah RJ, Sparagna GC, Khanna N, O'Shea KM, Hecker PA, Kristian T, Fiskum G, Des Rosiers C, Polster BM, Stanley WC. Dietary supplementation with docosahexaenoic acid, but not eicosapentaenoic acid, dramatically alters cardiac mitochondrial phospholipid fatty acid composition and prevents permeability transition. Biochim Biophys Acta. 2010;1797:1555–62.
166. Khairallah RJ, Kim J, O'Shea KM, O'Connell KA, Brown BH, Galvao T, Daneault C, Des Rosiers C, Polster BM, Hoppel CL, Stanley WC. Improved mitochondrial function with diet induced increase in either docosahexaenoic acid or arachidonic acid in membrane phospholipids. PLoS One. 2012;7:e34402.
167. O'Shea KM, Khairallah RJ, Sparagna GC, Xu W, Hecker PA, Robillard-Frayne I, Des Rosiers C, Kristian T, Murphy RC, Fiskum G, Stanley WC. Dietary omega 3 fatty acids alter cardiac mitochondrial phospholipid composition and delay Ca2+ induced permeability transition. J Mol Cell Cardiol. 2009;47:819–27.
168. Stanley WC, Khairallah RJ, Dabkowski ER. Update on lipids and mitochondrial function: impact of dietary n 3 polyunsaturated fatty acids. Curr Opin Clin Nutr Metab Care. 2012;15:122–6.
169. Chrysohoou C, Metallinos G, Georgiopoulos G, Mendrinos D, Papanikolaou A, N M, Pitsavos C, Vyssoulis G, Stefanadis C, Tousoulis D. Short term omega-3 polyunsaturated fatty acid supplementation induces favorable changes in right ventricle function and diastolic filling pressure in patients with chronic heart failure; a randomized clinical trial. Vascul Pharmacol. 2016;79:43–50.
170. Cicero AF, Ertek S, Borghi C. Omega-3 polyunsaturated fatty acids: their potential role in blood pressure prevention and management. Curr Vasc Pharmacol. 2009;7(3):330–7.
171. Wilk JB, Tsai MY, Hanson NQ, Gaziano JM, Djoussé L. Plasma and dietary omega-3 fatty acids, fish intake, and heart failure risk in the Physicians' Health Study. Am J Clin Nutr. 2012;96(4):882–8.
172. Bayer AL, Heidkamp MC, Patel N, Porter M, Engman S, Samarel AM. Alterations in protein kinase C isoenzyme expression and autophosphorylation during the progression of pressure overload-induced left ventricular hypertrophy. Mol Cell Biochem. 2003;242:145–52.
173. Djoussé L, Akinkuolie AO, Wu JH, Ding EL, Gaziano JM. Fish consumption, omega-3 fatty acids and risk of heart failure: a meta-analysis. Clin Nutr. 2012;31(6):846–53.
174. Tavazzi L, Maggioni AP, Marchioli R, Barlera S, Franzosi MG, Latini R, Lucci D, Nicolosi GL, Porcu M, Tognoni G, Gissi-HF Investigators. Effect of n-3 polyunsaturated fatty acids in patients with chronic heart failure (the GISSI-HF trial): a randomised, doubleblind, placebo-controlled trial. Lancet. 2008;372(9645):1223–30.
175. Ghio S, Scelsi L, Latini R, Masson S, Eleuteri E, Palvarini M, Vriz O, Pasotti M, Gorini M, Marchioli R, Maggioni A, Tavazzi L. GISSI-HF investigators.. Effects of n-3 polyunsaturated fatty acids and of rosuvastatin on left ventricular function in chronic heart failure: a substudy of GISSI-HF trial. Eur J Heart Fail. 2010;12(12):1345–53.
176. Maki KC, Palacios OM, Bell M, Toth PP. Use of supplemental long-chain omega-3 fatty acids and risk for cardiac death: an updated meta-analysis and review of research gaps. J Clin Lipidol. 2017;11(5):1152–1160.e2.
177. Dabkowski ER, O'Connell KA, Xu W, Ribeiro RF Jr, Hecker PA, Shekar KC, Daneault C, Des Rosiers C, Stanley WC. Docosahexaenoic acid supplementation alters key properties of cardiac mitochondria and modestly attenuates development of left ventricular dysfunction in pressure overload-induced heart failure. Cardiovasc Drugs Ther. 2013;27(6):499–510.
178. Moertl D, Hammer A, Steiner S, Hutuleac R, Vonbank K, Berger R. Dose-dependent effects of omega-3-polyunsaturated fatty acids on systolic left ventricular function, endothelial func-

tion, and markers of inflammation in chronic heart failure of non ischemic origin: a double-blind, placebo-controlled, 3-arm study. Am Heart J. 2011;161(5):915.e1–9.

179. Oikonomou E, Vogiatzi G, Karlis D, Siasos G, Chrysohoou C, Zografos T, Lazaros G, Tsalamandris S, Mourouzis K, Georgiopoulos G, Toutouza M, Tousoulis D. Effects of omega-3 polyunsaturated fatty acids on fibrosis, endothelial function and myocardial performance, in ischemic heart failure patients. Clin Nutr. 2018 May 3. pii: S0261–5614(18)30168-7.

180. Mehra MR, Lavie CJ, Ventura HO, Milani RV. Fish oils produce anti-inflammatory effects and improve body weight in severe heart failure. J Heart Lung Transplant. 2006;25:834–8.

181. Pepe S, McLennan PL. Cardiac membrane fatty acid composition modulates myocardial oxygen consumption and postischemic recovery of contractile function. Circulation. 2002;105:2303–8.

182. Cicero AF, Reggi A, Parini A, Borghi C. Application of polyunsaturated fatty acids in internal medicine: beyond the established cardiovascular effects. Arch Med Sci. 2012;8:784–93.

183. Trumbo P, Schlicker S, Yates AA, Poos M, Food and Nutrition Board of the Institute of Medicine, The National Academies. Dietary reference intakes for energy, carbohydrate, fiber, fat, fatty acids, cholesterol, protein and amino acids. J Am Diet Assoc. 2002;102:1621–30.

184. Nagatomo Y, Tang WH. Intersections between microbiome and heart failure: revisiting the gut hypothesis. J Card Fail. 2015;21(12):973–80.

185. Sandek A, Bjarnason I, Volk HD, Crane R, Meddings JB, Niebauer J, Kalra PR, Buhner S, Herrmann R, Springer J, Doehner W, von Haehling S, Anker SD, Rauchhaus M. Studies on bacterial endotoxin and intestinal absorption function in patients with chronic heart failure. Int J Cardiol. 2012;157(1):80–5.

186. Krack A, Sharma R, Figulla HR, Anker SD. The importance of the gastrointestinal system in the pathogenesis of heart failure. Eur Heart J. 2005;26(22):2368–74.

187. Wang Z, Klipfell E, Bennett BJ, Koeth R, Levison BS, Dugar B, Feldstein AE, Britt EB, Fu X, Chung YM, Wu Y, Schauer P, Smith JD, Allayee H, Tang WH, DiDonato JA, Lusis AJ, Hazen SL. Gut flora metabolism of phosphatidylcholine promotes cardiovascular disease. Nature. 2011;472:57–63.

188. Koeth RA, Wang Z, Levison BS, Buffa JA, Org E, Sheehy BT, Britt EB, Fu X, Wu Y, Li L, Smith JD, DiDonato JA, Chen J, Li H, Wu GD, Lewis JD, Warrier M, Brown JM, Krauss RM, Tang WH, Bushman FD, Lusis AJ, Hazen SL. Intestinal microbiota metabolism of l-carnitine, a nutrient in red meat, promotes atherosclerosis. Nat Med. 2013;19:576–85.

189. Wilson TWH, Zeneng W, Yiying F, Levison B, Hazen JE, Donahue LM, Wu Y, Hazen S. Prognostic value of elevated levels of intestinal microbe-generated metabolite trimethylamine-n-oxide in patients with heart failure. J Am Coll Cardiol. 2014;64(18):1908–14.

190. Shih DM, Wang Z, Lee R, Meng Y, Che N, Charugundla S, Qi H, Wu J, Pan C, Brown JM, Vallim T, Bennett BJ, Graham M, Hazen SL, Lusis AJ. Flavin containing monooxygenase 3 exerts broad effects on glucose and lipid metabolism and atherosclerosis. J Lipid Res. 2015;56(1):22–37.

191. Hartiala J, Bennett BJ, Tang WH, Wang Z, Stewart AF, Roberts R, McPherson R, Lusis AJ, Hazen SL, Allayee H, CARDIoGRAM Consortium. Comparative genome-wide association studies in mice and humans for trimethylamine Noxide, a proatherogenic metabolite of choline and L-carnitine. Arterioscler Thromb Vasc Biol. 2014;34(6):1307–13.

192. Costanza AC, Moscavitch SD, Faria Neto HC, Mesquita ET. Probiotic therapy with Saccharomyces boulardii for heart failure patients: a randomized, double-blind, placebo-controlled pilot trial. Int J Cardiol. 2015;179:348–50.

193. Gan XT, Ettinger G, Huang CX, Burton JP, Haist JV, Rajapurohitam V, Sidaway JE, Martin G, Gloor GB, Swann JR, Reid G, Karmazyn M. Probiotic administration attenuates myocardial hypertrophy and heart failure after myocardial infarction in the rat. Circ Heart Fail. 2014;7(3):491–9.

194. Khalesi S, Sun J, Buys N, Jayasinghe R. Effect of probiotics on blood pressure: a systematic review and meta analysis of randomized, controlled trials. Hypertension. 2014;64:897–903.

195. Wang L, Guo MJ, Gao Q, Yang JF, Yang L, Pang XL, Jiang XJ. The effects of probiotics on total cholesterol: a meta-analysis of randomized controlled trials. Medicine. 2018;97(5):e9679.
196. He M, Shi B. Gut microbiota as a potential target of metabolic syndrome: the role of probiotics and prebiotics. Cell Biosci. 2017;7:54.
197. Crommen S, Simon MC. Microbial regulation of glucose metabolism and insulin resistance. Gen. 2017;9(1) pii: E10
198. Robles-Vera I, Toral M, Romero M, Jiménez R, Sánchez M, Pérez-Vizcaíno F, Duarte J. Antihypertensive effects of probiotics. Curr Hypertens Rep. 2017;19(4):26.
199. Upadrasta A, Madempudi RS. Probiotics and blood pressure: current insights. Integr Blood Press Control. 2016;9:33–42.
200. Young RC, Blass JP. Iatrogenic nutritional deficiencies. Annu Rev Nutr. 1982;2:201–27.
201. Lonsdale D. Thiamin. Adv Food Nutr Res. 2018;83:1–56. https://doi.org/10.1016/bs.afnr.2017.11.001.
202. Pfitzenmeyer P, Guilland JC, d'Athis P, Petit-Marnier C, Gaudet M. Thiamine status of elderly patients with cardiac failure including the effects of supplementation. Int J Vitam Nutr Res. 1994;64(2):113–8.
203. Jain A, Mehta R, Al-Ani M, Hill JA, Winchester DE. Determining the role of thiamine deficiency in systolic heart failure: a metaanalysis and systematic review. J Card Fail. 2015;21(12):1000–7.
204. Katta N, Balla S, Alpert MA. Does long-term furosemide therapy cause thiamine deficiency in patients with heart failure? a focused review. Am J Med. 2016;129(7):753.e11.
205. Dabar G, Harmouche C, Habr B, Riachi M, Jaber B. Shoshin beriberi in critically-ill patients: case series. Nutr J. 2015;14(1):51.
206. Lei Y, Zheng M, Huang W, Zhang J, Lu Y. Wet beriberi with multiple organ failure remarkably reversed by thiamine administration: a case report and literature review. Medicine. 2018;97(9):e0010.
207. Jikrona R, Suharjono S, Ahmad A. Thiamine supplement therapy improves ejection fraction value in stage ii heart failure patients. Folia Medica Indon. 2017;53(2):139–43.
208. Shimon H, Almog S, Vered Z, Seligmann H, Shefi M, Peleg E, Rosenthal T, Motro M, Halkin H, Ezra D. Improved left ventricular function after thiamine supplementation in patients with congestive heart failure receiving long-term furosemide therapy. Am J Med. 1995;98(5):485–90.
209. Schoenenberger A, Schoenenberger-Berzins R, der Maur C, Suter P, Vergopoulos A, Erne P. Thiamine supplementation in symptomatic chronic heart failure: a randomized, double-blind, placebo-controlled, cross-over pilot study. Clin Res Cardiol. 2012;101(3):159–64.
210. Dinicolantonio JJ, Lavie CJ, Niazi AK, O'Keefe JH, Hu T. Effects of thiamine on cardiac function in patients with systolic heart failure: systematic review and metaanalysis of randomized, doubleblind, placebo-controlled trials. Ochsner J. 2013;13(4):495–9.
211. Mousavi M, Namazi S, Avadi M, Amirahmadi M, Salehifar D. Thiamine supplementation in patients with chronic heart failure receiving optimum medical treatment. J Cardiol Curr Res. 2017;9(2):00316.
212. Rocha RM, Silva GV, de Albuquerque DC, Tura BR, Albanesi Filho FM. Influence of spironolactone therapy on thiamine blood levels in patients with heart failure. Arq Bras Cardiol. 2008;90(5):324–8.
213. Kattoor AJ, Goel A, Mehta JL. Thiamine therapy for heart failure: a promise or fiction? Cardiovasc Drugs Ther. 2018;32(4):313–7. https://doi.org/10.1007/s10557-018-6808-8.
214. Bruckdorfer KR. Antioxidants and CVD. Proc Nutr Soc. 2008;67:214–22.
215. Wilcox BJ, Curb JD, Rodriguez B. Antioxidants in cardiovascular health and disease: key lessons from epidemiologic studies. Am J Cardiol. 2008;101(S):75D–86D.
216. Djoussé L, Driver JA, Gaziano JM. Relation between modifiable lifestyle factors and lifetime risk of heart failure. JAMA. 2009;302:394–400.
217. Levitan EB, Wolk A, Mittleman MA. Consistency with the DASH diet and incidence of heart failure. Arch Intern Med. 2009;169:851–7.

218. Wang Y, Tuomilehto J, Jousilahti P, Antikainen R, Mähönen M, Katzmarzyk PT, Hu G. Lifestyle factors in relation to heart failure among Finnish men and women. Circ Heart Fail. 2011;4:607–12.
219. Pfister R, Sharp SJ, Luben R, Wareham NJ, Khaw KT. Plasma vitamin C predicts incident heart failure in men and women in European Prospective Investigation into Cancer and Nutrition-Norfolk Prospective Study. Am Heart J. 2011;162:246–53.
220. Bingham SA, Welch AA, McTaggart A, Mulligan AA, Runswick SA, Luben R, Oakes S, Khaw KT, Wareham N, Day NE. Nutritional methods in the European Prospective Investigation of Cancer in Norfolk. Public Health Nutr. 2001;4:847–58.
221. Plantinga Y, Ghiadoni L, Magagna A, Giannarelli C, Franzoni F, Taddei S, Salvetti A. Supplementation with vitamins C and E improves arterial stiffness and endothelial function in essential hypertensive patients. Am J Hypertens. 2007;20:392–7.
222. Wannamethee SG, Bruckdorfer KR, Shaper AG, Papacosta O, Lennon L, Whincup PH. Plasma vitamin C, but not vitamin E, is associated with reduced risk of heart failure in older men. Circ Heart Fail. 2013;6(4):647–54.
223. Song EK, Kang SM. Vitamin C deficiency, high-sensitivity C-reactive protein, and cardiac event-free survival in patients with heart failure. J Cardiovasc Nurs. 2018;33(1):6–12.
224. Ashor AW, Lara J, Mathers JC, Siervo M. Effect of vitamin C on endothelial function in health and disease: a systematic review and meta-analysis of randomised controlled trials. Atherosclerosis. 2014;235(1):9–20.
225. Spoelstra-de Man AME, Elbers PWG, Oudemans-Van Straaten HM. Vitamin C: should we supplement? Curr Opin Crit Care. 2018;24(4):248–55. https://doi.org/10.1097/MCC.0000000000000510.
226. Holick MF. Vitamin D deficiency. N Engl J Med. 2007;357:266–81.
227. Wang Y, Zhu J, DeLuca HF. Where is the vitamin D receptor? Arch Biochem Biophys. 2012;523:123–33.
228. O'Connell TD, Simpson RU. Immunochemical identification of the 1,25dihydroxyvitamin D3 receptor protein in human heart. Cell Biol Int. 1996;20:621–4.
229. Simpson RU, Thomas GA, Arnold AJ. Identification of 1,25-dihydroxyvitamin D3 receptors and activities in muscle. J Biol Chem. 1985;260:8882–91.
230. Kim DH, Sabour S, Sagar UN, Adams S, Whellan DJ. Prevalence of hypovitaminosis D in cardiovascular diseases (from the National Health and Nutrition Examination Survey 2001 to 2004). Am J Cardiol. 2008;102(11):1540–4.
231. Anderson JL, May HT, Horne BD, Bair TL, Hall NL, Carlquist JF, Lappé DL, Muhlestein JB. Intermountain Heart Collaborative (IHC) Study Group. Relation of vitamin D deficiency to cardiovascular risk factors, disease status, and incident events in a general health care population. Am J Cardiol. 2010;106(7):963–8.
232. Pilz S, Marz W, Wellnitz B, Seelhorst U, Fahrleitner-Pammer A, Dimai HP, Boehm BO, Dobnig H. Association of vitamin D deficiency with heart failure and sudden cardiac death in a large cross-sectional study of patients referred for coronary angiography. J Clin Endocrinol Metab. 2008;93(10):3927–35.
233. Liu LC, Voors AA, van Veldhuisen DJ, van der Veer E, Belonje AM, Szymanski MK, Silljé HH, van Gilst WH, Jaarsma T, de Boer RA. Vitamin D status and outcomes in heart failure patients. Eur J Heart Fail. 2011;13:619–25.
234. Pourdjabbar A, Dwivedi G, Haddad H. The role of vitamin D in chronic heart failure. Curr Opin Cardiol. 2013 Mar;28(2):216–22. https://doi.org/10.1097/HCO.0b013e32835bd480.
235. Iqba lN, Ducharme J, Desai S, Chambers S, Terembula K, Chan GW, Shults J, Leonard MB, Kumanyika S. Status of bone mineral density in patients selected for cardiac transplantation. Endocr Pract. 2008;14(6):704–12.
236. Alsafwah S, Laguardia SP, Nelson MD. Hypovitaminosis D in African Americans residing in Memphis, Tennessee with and without heart failure. Am J Med Sci. 2008;335(4):292–7.

237. Arroyo M, Laguardia SP, Bhattacharya SK, Nelson MD, Johnson PL, Carbone LD, Newman KP, Weber KT. Micronutrients in African-Americans with decompensated and compensated heart failure. Transl Res. 2006;148(6):301–8.
238. Zittermann A, Schleithoff SS, Gotting C, Dronow O, Fuchs U, Kuhn J, Kleesiek K, Tenderich G, Koerfer R. Poor outcome in end stage heart failure patients with low circulating calcitriol levels. Eur J Heart Fail. 2008;10(3):321–7.
239. Shane E, Mancini D, Aaronson K, Silverberg SJ, Seibel MJ, Addesso V, McMahon DJ. Bone mass, vitamin D deficiency, and hyperparathyroidism in congestive heart failure. Am J Med. 1997;103(3):197–207.
240. Boxer RS, Dauser DA, Walsh SJ, Hager WD, Kenny AM. The association between vitamin D and inflammation with the 6-minute walk and frailty in patients with heart failure. J Am Geriatr Soc. 2008;56(3):454–61.
241. Boxer RS, Kenny AM, Cheruvu VK, Vest M, Fiutem JJ, Pina II. Serum 25-hydroxyvitamin D concentration is associated with functional capacity in older adults with heart failure. Am Heart J. 2010;160(5):893–9.
242. Schleithoff SS, Zittermann A, Tenderich G, Berthold HK, Stehle P, Koerfer R. Vitamin D supplementation improves cytokine profiles in patients with congestive heart failure: a doubleblind, randomized, placebo-controlled trial. Am J Clin Nutr. 2006;83:754–9.
243. Shedeed SA. Vitamin D supplementation in infants with chronic congestive heart failure. Pediatr Cardiol. 2012;33:713–9.
244. Gotsman I, Shauer A, Zwas DR, Hellman Y, Keren A, Lotan C, Admon D. Vitamin D deficiency is a predictor of reduced survival in patients with heart failure; vitamin D supplementation improves outcome. Eur J Heart Fail. 2012;14:357–66.
245. Witham MD, Crighton LJ, Gillespie ND, Struthers AD, McMurdo ME. The effects of vitamin D supplementation on physical function and quality of life in older patients with heart failure: a randomized controlled trial. Circ Heart Fail. 2010;3:195–201.
246. Robien K, Oppeneer SJ, Kelly JA, Hamilton-Reeves JM. Drug-vitamin D interactions: a systematic review of the literature. Nutr Clin Pract. 2013;28(2):194–208.
247. Sawyer DB. Oxidative stress in heart failure: what are we missing? Am J Med Sci. 2011;342:120–4.
248. Li F, Tan W, Kang Z, Wong CW. Tocotrienol enriched palm oil prevents atherosclerosis through modulating the activities of peroxisome proliferators-activated receptors. Atherosclerosis. 2010;211:278–82.
249. Rasool AH, Rahman AR, Yuen KH, Wong AR. Arterial compliance and vitamin E blood levels with a self emulsifying preparation of tocotrienol rich vitamin E. Arch Pharm Res. 2008;31:1212–7.
250. Prasad K. Tocotrienols and cardiovascular health. Curr Pharm Des. 2011;17:2147–54.
251. Loffredo L, Perri L, Di Castelnuovo A, Iacoviello L, De Gaetano G, Violi F. Supplementation with vitamin E alone is associated with reduced myocardial infarction: a meta-analysis. Nutr Metab Cardiovasc Dis. 2015;25:354–63.
252. Chae CU, Albert CM, Moorthy MV, Lee IM, Buring JE. Vitamin E supplementation and the risk of heart failure in women. Circ Heart Fail. 2012;5:176–82.
253. Sesso HD, Buring JE, Christen WG, Kurth T, Belanger C, MacFadyen J, Bubes V, Manson JE, Glynn RJ, Gaziano JM, Vitamins E. C in the prevention of cardiovascular disease in men: the Physicians' Health Study II randomized controlled trial. JAMA. 2008;300:2123–33.
254. Marchioli R, Levantesi G, Macchia A, Marfisi RM, Nicolosi GL, Tavazzi L, Tognoni G, Valagussa F, GISSI-Prevenzione Investigators. Vitamin E increases the risk of developing heart failure after myocardial infarction: results from the GISSI-prevenzione trial. J Cardiovasc Med. 2006;7:347–50.
255. Lonn E, Bosch J, Yusuf S, Sheridan P, Pogue J, Arnold JM, Ross C, Arnold A, Sleight P, Probstfield J, Dagenais G, HOPE and HOPE-TOO Trial Investigators. Effects of long-term vitamin E supplementation on cardiovascular events and cancer: a randomized controlled trial. JAMA. 2005;293:1338–47.

256. Wannamethee SG, Bruckdorfer KR, Shaper AG, Papacosta O, Lennon L, Whincup PH. Plasma vitamin C, but not vitamin E, is associated with reduced risk of heart failure in older men. Circ Heart Fail. 2013 Jul;6(4):647–54.
257. Finkel T, Holbrook NJ. Oxidants, oxidative stress and the biology of ageing. Nature. 2000;408:239–47.
258. Deveraj D, Jialei I. Failure of vitamin E in clinical trials: is γ-tocopherol the answer? Nutr Rev. 2005;63:290–3.
259. Hodge AM, Simpson JA, Fridman M, Rowley K, English DR, Giles GG, Su Q, O'Dea K. Evaluation of an FFQ for assessment of antioxidant intake using plasma biomarkers in an ethnically diverse population. Public Health Nutr. 2009;12:2438–47.
260. Redfield MM, Jacobsen SJ, Burnett JC Jr, Mahoney DW, Bailey KR, Rodeheffer RJ. Burden of systolic and diastolic ventricular dysfunction in the community: appreciating the scope of the heart failure epidemic. JAMA. 2003;289(2):194–202.
261. Ambrosy AP, Fonarow GC, Butler J, et al. The global health and economic burden of hospitalizations for heart failure: lessons learned from hospitalized. J Am Coll Cardiol. 2014;63(12):1123–33.
262. Tuppin P, Rivière S, Rigault A, et al. Prevalence and economic burden of cardiovascular diseases in France in 2013 according to the national health insurance scheme database. Arch Cardiovasc Dis. 2016;109(6-7):399–411.
263. Cook C, Cole G, Asaria P, Jabbour R, Francis DP. The annual global economic burden of heart failure. Int J Cardiol. 2014;171(3):368–76.
264. Yao G, Freemantle N, Flather M, et al. Long-term cost-effectiveness analysis of Nebivolol compared with standard care in elderly patients with heart failure: an individual patient-based simulation model. Pharmacoeconomics. 2008;26:879–89.
265. Ghio S, Scelsi L, Latini R, et al. GISSI-HF investigators. Effects of n-3 polyunsaturated fatty acids and of rosuvastatin on left ventricular function in chronic heart failure: a substudy of GISSI-HF trial. Eur J Heart Fail. 2010;12(12):1345–53.

Chapter 12
Cardiovascular Risk Factors Management in Pregnancy: A Role for Nutraceuticals?

Federica Fogacci and Silvia Fogacci

Background

Cardiovascular disorders are the leading cause of indirect maternal mortality in European countries [1]. However, drug treatment in pregnancy is a very specific and sensitive problem [2]. As a matter of fact, if untreated diseases can lead to harmful consequences for mothers and their children, the use of some drugs can negatively affect the correct embryonic and fetal development and, in some cases, lead to abortion or intrauterine death [3].

Though non-pharmacological treatments have always been considered marginal in the management of cardiovascular risk factors in pregnancy, their role should be taken into account from the most recent evidence. As a matter of fact, randomized controlled clinical trials testing the efficacy and the safety of dietary supplements in pregnancy are many and their results seem to be promising [4, 5]. For this reason, their use in clinical practice should be encouraged in order to prevent the development of the gestational diabetes mellitus (GDM) and/or of the hypertensive disorders and to support the drug treatment, when necessary [6, 7].

In this context, the present chapter aims to summarise the available evidence supporting, in clinical practice, the use of some active compounds available as dietary supplements and having significant effect in the management of the cardiovascular risk factors in pregnancy.

F. Fogacci (✉)
Medical and Surgical Sciences Department, University of Bologna, Bologna, Italy

S. Fogacci
Medical and Surgical Sciences Department, University of Bologna, Bologna, Italy

© Springer Nature Switzerland AG 2021
A. F.G. Cicero, M. Rizzo (eds.), *Nutraceuticals and Cardiovascular Disease*,
Contemporary Cardiology, https://doi.org/10.1007/978-3-030-62632-7_12

Active Compounds

Calcium During pregnancy, the risk of hypertensive disorders can be prevented through an adequate calcium intake [8].

A meta-analysis by the Cochrane Collaboration showed that calcium supplementation compared to placebo decreased the overall risk of pre-eclampsia in pregnancy (n = 15,730 women; RR = 0.45, 95%CI: 0.31; 0.65) [8], with an even greater reduction in women clinically diagnosed at high risk (n = 587 women; RR = 0.22, 95%CI: 0.12; 0.42) [8]. Similar findings were found in an even more recent meta-analysis of 27 clinical studies, including 28.492 pregnant women (RR = 0.51, 95%CI: 0.40; 0.64) [9].

What is still unclear is the mechanism by which calcium may have an effect on blood pressure; one hypothesis is that low calcium intakes increase the parathyroid hormone and 1,25-dihydroxy vitamin D levels, that are required to maintain specific calcium concentrations in extracellular fluids. Higher blood concentrations of 1,25-dihydroxy vitamin D and parathyroid hormone stimulate calcium influx into different cell types and increase intracellular calcium into the vascular smooth muscle cell, consequently increasing the peripheral vascular resistance and, then, the blood pressure [10, 11].

However, some concerns have been raised as regards the safety profile of calcium during gestation – as it may cause rebound postnatal bone demineralisation and increase the HELLP syndrome occurrence, with hemolysis, elevated liver enzymes and a low platelet count [12–14].

Calcium supplementation is recommended by the most recent ACOG, World Health Organization (WHO), and ESC Guidelines to be prescribed in deficiency during pregnancy in order to reduce the risk of pre-eclampsia [15–17]. The suggested scheme for calcium supplementation is 1.5–2.0 g daily, with the total dosage divided into three dosages, preferably taken at mealtimes [17].

Omega-3 Polyunsaturated Fatty Acids (PUFAs) Observational studies suggest that both GDM and pre-eclampsia are associated with low intake of PUFAs from diet [18–20].

In patients with GDM, PUFAs supplementation is associated with an improved metabolic function, by increasing insulin sensitivity and decreasing inflammation [21]. However, it seems not to exert a detectable effect on hypertensive disorders [22–24].

Vitamin D Vitamin D deficiency, as measured by circulating 25(OH)-vitamin D concentrations, is reported to be as high as 40% among pregnant women and is also very common during lactation [25]. As pregnancy progresses, the requirements of vitamin D increase and, as a consequence, any preexisting vitamin D deficiency can worsen [26].

Accordingly to the findings of a recent meta-analysis, vitamin D supplementation (1000–4762 IU/day) is able to promote the glycaemic control in women with GDM [27]. Furthermore, vitamin D supplementation in women with GDM reduces the incidence of newborn complications such as polyhydramnios (RR = 0.17, 95%CI: 0.03; 0.89) and hyperbilirubinemia (RR = 0.4, 95%CI: 0.23; 0.68) and the need for maternal hospitalization (RR = 0.13, 95%CI: 0.02; 0.98) and infant hospitalization (RR = 0.4, 95%CI: 0.23; 0.69) [28].

Vitamin D supplementation was also demonstrated to potentiate nifedipine treatment for preeclampsia, shortening the time to control blood pressure and prolonging time before subsequent hypertensive crisis, probably via an immunomodulatory mechanism [29].

A lately meta-analysis by Fogacci et al. carried out on 4777 women suggests that the ones in treatment with vitamin D have a lower risk of pre-eclampsia compared to those that receive no intervention or placebo (OR = 0.37, 95%CI: 0.26; 0.52), being the effect largely independent of the supplementation duration and the co-administration of calcium and enhanced for increasing vitamin D doses [5]. Adequate vitamin D intake might help with the maintenance of the calcium homeostasis – which is inversely related to blood pressure levels – [30] or may directly suppress the proliferation of the vascular smooth muscle cells [31]. Furthermore, vitamin D might be a powerful endocrine suppressor of renin biosynthesis and could act on the regulation of the renin-angiotensin system, which plays a critical role in blood pressure control [31]. Finally, vitamin D may also act on the synthesis of adipokines related to endothelial and vascular health [32].

Folic Acid   Epidemiological studies of the association between folic acid supplementation and the incidence of pre-eclampsia showed a potential protective effect [33]. On the contrary, higher plasma folate was found to be associated with higher risk of GDM [34].

Findings from the Ottawa and Kingston (OaK) Birth Cohort suggested a 60% reduction in the risk of pre-eclampsia (n = 8085; OR = 0.37, 95%CI: 0.18; 0.75) and a dose-response association between folic acid and pre-eclampsia events in women with identified risk factors [33, 35]. The possible reason can be found on folic acid action affecting levels of hyperhomocysteinemia, which is known to damage the vascular endothelium of the developing placenta [36].

However, a recent analysis from the Tongji Maternal and Child Health Cohort (TMCHC) involving 4353 pregnant women recently showed that folic acid supplementation (≥800 μg/day) from prepregnancy through midpregnancy is associated with a higher risk for GDM after adjustment for potential confounders (OR = 2.36, 95%CI: 1.51; 3.69) [37]. Certainly, the potential risk of excess folic acid intake is a concern which will require further evaluation to examine the underlying mechanism.

Resveratrol   Resveratrol (3,5,4'-trihydroxystilbene) belongs to a family of polyphenolic compounds known as stilbenes, which are particularly concentrated in grapes, berries and nuts [38].

Findings from a recent meta-analysis showed that the combination treatment nifedipine/resveratrol is able, in pregnancy, to shorten the time for achieving target BP with a relative risk (RR) reduction of -13.9 (95%CI: -22.6; -5.2), compared to nifedipine alone (RR $= -3.5$, 95%CI: -26.5; 19.7) and labetalol (RR $= -1$, 95%CI: -22.2; 23) [39], which are the recommended treatments from the International Guidelines for the management of pre-eclampsia [16, 40, 41].

Alpha-Lipoic Acid Alpha-lipoic acid (ALA) is a natural antioxidant lipophilic compound which acts as an essential cofactor for mitochondrial enzymes [42]. A randomized double-blind clinical placebo-controlled clinical trial recently showed that supplementation with 100 mg/day of ALA for 8 weeks is able to exert some beneficial effects on glucose metabolism and liver function in women with GDM, by decreasing the circulating levels of fasting blood glucose (P < 0.001 *versus* baseline and *versus* control), gamma-glutamyltransferase (P < 0.001 *versus* baseline and *versus* control) and alanine trantaminase (P < 0.05 *versus* baseline) [43]. A further clinical trial carried out on 60 women diagnosed with GDM showed that supplementation with 100 mg/day of ALA for 8 weeks significantly decreases not only maternal fasting plasma glucose, but also the homeostatic model assessment for insulin resistance (HOMA-IR) [44].

Recently, some studies have finally evaluated the protective effect of ALA on fetal outcome of diabetic mothers, leading to interesting though preliminary results [45].

An observational retrospective study carried out analyzing data regarding 610 expectant mothers provided a reassuring picture about the safety of ALA oral treatment during pregnancy, with no treatment-related adverse events occurred in mothers or newborns [46].

Zinc Zinc supplementation has valuable anti-inflammatory effects, which may provide important benefits to metabolic status of gestational diabetes [47]. Accordingly to the most recent evidence, zinc supplementation is able to improve metabolic status in GDM by significantly reducing fasting plasma glucose, insulin and improving HOMA and QUICKI indexes [48].

Low maternal circulating zinc concentrations was also associated with incidence of pre-eclampsia [49, 50]. However, attempts to modify the incidence of pre-eclampsia with zinc supplementation was not successful. A meta-analysis from the Cochrane Collaboration Group involving 7 randomized clinical trials with 2975 enrolled women failed to show that zinc supplementation might significantly decrease the risk of hypertension or pre-eclampsia (RR $= 0.83$, 95%CI: 0.64; 1.08) [47].

Inositol Myo-inositol is able to improve metabolic disorders in pregnancy [51]. Myo-inositol supplementation leads pregnant women at high risk of developing GDM to a lower incidence of GDM [52]. In particular, its supplementation is able to reduce the occurrence of GDM-related complications, such as shoulder dystocia, respiratory distress syndrome, neonatal hypoglycemia, preterm delivery and poly-hydramnios [53, 54].

Probiotics A 6-week probiotic supplementation has shown to have beneficial effects on gene expression related to insulin and inflammation, glycemic control, inflammatory markers and oxidative stress in patients with GDM [55]. A recent meta-analysis carried out on 10 RCTs overall including 1139 pregnant women showed that probiotics supplementation effectively reduces fasting plasma glucose [mean difference (MD) = −0.11 mmol/L, $P < 0.001$], serum insulin levels (MD = −2.06 μU/mL, $P < 0.001$) and HOMA-IR (MD = −0.38, $P < 0.001$) [56].

Other Functional Foods and Nutraceuticals Pre-clinical data suggest that supplementation with ergothioneine (ERG) –a water-soluble amino acid- might be a viable therapeutic agent in pre-eclampsia [57]. On the other hand, dietary inorganic nitrate supplements should be avoided during pregnancy. As a matter of fact, even though they might be useful in attenuating hypertension and pre-eclampsia by improving the placental blood flow, their use was associated with a wide range of unexpected maternal and fetal adverse events outcomes, such as methemoglobin-emia, alteration in embryonic cells and malignant transformation, as well as thyroid disorders [58].

Finally, lycopene supplementation recently failed to decrease the risk of pre-eclampsia, though it may mitigate fetal complications [59]. The potential effect of supplementation of vitamin C and vitamin E on pre-eclampsia was also refused from lately published meta-analysis [60, 61].

Conclusions

In consideration on the available evidence, the use of nutraceuticals with a good safety profile and well-established effect in pregnancy might represent a good thera-peutic alternative to prevent the hypertensive disorders or it may be an adjuvant for their treatment together with the traditional drugs.

Certainly, we still need data on long-term safety regarding many of the above-discussed active compounds, particularly when they are supplemented at a high dosage. In particular, further clinical research is advisable to identify, from the available active nutraceuticals, those with the best cost-effectiveness and risk–ben-efit ratio for widespread use in the clinical practice.

References

1. Lameijer H, Schutte JM, Schuitemaker NWE, van Roosmalen JJM, Pieper PG. Dutch maternal mortality and morbidity committee. Maternal mortality due to cardiovascular disease in the Netherlands: a 21-year experience. Neth Heart J. 2019 Nov;27 https://doi.org/10.1007/s12471-019-01340-w. [Epub ahead of print]
2. Raganova A, Petrova M, Gazova A, Kriska M, Kristova V. Drug usage analysis in pregnant women. Bratisl Lek Listy. 2019;120(11):867–71. https://doi.org/10.4149/BLL_2019_145.
3. Lai T, Xiang L, Liu Z, Mu Y, Li X, Li N, Li S, Chen X, Yang J, Tao J, Zhu J. Association of maternal disease and medication use with the risk of congenital heart defects in offspring: a case-control study using logistic regression with a random-effects model. J Perinat Med. 2019 May 27;47(4):455–63. https://doi.org/10.1515/jpm-2018-0281.
4. Poon LC, Shennan A, Hyett JA, Kapur A, Hadar E, Divakar H, McAuliffe F, da Silva CF, von Dadelszen P, McIntyre HD, Kihara AB, Di Renzo GC, Romero R, D'Alton M, Berghella V, Nicolaides KH, Hod M. The International Federation of Gynecology and Obstetrics (FIGO) initiative on pre-eclampsia: a pragmatic guide for first-trimester screening and prevention. Int J Gynaecol Obstet. 2019 May;145(Suppl 1):1–33. https://doi.org/10.1002/ijgo.12802. Erratum in: Int J Gynaecol Obstet 2019 Sep;146(3):390–391
5. Fogacci S, Fogacci F, Banach M, Michos ED, Hernandez AV, Lip GYH, Blaha MJ, Toth PP, Borghi C, Cicero AFG; Lipid and Blood Pressure Meta-analysis Collaboration (LBPMC) Group. Vitamin D supplementation and incident preeclampsia: A systematic review and meta-analysis of randomized clinical trials. Clin Nutr. 2019 Sep 4. pii: S0261–5614(19)33027-4. https://doi.org/10.1016/j.clnu.2019.08.015. [Epub ahead of print].
6. Dolatkhah N, Hajifaraji M, Abbasalizadeh F, Aghamohammadzadeh N, Mehrabi Y, Abbasi MM. Is there a value for probiotic supplements in gestational diabetes mellitus? A randomized clinical trial. J Health Popul Nutr. 2015 Nov 25;33:25. https://doi.org/10.1186/s41043-015-0034-9.
7. Ding J, Kang Y, Fan Y, Chen Q. Efficacy of resveratrol to supplement oral nifedipine treatment in pregnancy-induced preeclampsia. Endocr Connect. 2017 Nov;6(8):595–600. https://doi.org/10.1530/EC-17-0130.
8. Hofmeyr GJ, Lawrie TA, Atallah ÁN, Torloni MR. Calcium supplementation during pregnancy for preventing hypertensive disorders and related problems. Cochrane Database Syst Rev. 2018;10:CD001059. https://doi.org/10.1002/14651858.CD001059.pub5.
9. Sun X, Li H, He X, Li M, Yan P, Xun Y, Lu C, Yang K, Zhang X. The association between calcium supplement and preeclampsia and gestational hypertension: a systematic review and meta-analysis of randomized trials. Hypertens Pregnancy. 2019 May;38(2):129–39. https://doi.org/10.1080/10641955.2019.1593445.
10. Repke JT, Villar J, Anderson C, Pareja G, Dubin N, Belizan JM. Biochemical changes associated with blood pressure reduction induced by calcium supplementation during pregnancy. Am J Obstet Gynecol. 1989 Mar;160(3):684–90.
11. Cormick G, Ciapponi A, Cafferata ML, Belizán JM. Calcium supplementation for prevention of primary hypertension. Cochrane Database Syst Rev. 2015 Jun 30;6:CD010037. https://doi.org/10.1002/14651858.CD010037.pub2.
12. Hofmeyr GJ, Manyame S. Calcium supplementation commencing before or early in pregnancy, or food fortification with calcium, for preventing hypertensive disorders of pregnancy. Cochrane Database Syst Rev. 2017 Sep 26;9:CD011192. https://doi.org/10.1002/14651858.CD011192.pub2.
13. Jarjou LM, Laskey MA, Sawo Y, Goldberg GR, Cole TJ, Prentice A. Effect of calcium supplementation in pregnancy on maternal bone outcomes in women with a low calcium intake. Am J Clin Nutr. 2010;92(2):450–7.
14. Hofmeyr GJ, Lawrie TA, Atallah ÁN, Duley L, Torloni MR. Calcium supplementation during pregnancy for preventing hypertensive disorders and related problems. Cochrane Database Syst Rev. 2014, Issue 6. https://doi.org/10.1002/14651858.CD001059.pub4.

15. Regitz-Zagrosek V, Roos-Hesselink JW, Bauersachs J, et al.; ESC Scientific Document Group. 2018 ESC Guidelines for the management of cardiovascular diseases during pregnancy. Eur Heart J. 2018;39:3165–3241. https://doi.org/10.1093/eurheartj/ehy340.
16. ACOG Practice Bulletin No. 202. Gestational hypertension and preeclampsia. Obstet Gynecol. 2019 Jan;133:e1–25. https://doi.org/10.1097/AOG.0000000000003018.
17. WHO. WHO recommendation: Calcium supplementation during pregnancy for the prevention of pre-eclampsia and its complications. Geneva: World Health Organization; 2018.
18. Williams MA, Zingheim RW, King IB, Zebelman AM. Omega-3 fatty acids in maternal erythrocytes and risk of preeclampsia. Epidemiology. 1995 May;6(3):232–7.
19. Velzing-Aarts FV, van der Klis FR, van der Dijs FP, Muskiet FA. Umbilical vessels of pre-eclamptic women have low contents of both n-3 and n-6 long-chain polyunsaturated fatty acids. Am J Clin Nutr. 1999 Feb;69(2):293–8.
20. Devarshi PP, Grant RW, Ikonte CJ, Hazels MS. Maternal omega-3 nutrition, placental transfer and fetal brain development in gestational diabetes and preeclampsia. Nutrients. 2019 May 18;11(5):pii: E1107. https://doi.org/10.3390/nu11051107.
21. McGregor JA, Allen KG, Harris MA, Reece M, Wheeler M, French JI, Morrison J. The omega-3 story: nutritional prevention of preterm birth and other adverse pregnancy outcomes. Obstet Gynecol Surv. 2001 May;56(5 Suppl 1):S1–13.
22. Zhou SJ, Yelland L, McPhee AJ, Quinlivan J, Gibson RA, Makrides M. Fish-oil supplementation in pregnancy does not reduce the risk of gestational diabetes or preeclampsia. Am J Clin Nutr. 2012 Jun;95(6):1378–84. https://doi.org/10.3945/ajcn.111.033217.
23. Freeman MP, Sinha P. Tolerability of omega-3 fatty acid supplements in perinatal women. Prostaglandins Leukot Essent Fatty Acids. 2007 Oct–Nov;77(3–4):203–8.
24. Elshani B, Kotori V, Daci A. Role of omega-3 polyunsaturated fatty acids in gestational diabetes, maternal and fetal insights: current use and future directions. J Matern Fetal Neonatal Med. 2019 Mar;27:1–13. https://doi.org/10.1080/14767058.2019.1593361. [Epub ahead of print].
25. Wheeler BJ, Taylor BJ, de Lange M, et al. A longitudinal study of 25-hydroxy vitamin D and parathyroid hormone status throughout pregnancy and exclusive lactation in New Zealand mothers and their infants at 45° S. Nutrients. 2018;10:pii: E86. https://doi.org/10.3390/nu10010086.
26. Heyden EL, Wimalawansa SJ. Vitamin D: Effects on human reproduction, pregnancy, and fetal well-being. J Steroid Biochem Mol Biol. 2018;180:41–50. https://doi.org/10.1016/j.jsbmb.2017.12.011.
27. Ojo O, Weldon SM, Thompson T, Vargo EJ. The effect of vitamin D supplementation on glycaemic control in women with gestational diabetes mellitus: a systematic review and meta-analysis of randomised controlled trials. Int J Environ Res Public Health. 2019 May 16;16(10):pii: E1716. https://doi.org/10.3390/ijerph16101716.
28. Rodrigues MRK, Lima SAM, Mazeto GMFDS, Calderon IMP, Magalhães CG, Ferraz GAR, Molina AC, Costa RAA, Nogueira VDSN, Rudge MVC. Efficacy of vitamin D supplementation in gestational diabetes mellitus: systematic review and meta-analysis of randomized trials. PLoS One. 2019 Mar 22;14(3):e0213006. https://doi.org/10.1371/journal.pone.0213006.
29. Shi DD, Wang Y, Guo JJ, Zhou L, Wang N. Vitamin D enhances efficacy of oral nifedipine in treating preeclampsia with severe features: a double blinded, placebo-controlled and randomized clinical trial. Front Pharmacol. 2017;8:865. https://doi.org/10.3389/fphar.2017.00865.
30. Sablok A, Batra A, Thariani K, et al. Supplementation of vitamin D in pregnancy and its correlation with feto-maternal outcome. Clin Endocrinol (Oxf). 2015;83:536–41. https://doi.org/10.1111/cen.12751.
31. Evans KN, Bulmer JN, Kilby MD, Hewison M. Vitamin D and placental-decidual function. J Soc Gynecol Investig. 2004;11:263–71.
32. Dinca M, Serban MC, Sahebkar A, et al. Lipid Blood Pressure Meta-analysis Collaboration LBPMC Group. Does vitamin D supplementation alter plasma adipokines concentrations? a systematic review and meta-analysis of randomized controlled trials. Pharmacol Res. 2016;107:360 371.

33. Wen SW, Chen XK, Rodger M, White RR, Yang Q, Smith GN, Sigal RJ, Perkins SL, Walker MC. Folic acid supplementation in early second trimester and the risk of preeclampsia. Am J Obstet Gynecol. 2008 Jan;198(1):45.e1–7. https://doi.org/10.1016/j.ajog.2007.06.067.

34. Lai JS, Pang WW, Cai S, Lee YS, Chan JKY, Shek LPC, Yap FKP, Tan KH, Godfrey KM, van Dam RM, Chong YS, Chong MFF. High folate and low vitamin B12 status during pregnancy is associated with gestational diabetes mellitus. Clin Nutr. 2018 Jun;37(3):940–7. https://doi.org/10.1016/j.clnu.2017.03.022.

35. Walker MC, Finkelstein SA, Rennicks White R, Shachkina S, Smith GN, Wen SW, Rodger M. The Ottawa and Kingston (OaK) birth cohort: development and achievements. J Obstet Gynaecol Can. 2011 Nov;33(11):1124–33.

36. Roberts JM, Cooper DW. Pathogenesis and genetics of pre-eclampsia. Lancet. 2001 Jan 6;357(9249):53–6.

37. Li Q, Zhang Y, Huang L, Zhong C, Chen R, Zhou X, Chen X, Li X, Cui W, Xiong T, Gao Q, Xu S, Wu Y, Wang X, Zhang G, Zhang X, Lin L, Gao D, Xiao M, Xiong G, Yang H, Yang N, Yang X, Hao L, Jin Z, Yang N. High-dose folic acid supplement use from prepregnancy through midpregnancy is associated with increased risk of gestational diabetes mellitus: a prospective cohort study. Diabetes Care. 2019 Jul;42(7):e113–5. https://doi.org/10.2337/dc18-2572.

38. Cicero AFG, Fogacci F, Banach M. Botanicals and phytochemicals active on cognitive decline: the clinical evidence. Pharmacol Res. 2018 Apr;130:204–12. https://doi.org/10.1016/j.phrs.2017.12.029.

39. Sridharan K, Sequeira RP. Drugs for treating severe hypertension in pregnancy: a network meta-analysis and trial sequential analysis of randomized clinical trials. Br J Clin Pharmacol. 2018 Sep;84(9):1906–16. https://doi.org/10.1111/bcp.13649.

40. Regitz-Zagrosek V, Roos-Hesselink JW, Bauersachs J, Blomström-Lundqvist C, Cífková R, De Bonis M, Iung B, Johnson MR, Kintscher U, Kranke P, Lang IM, Morais J, Pieper PG, Presbitero P, Price S, Rosano GMC, Seeland U, Simoncini T, Swan L, Warnes CA; ESC Scientific Document Group. 2018 ESC Guidelines for the management of cardiovascular diseases during pregnancy. Eur Heart J. 2018 Sep 7;39(34):3165–3241. https://doi.org/10.1093/eurheartj/ehy340.

41. Bushnell C, McCullough LD, Awad IA, Chireau MV, Fedder WN, Furie KL, Howard VJ, Lichtman JH, Lisabeth LD, Piña IL, Reeves MJ, Rexrode KM, Saposnik G, Singh V, Towfighi A, Vaccarino V, Walters MR, American Heart Association Stroke Council; Council on Cardiovascular and Stroke Nursing; Council on Clinical Cardiology; Council on Epidemiology and Prevention; Council for High Blood Pressure Research. Guidelines for the prevention of stroke in women: a statement for healthcare professionals from the American Heart Association/American Stroke Association. Stroke. 2014 May;45(5):1545–88. https://doi.org/10.1161/01.str.0000442009.06663.48.

42. Bast A, Haenen GR. Lipoic acid: a multifunctional antioxidant. Biofactors. 2003;17(1–4):207–13.

43. Aslfalah H, Jamilian M, Rafiei F, Khosrowbeygi A. Reduction in maternal serum values of glucose and gamma-glutamyltransferase after supplementation with alpha-lipoic acid in women with gestational diabetes mellitus. J Obstet Gynaecol Res. 2019 Feb;45(2):313–7. https://doi.org/10.1111/jog.13842.

44. Aslfalah H, Jamilian M, Khosrowbeygi A. Elevation of the adiponectin/leptin ratio in women with gestational diabetes mellitus after supplementation with alpha-lipoic acid. Gynecol Endocrinol. 2019 Mar;35(3):271–5. https://doi.org/10.1080/09513590.2018.1519795.

45. Di Tucci C, Di Feliciantonio M, Vena F, Capone C, Schiavi MC, Pietrangeli D, Muzii L, Benedetti PP. Alpha lipoic acid in obstetrics and gynecology. Gynecol Endocrinol. 2018 Sep;34(9):729–33. https://doi.org/10.1080/09513590.2018.1462320.

46. Parente E, Colannino G, Picconi O, Monastra G. Safety of oral alpha-lipoic acid treatment in pregnant women: a retrospective observational study. Eur Rev Med Pharmacol Sci. 2017 Sep;21(18):4219–27.

47. Ota E, Mori R, Middleton P, Tobe-Gai R, Mahomed K, Miyazaki C, Bhutta ZA. Zinc supplementation for improving pregnancy and infant outcome. Cochrane Database Syst Rev. 2015 Feb 2;2:CD000230. https://doi.org/10.1002/14651858.CD000230.pub5.
48. Li X, Zhao J. The influence of zinc supplementation on metabolic status in gestational diabetes: a meta-analysis of randomized controlled studies. J Matern Fetal Neonatal Med. 2019 Sep;12:1–6. https://doi.org/10.1080/14767058.2019.1659769. [Epub ahead of print].
49. Wilson RL, Grieger JA, Bianco-Miotto T, Roberts CT. Association between maternal zinc status, dietary zinc intake and pregnancy complications: a systematic review. Nutrients. 2016 Oct 15;8(10):pii: E641.
50. He L, Lang L, Li Y, Liu Q, Yao Y. Comparison of serum zinc, calcium, and magnesium concentrations in women with pregnancy-induced hypertension and healthy pregnant women: a meta-analysis. Hypertens Pregnancy. 2016 May;35(2):202–9. https://doi.org/10.3109/10641955.201 5.1137584.
51. Croze ML, Soulage CO. Potential role and therapeutic interests of myo-inositol in metabolic diseases. Biochimie. 2013 Oct;95(10):1811–27. https://doi.org/10.1016/j.biochi.2013.05.011.
52. Guardo FD, Currò JM, Valenti G, Rossetti P, Di Gregorio LM, Conway F, Chiofalo B, Garzon S, Bruni S, Rizzo G. Non-pharmacological management of gestational diabetes: the role of myo-inositol. J Complement Integr Med. 2019 Sept 17; pii: /j/jcim.ahead-of-print/jcim-2019-0111/ jcim-2019-0111.xml; https://doi.org/10.1515/jcim-2019-0111. [Epub ahead of print]
53. Santamaria A, Alibrandi A, Di Benedetto A, Pintaudi B, Corrado F, Facchinetti F, D'Anna R. Clinical and metabolic outcomes in pregnant women at risk for gestational diabetes mellitus supplemented with myo-inositol: a secondary analysis from 3 RCTs. Am J Obstet Gynecol. 2018;219(3):300.e1–6. https://doi.org/10.1016/j.ajog.2018.05.018.
54. Howlett A, Ohlsson A, Plakkal N. Inositol in preterm infants at risk for or having respiratory distress syndrome. Cochrane Database Syst Rev. 2019 Jul 8;7:CD000366. https://doi.org/10.1002/14651858.CD000366.pub4.
55. Babadi M, Khorshidi A, Aghadavood E, Samimi M, Kavossian E, Bahmani F, Mafi A, Shafabakhsh R, Satari M, Asemi Z. The effects of probiotic supplementation on genetic and metabolic profiles in patients with gestational diabetes mellitus: a randomized, double-blind, Placebo-Controlled Trial. Probiotics Antimicrob Proteins. 2018 Dec 8; https://doi.org/10.1007/ s12602-018-9490-z. [Epub ahead of print]
56. Han MM, Sun JF, Su XH, Peng YF, Goyal H, Wu CH, Zhu XY, Li L. Probiotics improve glucose and lipid metabolism in pregnant women: a meta-analysis. Ann Transl Med. 2019 Mar;7(5):99. https://doi.org/10.21037/atm.2019.01.61.
57. Kerley RN, McCarthy C, Kell DB, Kenny LC. The potential therapeutic effects of ergothioneine in pre-eclampsia. Free Radic Biol Med. 2018 Mar;117:145–57. https://doi.org/10.1016/j. freeradbiomed.2017.12.030.
58. Bahadoran Z, Mirmiran P, Azizi F, Ghasemi A. Nitrate-rich dietary supplementation during pregnancy: the pros and cons. Pregnancy Hypertens. 2018 Jan;11:44–6. https://doi. org/10.1016/j.preghy.2017.12.010.
59. Antartani R, Ashok K. Effect of lycopene in prevention of preeclampsia in high risk pregnant women. J Turk Ger Gynecol Assoc. 2011 Mar 1;12(1):35–8. https://doi.org/10.5152/ jtgga.2011.08.
60. Rumbold A, Ota E, Nagata C, Shahrook S, Crowther CA. Vitamin C supplementation in pregnancy. Cochrane Database Syst Rev. 2015 Sep 29;9:CD004072. https://doi. org/10.1002/14651858.CD004072.pub3.
61. Rumbold A, Ota E, Hori H, Miyazaki C, Crowther CA. Vitamin E supplementation in pregnancy. Cochrane Database Syst Rev. 2015 Sep 7;9:CD004069. https://doi. org/10.1002/14651858.CD004069.pub3.

Chapter 13
Nutraceuticals for Cardiovascular Risk Factors Management in Children: An Evidence Based Approach

Ornella Guardamagna and Giulia Massini

Introduction

Dyslipidemias represent a primary health concern as a major risk factor for atherosclerosis. Increased serum total cholesterol (TC), LDL cholesterol (LDL-C), low levels of HDL cholesterol (HDL-C), and/or elevated triglyceride (TG) levels impact negatively on the cardiovascular outcome and precociously since pediatric age [1]. Children or adolescents showing phenotypes related to primary or secondary dyslipidemia, including overweight, should undergo a treatment aimed to improve their lipid profile, in order to achieve LDL-C targets according to the American Academy of Pediatrics guidelines [2]. LDL-C serum levels are considered acceptable or safe when ≤130 or ≤ 110 mg/dl respectively [3]. Therapy steps include firstly the dietary regimen aimed to provide adequate calories and nutrients intake before driving to hypolipidemic drugs. Nutraceuticals represent the intermediate option to be considered in the pediatric practice [4].

The nutraceutical experience in pediatrics is so far rather limited as scanty, short-term, randomized, controlled studies have been performed. These mainly concern the administration of Fibre and Phyto-sterol/stanol while sporadic reports include Red Yeast Rice (RYR) extract, Soy Protein, Probiotic, Omega 3, Omega 6 PoliUnsatured Fatty Acids (PUFAs) and Nut. This review summarizes results from Pub-Med source that have been reached by intervention trials performed in hyperlipidemic children and adololescents. The objective of this review is to update benefits and limitations of nutraceuticals in this selected population and to demonstrate the lipid-lowering activity based on evidences from clinical trials.

O. Guardamagna (✉) · G. Massini
Department of Public Health and Pediatric Sciences, Università di Torino, Torino, Italy
e-mail: ornella.guardamagna@unito.it

© Springer Nature Switzerland AG 2021
A. F.G. Cicero, M. Rizzo (eds.), *Nutraceuticals and Cardiovascular Disease*,
Contemporary Cardiology, https://doi.org/10.1007/978-3-030-62632-7_13

Fibre

Fibres consist of edible part of plants not digested in the human small intestine including complex carbohydrates indigestible as non-starch polysaccharides (cellulose, hemi-cellulose, gums, pectins, oat bran, wheat bran), oligosaccharides (inulin, fructo-oligosaccharides) and lignin (a noncarbohydrate substance bound to fiber), which are intact in plants and have been linked to positive health outcome, including cardiovascular disease (CVD) and obesity prevention [5]. Fibre contained in cereals, fruits, and vegetables, as part of a correct dietary regimen, ameliorates lipid profile [6] reducing TC and LDL-C blood levels around 5–15% and 9–22% in adults, respectively [7, 8]. Evidences allowed the regulatory Agencies to issue Health Claims of food fiber intake [9], Oat β-glucan and their LDL-C lowering effect or CVD risk reduction [10, 11].

The need of fibre in children is still critical and not finally solved [12]. There is no agreement in terms of quantity as guidelines relate the need to the intake of Calories (12 g/1000 calories), as FDA suggests, or to the weight or to the age as established by the American Academy of Pediatrics (AAP) [13]. It should then be mentioned that recommendations in pediatrics vary widely depending on countries and the evidence base used [14]. Overall, in practice the most pediatricians apply the formula that correspond, in grams per day, to the sum of the age (in children >3 years old) plus 5 [15]. This intake is respected when mediterranean dietary style or vegetables enriched diet is pursued, but this condition is rarely satisfied. Most children living in West Countries typically consume less vegetables and fruits which contribute to the lower dietary fibre intake than appropriate and to a calorically dense, highly refined, high fat diet despite the dietary guidelines provided [16]. The consequences of the uncorrect food intake include metabolic changes and hyperlipidemia, sometimes related to overweight/obesity. In the Healthy Start Preschool Study of Cardiovascular disease risk factors and Diet a follow up of children demonstrates the beneficial effect on blood lipids of dietary fibre besides that of monounsaturated fatty acids (MUFAs) [17].

Soluble fibres comprising mainly Psyllium (soluble, viscous, non-fermentable fibre), Glucomannan, Oat, Pectin, and Guar Gum (soluble, viscous, fermentable fibre) are commercially available as unprocessed and additionable to food, or as flavored powder or capsule as well. Psyllium is one of the richest sources of soluble mucilaginous dietary fibre. It is derived from the seed husk of *Plantago ovata* and is considered a proper supplement to dietary therapy [18]. Glucomannan, the main polysaccharide obtained from the tuber *Amorphophallus Konjac,* (a member of the Araceae family, found in East Asia) is a palatable soluble fibre. In the Asian Continent, people have been consuming glucomannan for thousands of years; its use is also increasing in West Countries. The chemical structure of glucomannan consists in a mannose:glucose 8:5 ratio, linked by *B*-glycosidic bonds. Glucomannan has the highest molecular weight and viscosity of any other known dietary fibre [19]. Oat is a cereal containing a complex array of compounds, the main is *B*-glucan constituent, consisting of glucose molecules. It is a viscous, soluble fibre found in the endosperm of the *Avena sativa* plant [20]. Isabgol husk is included under the mucilage component of fiber and derives from the seeds of *Plantago ovata Forsk,* of which it represents the 30%. It acts as a gel forming polysaccharides, simil to Guar Gum and Pectin. Locust bean gum is a white and odorless powder extract from the endosperm of the bean without a distinctive taste. Interestingly it was used by Greeks as a laxative but if taken in a non-hydrated form it should cause intestinal bolus and obstruction. It is less viscous than Guar Gum but is similar to Ash and Galactomannan moisture protein content and is more palatable [21]. The lipid-lowering ability of fibre depends on their physical-chemical properties and different levels of viscosity. Among all fibre types Glucomannan is considered one of the most viscous, its water content being eight times more than the Oat one. Glucomannan significantly lowers LDL-C and more than Psyllium and Wheat Bran, even if administered at half dosage [22].

Soluble fibres act mainly forming viscous solutions that slow down gastric emptying and reduce fat absorption, then modulating the lipoprotein metabolism. In the small intestine the gelling process binds dietary fats, hinders the absorption of cholesterol and the reabsorption of bile acids increasing their excretion in feces. The consequence is the reduced chylomicron circulation and the intestinal cholesterol uptake, increases the liver bile synthesis with the consequent hypocholesterolemic effect. A further mechanism consists in the bacterial fermentation, taking part in the colon (except lignin) and resulting in the production of short-chain fatty acids (acetate, propionate and butyrate). The propionate is postulated to inhibit the cholesterol synthesis [23, 24].

Reports

The largest study was performed in a cohort of Japanese children, 10–11 years old, from the general population (n = 5873) and found dietary fiber consumption to be inversely associated with TC, overweight, and obesity then confirming data from adult trials [25].

Fibres are commonly added to diet in children and adolescents affected by primary hyperlipidemias, then to familial hypercholesterolemia (FH), hypertrygliceridemia and poligenic hypercholesterolemia, including subjects affected by familial combined hyperlipidemia (FCH) and obese children, to promote TC and LDL-C reduction. Implications related to physiopatologic differences underlying these disorders could be a relevant topic when considering the fibre choice. For example if we consider that psyllium should possibly reduce chylomicron intestinal absorption and Very Low Density Lipoproteins (VLDL) liver synthesis it is presumed a more pronounced effect on familial combined hyperlipidemia disorder with respect to other conditions. A number of studies focused on the short term efficacy and tolerance of different type of fibre on LDL-C levels in hyperlipidemic children and adolescents. Most trials were performed in the 90's with results greatly variable from no change to 30% decrease [21, 26–34], (Table 13.1).

Table 13.1 Randomized controlled trials in children on the lipid-lowering effects of different types of fibre

Nutraceutical	Type of study	Subjects	Aim of the study	Intervention	Intolerance and/or side effect	Compliance	Observed effects	Ref.
Psyllium	RCT	n.36 FH children	Determine TC and LDL-C drop in children	n.14 pre-treated with Step-One-Diet	No side effects	Good compliance	↓ TC: −18%	Glassman et al. American Journal of Diseases of Children 1990
		Age: 3–17 years		Duration: 8.0 ± 1.1 months				
		Inclusion criteria: children, primary type IIa hypercholesterolemia		Intervention			↓ LDL-C: −23%	
				Children <7 years: 5 g/day psyllium				
				Children >7 years: 10 g/day psyllium			No significant changes in HDL-C levels or TG concentrations	
				Duration: 8 ± 2.4 months				
	DB-PLACEBO-CO-RCT	n. 20 children	Efficacy of psyllium in lowering LDL-C levels in HyperCT children	Diet counselling	No side effects	Good compliance (80%)	No clinically significant differences in TC, LDL-C, or HDL-C	BA Dennison et al. J Pediatr. 1993
		Age: 5–17 years		Duration: 3 months			TG levels increased in the control group in comparison with the psyllium group	
		Inclusion criteria: subjects with LDL-C levels >110 mg/dl after at least 3 months of controlled diet		Intervention: 6 g/day ready-to-eat cereals, with water-soluble psyllium fiber or placebo without psyllium				
				Duration: 4 to 5 weeks each stage				
				Wash out phase: 2-weeks				

	Study type	Population	Aim	Intervention/Duration	Side effects	Compliance	Results	Reference
Psyllium	SB-PLACEBO-RCT	n.50 children. Age: 2–11 years. Inclusion criteria: children with two baseline LDL-C levels > or = 110 mg/dL	Psyllium effectiveness in lowering TC and LDL-C in HyperCT children	Step 1 diet: All groups. Intervention: Psyllium-enriched cereal containing 3.2 g of soluble fiber, each box of placebo cereal containing less than 0.5 g of soluble fiber. Duration: 12 weeks	No side effects	Good compliance	↓ TC: −9.6% ↓ LDL-C: −15.7% ↑ HDL-C: +9.96% ↓ TC/HDL-C: −17.9% ↓ LDL-C/HDL-C: −21.1%	CL Williams et al. J Am Coll Nutr. 1995
	DB-CO-RCT	n. 32 children. n. 7 drop-out. TOT: n.25. Age: 6–18 years. Inclusion criteria: LDL-C concentrations greater than the 90th percentile for age and sex at baseline	Hypocholesterolemic effect of a psyllium-enriched breakfast cereal in children with hyperlipidemia	8-weeks diet period. Intervention: 58 g of a psyllium enriched cereal/day, for a total daily dose of 6.4 g soluble fiber from psyllium or placebo. Duration: 6 weeks	n. 1 child with slight abdominal bloating	Good compliance	↓ TC: −5% ↓ LDL-C: −6,8% No significant changes in HDL-C or TG concentrations	Michael H Davidson et al. Am J Clin Nutr 1996
	DB-PLACEBO-RCT	n.51 dyslipidaemic children (mild to moderate). n. 25 control group. n.26 intervention group − 2 drop-out. TOT: n.49. Age: 6–19 years. Inclusion criteria: TC > 4.40 mmol/l	Investigate the LDL-C lowering effects of psyllium in Brazilian dyslipidaemic children and adolescents	Step 2 diet: 6 weeks. Intervention group: 7.0 g/day psyllium. Control group: 7.0 g/day cellulose. Duration: 8 weeks	No side effects	Control group: n.2 drop-out during follow up	↓ TC: −7.7% ↓ LDL-C: −10.7% Psyllium treatment had no significant effect on HDL-C concentrations and LDL-C/HDL-C	Simone Augusta Ribas et al. British Journal of Nutrition 2015

(continued)

Table 13.1 (continued)

Nutraceutical	Type of study	Subjects	Aim of the study	Intervention	Intolerance and/or side effect	Compliance	Observed effects	Ref.
GLUCOMANNAN	RCT	n. 51 children	Effect of glucomannan to a Step-One-Diet in HyperCT children, to reduce TC and LDL-C	Capsules containing 0.5 g of active glucomannan: Children ≤6 years 2 g/day Children >6 years 3 g/day	No side effects	Good compliance	↓ TC (F:−24%; M:−9%)	Francesco Martino et al. Nutrition, Metabolism & Cardiovascular Diseases 2005
		n. 11 drop-out						
		TOT: n.40					↓ LDL-C (F:−30%; M: −9%)	
		Inclusion criteria: TC levels higher than age and sex-specific 90th percentile at baseline, in 2 determinations. No dietary treatment in previous 3 months. One parent with TC higher than 6.2 mmol/L or family anamnesis for CVD in first- or second degree relatives		Duration: 8 weeks				
	DB- PLACEBO-CO-RCT	n. 36 FH children Age: 6–15 years	Efficacy and tolerability of a short-term treatment with glucomannan in FH children.	Dietary counselling	No side effects	Compliance 92% and 90% for supplement and placebo, respectively	↓ TC: −5.1%	Ornella Guardamagna et al. Nutrition 2013
		Inclusion criteria: TC levels higher than age and sex-specific 90th percentile		Duration: 4 weeks			↓ LDL-C: −7.3%	
				2/weeks capsule administration containing: 500 mg of glucomannan (dietary supplement) or placebo.			↓ non-HDL-C: −7.2%	
				Duration: 8 weeks			No significant differences in TG, HDL-C, ApoA-I and ApoB levels	
				Washout period: 4 weeks				

GUM	CO-RCT	n. 17 adults n. 11 children TOT n.18 FCH + n.10 normal subjects Age adults: 22–53 years Age children: 10–18 years Inclusion criteria: one parent and one child and at least one additional first degree relative with FCH. Families with increased incidence of premature CVD	Assess the hypolipidemic effect of Locust Bean Gum (LBG)	Group A: ECE Group B: CEE Children: 10–20 g/day LBG Adult M: 25–35 g/day LBG Adult F: 10–25 g/day LBG Duration: 8 weeks	No side effects	Good compliance	Group A: FCH ↓TC: −10% ↓LDL-C: −11% Normal subjects ↓TC: −6% ↓LDL-C: −10% Group B: FCH ↓TC: −17% ↓LDL-C: −19% Normal subjects ↓TC: −11% ↓LDL-C: −6%	JH Zavoral et al. Am J Clin Nutr 1983
PECTIN	No randomization, no placebo	n. 53 children with elevated serum LDL-C levels (>135 mg/dl) n.2 children drop-out Age: 4–18 years Control group: n.33 children (only diet) Age: 5–16 years Inclusion criteria: LDL-C serum levels >135 mg/dl after 6 month of dietary counselling	Effects of fiber supplements on lipid concentrations in cyslipidemic children on dietary treatment	Dietary counselling + supplementation: 50% wheat bran +50% of pectin, 2–3 tablets/day (50mg/Kg/day) Duration: 3 months	n.2 children abdominal discomfort and soft stools	Good compliance	↓TC: −15% ↓LDL-C: −17% ↓TG: −18% ↓ApoB: −14% No significant differences in HDL-C, ApoA-1 levels	Marciano Sanchez-Bayle et al. Clinical Pediatrics 2001

(continued)

Table 13.1 (continued)

Nutraceutical	Type of study	Subjects	Aim of the study	Intervention	Intolerance and/or side effect	Compliance	Observed effects	Ref.
GLUCOMANNAN + POLICOSANOL OR CHROMIUM-POLYNICOTINATE	DB-RCT	n.132 children CT↑	Effects of low-dose CP or PC and their glucomannan combination in HyperCT children	Step-One-Diet: 1 week Control group: capsules containing resistant starch as placebo	No side effects	n. 6 children refused diet n. 6 children refused capsules	GM+ CP group: ↓LDL-C: −16% No change in HDL-C or TG concentrations	Francesco Martino et al. Atherosclerosis 2013
		n.12 dropouts		GM + CP group: GM 500 mg + CP 0.2 mg				
		TOT: n.120 children		CP group: CP 0.2 mg + starch 500 mg			GM + PC group: ↓LDL-C: −10% No change in HDL-C, TG.	
		Age: 3–16 years		GM + PC group: GM 500 mg + policosanol 1.2 mg				
		M: n.60		PC group: policosanol 1.2 mg + starch 500 mg				
		F: n. 60		GM group: GM 500 mg + starch 500 mg			PC group: No lipid lowering effects	
		Inclusion criteria: TC > 170 mg/dl in two measurements, no drug treatment before enrollment.		Children ≤6 years: 2 capsules at lunch and 2 at dinner				
		No dietary treatment in the previous 3 months. 1 parent with TC >240 mg/dL or a family history of CVD in first- or second-degree relatives		Children >6 years: 3 capsules at lunch and 3 at dinner				
				Duration: 8 weeks				

↑: increase, ↓: decrease, *HDL-C*: HDL-cholesterol, *LDL-C*: LDL-cholesterol, *TC*: total cholesterol, *ApoB*: Apolipoprotein B, *ApoA1*: Apolipoprotein A-1, *RCT*: randomized controlled trials, *DB*: double-blind, *SB*: single-blind, *CO*: crossover, *FH*: familial hypercholesterolemia, *HyperCT*: Hypercholesterolemia, *FCH*: familial combined hypertlipidemia, *GM*: Glucomannan, *PC*: Policosanols, *CP*: chromium-polynicotinate, *y*: years, *ECE*: Experimental, control, experimental, *CEE*: Control, experimental, experimental

Fibre supplied in children studies were preferably Psyllium but also Glucomannnan, Oat and Gum were added to STEP I (Daily Fat intake<30%, Satured fatty acids<10%, Cholesterol<300 mg) or STEP II (Satured fatty Acids 7%, Cholesterol <200 mg.) diets (more recently nominated as CHILD I diet and CHILD II diet but here, to simplify, indicated as in trials) [3]. Balancing the intake of fibre from food, nutraceutical or fibre added-food is relevant to the compliance and outcome. A very restricted diet, as required by STEP II diet, although safe [35, 36] is not always agreed by children then the combination of STEP I diet added to food fibre-enriched or capsules containing fibre is considered more effective at reducing serum LDL-C levels.

The efficacy of Psyllium was demonstrated in most studies [31, 37, 26, 38] but one [33]. A 12 weeks randomized controlled study conducted on 50 mildly hypercholesterolemic children on STEP I diet and supplemented with Psyllium 3.2 g/day showed a 8.9% LDL-C decrease when compared to the control group [37]. A further success was demonstrated in 36 children, FCH affected, showing 11.9% TC and 13.8% LDL-C decrease. This latter group when assumed Psyllium 2.5 g–10 g day (depending on the age) showed a final TC and LDL-C levels reduction of 18% and 23% respectively [31]. Moreover it should be mentioned the success of Psyllium in further reducing LDL-C in hyperlipidemic children on STEP II diet, as more recently demonstrated [38]. By contrast a randomized double blind, placebo controlled, cross-over study employing 6 g/day of Psyllium in 20 mild hypercolesterolemic children, already on STEP II diet, did not demonstrate any significant effect on CT but on TG. Minerals (Calcium, Iron and Zinc) and fat-soluble vitamins (A; D; E) were unchanged at the end of the study [33].

In 2010, the European Food Safety Authority approved health claims related to Konjac Glucomannan and reductions in body weight, postprandial glycemia, and blood cholesterol [39].

Glucomannan have been tested with success on 36 hyperlipidemic children who underwent a double-blind, randomized, placebo-controlled, cross-over trial 24 week long dutation. This cohort, affected by primary dyslipidemia, was on dietary control CHILD I diet since at least 1 month. Capsules containing Glucomannan 500 mg were administered at the dose of 1–1.5g/day depending on the proband weight. TC, LDL-C and non-HDL-C decreased significantly by 5.1%, 7.3%, and 7.2% respectively [40]. These results were more pronounced in female while in males just non-HDL-C decreased significantly and in agreement with previously results [28]. Two metanalysis on Glucomannan, including children, have been done. The first considered 531 subjects from the 3 studies in children and did not found any significant change of LDL-C but of TG in obese children [41, 42]. The second estimated that the degree of lipid lowering effect was consistent and similar in adults and children therefore concluding that dose, follow-up duration, baseline cholesterol concentration, or the matrix of Glucomannan administration, did not modify the estimate effect on LDL-C [43].

Other sporadic studies concerning Oat Bran demonstrated the significant increase of HDL-C and decrease of LDL-C after 7 months of consumption (dosage: 1 g/kg body weight/day) if compared with Soy Derivatives [44] in 20 hypercholesterolemic children (5–12 years old). These results may suggest that a long duration of Oat Bran consumption may improve lipid profile in children with high cholesterol levels. Anyway at present no recommendation could be made for Oat Bran in children as a supplement to diet [23]. Isabogol husk, (25 g/day for 3 weeks), decreased LDL-C (7%), free fatty acids, and phospholipids in 11 borderline hypercholesterolemic adolescents [32]. Furthermore Locust bean gum (Carruba), 8–30 g/day, showed a significant 11% to 19% LDL-C decrease when comparing active and placebo groups undergoing a 16-weeks, cross-over trial including 11 FCH children, 10 controls and 17 adults [21].

A critical topic concerns Apolipoprotein B (ApoB), recognized as a relevant cardiovascular risk marker [45], then the relationship between ApoB/non-HDL-C and Glucomannan was considered. ApoB levels were not influenced by Glucomannan supplementation [40] and this result was further confirmed as unchanged in the recent metanalysis of 12 trials involving 370 individuals, children included [43]. The metanalysis focused on ApoB from 6 studies including 2 pediatric reports and 96 children [40, 46]. While the robust effect on LDL-C (−10%) and non-HDL-C (−7%) was proven there was no impact on ApoB levels. The utility of ApoB is important in subjects showing increased CVD risk, but normal or slightly elevated LDL-C [43]. As regard to Oat bran a study conducted on 49 hypercholesterolemic children, (mean age 10 years), supplemented 38 g/day of Oat bran for 4 weeks, demonstrated that while the lipid profile did not differ significantly, ApoB decreased (P = 0.05) if compared to controls [29]. On the contrary positive effects were confimed on LDL-C but not on ApoB [47]. Therefore, as results are conflicting more studies are required to better understand the role of Glucomannan on ApoB.

There are no great safety issues to underline but Psillium intake should be related to allergies then attention should be paid in giving this type of fiber to allergic subjects [26]. It should be added to cereals without affecting taste or texture then tolerance is good. Most of children undergoing trials showed just occasionally intestinal disturbances and found both Psyllium and Glucomanan palatable [38, 40] while reports on B-Glucan, Guar Gum and Pectin do not always confirm this acceptance [48]. Concerning the tolerability diarrhea and abdominal discomfort were the most commonly reported symptoms, while a paucity of data exists on the long-term safety of Glucomannan. Glucomannan does not exhibit adverse effects on the absorption of oligoelements such as iron, calcium, copper, and zinc, as demonstrated in children [42]. It should be considered that the FDA issued warnings about consuming products containing Glucomannan as "jelly cup type candies" stating they posed a serious choking risk, particularly to children [49].

The reduction of LDL-C ranges between 7–10% across different type of fibre, which indicate a class effect of soluble fibre [41]. The cholesterol drop varies with viscous fibre types and each gram of Glucomannan reduces LDL-C by 0.12 mmol/L

[43], more than double if compared to *B*-Glucans from Oats and Barley [50] suggesting that smaller quantities of glucomannan are required to reduce LDL-C.

Studies considered show a wide range of effects, possibly related to the quality of dietary intervention and dietary intake evaluation method, to different study designs and randomisation methods as well as to laboratory measurement and overall to the small number of subject recruited that should not exceeds n°480. It should then be considered that fibre intake needs to be respected primarily pursuing a correct mediterranean style diet but in the presence of persistent high LDL-C, TC and/ or TG levels soluble fibre added to diet should help in ameliorating lipid profile without relevant adverse effects.

Plant Sterols

Plant sterols (phytosterols or non-cholesterol sterols) are naturally occurring plant compounds commonly taken by food, through vegetable oils and nuts in amount corresponding to that of cholesterol (200–400 mg/die) as cannot be synthetized in humans. Plant sterols safely and effectively reduce serum cholesterol concentrations inhibiting cholesterol absorption [51] and since 2001, NCEP Guidelines have included plant sterol–enriched food as part of a dietary strategy aimed at reducing LDL-C levels [52].

Non-cholesterol sterols or stanols (or sterol ester), are commercially available added to bread, cereals, salad dressing, milk, margarine or yoghurt with different flavors and good palatability. These factors are likely to increase acceptability and favor the compliance [53]. Milk, as a vehicle for phytosterols, is a good option as 2 cups of phytosterol-enriched milk ensure 150% and 60% of the dietary calcium needs for children and adolescents, respectively [16]. Furthermore it was evidenced in adults that milk matrix provide better results than cereals then LDL-C decreased 15.9% versus 5.4% respectively [54]. Although the efficacy of stanols was ascertained as greater in lowering cholesterol levels, compared to sterols, most studies administered sterols at variable doses of 1.6–2 g/day.

Plant sterols inhibit the cholesterol absorption at the intestinal level then reducing its serum concentration [55] but the exact mechanism is not fully understood [56]. Phytosterols, and mainly sitostanol, compete with cholesterol for intestinal absorption displaying cholesterol from micelle (Fig. 13.1). This event is enhanced by the hydrophobic properties of phytosterols, higher than that of cholesterol, which make phytosterols more susceptible to mixed micelles. Both cholesterol and phytosterols require the Niemann-Pick C1 Like 1 Protein (NPC1L1) to enter enterocytes. Non-esterified cholesterol and phytosterols are pumped back into the intestine lumen through the ABCG5/G8 complex. Finally about 50% of cholesterol, but less than 5% of plant sterols, is absorbed [57, 58]. Phytosterols in their free form are absorbed in a low percentage < 10% while stanols are unabsorbable [59]. The decreased entry of intestinal cholesterol and transport by chylomicrons to the liver reduce the levels of Intermediate Density Lipoprotein besides LDL [60].

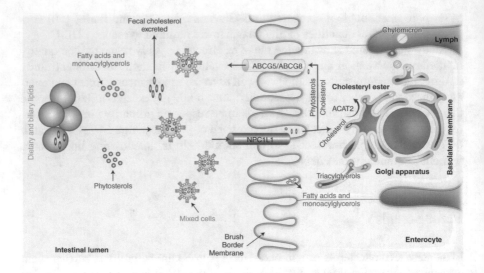

Fig. 13.1 Phytosterols and colesterol interaction at the enterocyte level. Phytosterols enter the mixed cells and display cholesterol which is only partially absorbed and enter chylomicrons while phytosterols are secreted into the intestinal lumen as only partially absorbed

Reports

Data concerning Phytosterol use in children are limited despite a great number of studies have been performed in adults. Plant Sterols have been demonstrated useful in decreasing cholesterol levels in mild affected hypercholesterolemic children [61, 62] and in FH children as confirmed in a series of paper [60, 63–69] (Table 13.2).

Subjects more commonly submitted to sterol treatment (1.2–2.0 g/day) were FH children, already on STEP I or II diet. They showed an approximate reduction of LDL-C by 10% [63, 65, 67] in a period range of 2–12 months and about 2l3 of FH children randomized were responders [65, 67]. An higher intake of 2.3 g/day of plant sterols decreased TC (11%) and LDL-C (14%) as compared to placebo spread in FH children [69] while higher decreases were observed in stanol added diet 3 g/day [60]. ApoB was reduced significantly by phytosterols (7–10%) [63, 65, 69]. The efficacy of plant sterols was further demonstrated in mild affected hypercholesterolemic (mean values TC > 197 mg and LDL >125 mg/dl) non FH children, already on STEP II diet. The intake of 1.2 g/day in two doses reduced TC (7–11%) and LDL-C (9–14%) significantly compared to the control group [61].

The well-tolerated plant stanol ester margarine reduced TC and LDL-C by 9% and 12% respectively in FH children after 1.6 g/day for 5–6 weeks [66, 68] and 15% on 3.0 g/day of margarine stanol enriched for 6 weeks (60). In mild elevated cholesterol 6 yrs. old children, from the STRIP Study, serum TC and LDL-C dropped significantly by 5.4% and 7.5%, respectively [57].

Table 13.2 Randomized controlled trials in children on the lipid-lowering effects of different types of phyto-sterol/stanol

Nutraceutical	Type Of Study	Subjects	Aim of the study	Intervention	Intolerance And/Or Side Effect	Compliance	Observed Effects	Ref.
Phytosterols/Phytostanols	DB-Co-RCT	n. 30 dyslipidemic children n. 14: Group A n. 16: Group B n. 25 completed trial Age: 6–9 years Inclusion criteria: fasting plasma TC concentration > 170 mg/dL, LDL-C concentrations >110 mg/dL	Demonstrate the lipid-lowering effect of plant sterols	Intervention group: milk enriched with 1.2 g/day of plant sterol. Control group: skim milk Duration: 8 weeks	No serious adverse events, 1 child presented nausea	Good compliance	Intervention group: ↓TC: −4.5% ↓LDL-C: −11.1% Control group: ↓TC: −5.9% ↓LDL-C: −10.2%	Ribas et al. Nutr Metabol Cardiovasc Dis. 2017
	CT	n. 64 HyperCT children n. 5 drop-out TOT: n. 59 children n. 25 LDL-C ≥ 130 mg/dl n. 34 LDL-C < 130 mg/dl Age: 4.5–15.9 years	effect of the daily consumption of 2 g of plant sterols on sdLDL-C levels in children with hypercholesterolemia	Step II Diet Intervention: yoghurt-drink (2 g/day plant sterols) Duration: 6–12 months	No serious adverse events	Compliance rate 86.6%	Intervention group: ↓sdLDL-C: −16.6% ↓LDL-C: −13% No changes in serum HDL-C, TG, Lp(a) levels	A. Garoufi et al. Ital J Pediatr. 2014

(continued)

Table 13.2 (continued)

Nutraceutical	Type Of Study	Subjects	Aim of the study	Intervention	Intolerance And/Or Side Effect	Compliance	Observed Effects	Ref.
	RCT	n. 32 HeFH	Efficacy, tolerability and safety of plant sterol supplementation in children with primary hyperlipidemias	Plant sterol-enriched yoghurt (100 ml, 1.6–2.0 g/day of sterol)	n. 1 Abdominal discomfort	n. 2 had difficulties in drinking yoghurt n. 2 had poor adherence to diet program	Reduction in LDL-C: -10.7% FH; -14.2% FCH; -16% HyperCTH	O. Guardamagna et al. Acta Diabetol. 2011
		n. 13 FCH		Biochemical and clinical evaluation after 12-weeks treatment			Lathosterol unchanged. Sitosterol slight increased. Significant decrease in CT and ApoB.	
		n. 13 HyperCT					TG, HDL-C and ApoA-1 unmodified	
		n. 6 drop-out						
		TOT: n. 52 children						
		Age: 8–16 years						
		Inclusion criteria: Outpatients affected by primary hyperlipidemia						
	DB-RCT	n. 42 FH children	Effect of plant stanols on lipids and endothelial function in pre-pubertal FH children	500 mL of a low-fat yoghurt enriched with 2.0 g of plant stanols	No serious adverse events	Compliance was 98% during plant stanol consumption and 96% in the control period.	↓ TC: -7.5%	L. Jakulj et al. J Pediatr. 2006
		n. 1 drop-out as not able to drink the yoghurt.		500 mL of a low-fat placebo yoghurt			↓ LDL-C: -9.2%	
		n.1 reached menarche during the study		Duration: 4 weeks			No significant changes in HDL-C and TG	
		TOT: n. 40 FH children		Washout period: 6-weeks			The reduction of LDL-C levels did not improve FMD	
		Age: 7–12 years						
		Inclusion criteria: personal diagnosis of FH by detection of mutation or a LDL-C > 95th percentile for age and sex and 1 FH parent						

CO-RCT	n. 37 He-FH children	Compliance and changes in plasma lipids, plant sterols, fat-soluble vitamins and carotenoids in children and parents with FH consuming PSE spread	13.7 g/days of PSE spread (1.2 g of plant sterols) in children + lipid-lowering diet	No serious adverse events	Good compliance	↓ TC: −9.1% in children and parents	Å. L. Amundsen et al. Eur J Nutr. 2004
			16.5 g/days of PSE spread (1.5 g of plant sterols) in parents + lipid-lowering diet			↓ LDL-C: −11.4% in children	
	Age children: 7–13 y		Follow-up: 26-weeks			↓ LDL-C: −11.0% in parents	
	Age parents: 32–51 y					↑ serum lathosterol, campesterol and sitosterol: +31, 96, 48% respectively (in children)	
	Inclusion criteria: diagnosis "definite" or "possible" HeFH					↓ serum α- and β-carotene: −17.4% and 10.9% respectively	
DB-Co-RCT	TOT: n. 38 HeFH children	Effect of SE enriched spread on serum lipids, lipoproteins, carotenoids, fat-soluble vitamins, and physiologic variables in FH children	18.2 ± 1.5 g SE spread/d (1.60 ± 0.13 g SEs) or a control spread + Child 1 Diet	No serious adverse events	The children consumed 90.9% of the control spread and 91.7% of the SE spread	↓ LDL-C: −10.2%	Å. L. Amundsen et al. Am J Clin Nutr. 2002
			Duration: 8 weeks			↓ TC and ApoB: −7.4%	
	Age: 7–12 years					No significant changes in HDL-C, TG and ApoA1 levels	
	Inclusion criteria: diagnosis "definite" or "possible" HeFH					↓ Serum lycopene: −8.1%	
						↑ Serum retinol and α-tocopherol: +15.6% and +7.1% respectively	

(continued)

Table 13.2 (continued)

Nutraceutical	Type Of Study	Subjects	Aim of the study	Intervention	Intolerance And/Or Side Effect	Compliance	Observed Effects	Ref.
	DB-placebo-Co-RCT	n. 81 normocholesterolaemic children Age: 6 years Inclusion criteria: children recruited from the STRIP study	Effects of gender, Apolipoprotein E phenotype, cholesterol absorption and synthesis on the cholesterol-lowering effect of PSE in children.	Intervention: dietary fat intake was replaced with 20 g/day of PSE margarine or control margarine. Duration: 3-months separated by 6-weeks wash-out period	No serious adverse events	Good compliance	Plant ester stanols group Boys: ↓ TC: −6% ↓ LDL-C: −9% Girls: ↓ TC: −4% ↓ LDL-C: −6% No gender differences Cholesterol absorption decreased in both apoE4+ and in apoE4−, cholesterol synthesis increased only in the apoE4+ children	A. Tammi et al. Acta Pediatr. 2002
	DB-placebo-Co-RCT	n. 41 FH children n. 20 non-FH children (control group) Age: 5–12 years Inclusion criteria: LDL-C > 95° percentile for age and gender; family history of HyperCT and LDL-C levels >95th percentile for age and gender before treatment or FH diagnosis by detection of a mutation in the LDL receptor gene	Effect of plant sterols on cholesterol and vascular function in prepuberal FH children.	Diet Step I Intervention: 15 g of plant sterol (2.3 g) spread or 15 g placebo spread Duration: 4 weeks separated by 6-weeks washout period.	No serious adverse events	Good compliance	↓ TC: −11% ↓ LDL-C: −14% The reduction of LDL in FH children not improve FMD (placebo: 7.2% ± 3.4% versus plant sterols: 7.7% ± 4.1%)	S. De Jongh et al. J Inherit Metab Dis. 2003

| DB-co-RCT | n.23 HyperCT children

Age: 2–9 years

Inclusion criteria:
TC > 194 mg/dl and
TG < 176 mg/dl | Evaluation of plant sterol and stanol effects in HyperCT children | Intervention: 19.9 g/day stanol ester (1.6 g) spread and 21 g/day of sterol ester (1.7 g) spread

Duration: 5-weeks periods separated by 5-weeks wash-out period | No serious adverse events | Good compliance | Stanol:
↓ TC: −9%
↓ LDL-C: −12%

Sterol:
↓ TC: −6%
↓ LDL-C: −9%

No significant changes HDL-c or serum Tg concentrations and on red cell cholesterol | A. M. Ketomäki et al. J Pediatr. 2003 |
| DB-RCT | n. 14 HeFH children
n. 1 HoFe children

Age: 2–15 years

Inclusion criteria:
FH diagnosis established in children and in parents by DNA technique | Effects of sitostanol (3 g/day) ester dissolved in rapeseed oil margarine as a hypocholesterolemic agent in 1 HoFH and 14 He-FH children on low cholesterol diet for 6 weeks | Intervention: 24 g of rapeseed oil-rich margarine without or with sitostanol ester (mean sitostanol intake 2.76 ± 0.15 g/d)

Duration: 6 weeks | No serious adverse events | Good compliance | ↓ TC: −10.6%

↓ IDL: −25.9%

↓ LDL-C: −15%

↑ HDL/LDL: +27%

↑ serum Δ-cholesterol, lathosterol, and desmosterol: +9, +42 and +29% respectively | H. Gylling et al. J Lipid Res. 1995 |

↑: increase, ↓: decrease, *HDL-C*: HDL-cholesterol, *HyperCT*: Hypercholesterolemia, *LDL-C*: LDL-cholesterol, *TG*: triglycerides, *TC*: total cholesterol, *IDL*: intermediate density lipoprotein, *sdLDL-C*: small dense low density lipoprotein-cholesterol, *CT*: controlled trial, *RCT*: randomized controlled trial, *DB*: double-blind, *CO*: crossover; *He*: heterozygous; *Ho*: homozygous; *FH*: familial hypercholesterolemia, *FMD*: flow-mediated dilation, *PSE*: plant sterol ester-enriched, *FMD*: £ow-mediated dilation

An additive benefit to the above described changes is the significant decrease of small dense LDL-C (sdLDL-C) levels after a daily consumption of 2 g of plant sterols in children and adolescents with dyslipidemia. This topic is of great relevance, and never described before, as sdLDL-C particles characterize the phenotypeB described in subjects affected by metabolic syndrome. Reducing sdLDL-C concentrations means to reduce a marker of cardiovascular risk then to improve benefits [65].

Data are concordant on the lack of significant effect on TG concentrations, at times reduced but not significantly [70] while HDL-C did not change [71].

Variations in carotenoids and fat-soluble vitamins were reported by investigators using plant sterol– or stanol ester–enriched spreads in both adults and children. In FH children lipid-adjusted lycopene decreased by 8.1% (P = 0.015) when on stanol period but this reduction was not confirmed as statistically significant at 6 month follow-up. As well alfa- and beta-carotene dropped down significantly by 17.4% and 10.9%, respectively, in FH children, after daily consumption of 1.2 g of plant sterols for 2 months, but recovered at 6 month follow-up [64]. In the STRIP study the administration of 1.5 phytostanols to mild hypercholesterolemic children decreased the serum beta-carotene to LDL-C ratio by 19% (P = 0.003), while alpha-tocopherol to LDL-C ratio remained unchanged [57]. No changes in other carotenoids or fat soluble vitamins occurred [63]. Anyway, as results in children are numerically poor it should be suggested to improve the intake of vegetables and fruits, when on phytosterol added to the dietary regimen, to compensate any possible carotenoid reduction also possibly related to seasonal dietary variation.

To establish if the LDL-C change on phytosterol addiction ameliorate the endothelial function in children, a marker related to future cardiovascular events, flow mediated dilation was assessed in two different studies on FH children with no benefit [69, 68]. Two ocurrences were considered: the lack of a direct effect on the endothelium, independent of LDL-C levels or the failure to reach a threshold level, as the endothelial function is strictly related to LDL-C [68]. Finally the Apolipoprotein E4 or Apolipoprotein E3 genotypes do not impact on biochemical effects of sterols or stanols addiction in children [62], but this topic is controversial as several studies demonstrate in adults [63].

Children undergoing statin therapy show commonly homeostasic changes characterized by increased cholesterol absorption and increased plant sterol levels. In this condition phytostanol supplementation was demonstrated to reverse these changes then it should be considered advantageous to ameliorate the metabolic balance [72, 73].

Although most studies demonstrate the benefits of sterol/stanol administration, by contrast two studies showed no improvement when conducted for 8 weeks [74] or 12 months [75]. These observations are supposed to be related to critical and still questionable points. These include the administration vehicle (i.e. milk, yoghurt, and margarine), the administration frequency and the dosage of daily intake [54, 76]. Moreover the lipid drop seems independent of baseline levels, the effects are similar in adults and children and the maximum effect is reached in a short time, generally 2 weeks [77]. The administration for a longer period did not reduce LDL-C levels further [78] and not only it should be considered that the compliance reduces with time. The latter, as demonstrated in a 6 months follow-up, the longest conducted in FH children, dropped from 92% to 65% then lowering the intake of spread of 25% [64].

Adverse Effects

The experts agree with no relevant adverse events on the short and mean term as children did not referred any side effects, or any other difficulties in complying to the diet and to phyto-sterols/stanols intake, [63] as functional food were well tolerated. Furthermore plant stanols have been evaluated for safety for as long as 5 years without any reported adverse events [79].

The long term safety, on the contrary, was questioned as phytosterol levels were demonstrated to increase the incidence of atherosclerosis [80]; it should be related to increased cardiovascular events, as described in the large epidemiological cohort of the PROCAM Study [81]. Furthermore, in the MONICA/KORA study, campesterol correlated with the incidence of acute myocardial infarction [82]. Controversies concerning the role of beta-sitosterol as a causative agent of premature atherosclerosis in the autosomal recessive familial form of sitosterolemia is well known [83] but other reports seem to contradict this finding [84, 85]. The mild increase in sitosterol, as relevant to cardiovascular risk remains a matter of debate. Campesterol and sitosterol increased but were still less than 8% [64] of that observed in subjects with homozygous phytosterolemia [86] and did not exceed 1% of total serum sterols, while cholesterol accounts for more than 99% of serum sterols [64]. Lathosterol, a marker of liver cholesterol synthesis, was unmodified after a 12-weeks sterol intake [67] while it increased by 259% after 6 months follow-up on sterol ester supplementation [64]. Discussion underline that plant sterol homeostasis is still unsolved [66] then long-term trials with plant sterol–enriched foods are mandatory for solving the question.

The administration of phyto-sterols/stanols has been demonstrated an efficacious tool in order to reduce cholesterol levels in children with hyperlipidemia and at high risk of premature atherosclerotic disease. In addition, plant sterols do not decrease HDL-C concentration and overall their complementary effects to diet can represent a choice to be considered under strict dietician and medical follow-up.

Other Nutraceuticals

Children suffering dyslipidemias have been investigated for other nutraceuticals including RYR, Probiotics, Omega-3 and Omega-6 PUFA, Soy Protein and Nuts recognized safe for cardiovascular prevention (Table 13.3). These trials, although randomized and controlled, are sporadic then observations need confirmations on wider and well selected cohort.

Table 13.3 Randomized controlled trials in children on the lipid-lowering effects of other nutraceuticals

Nutraceutical	Type of study	Subjects	Aim of the study	Intervention	Intolerance AND/OR side effect	Compliance	Observed effects	Ref.
RED YEAST RICE EXTRACT + POLICOSANOLS	DB-PLACEBO-CO-RCT	n. 40 HyperCT children FH: n.24 FCH: n.16 Age: 8–16 years	Evaluation of efficacy tolerability and safety of treatment with a dietary supplement containing red yeast rice extract and policosanols in a group of FH and FCH children	Dietary advice: 4 weeks	n.2 children on placebo: mild flu-like symptoms	Good compliance	↓CT: - 18.5% ↓LDL-c: - 25.1% ↓ApoB: 25.3%	O. Guardamagna et al. Nutrition, Metab & Cardiovasc Diseases. 2011
				200 mg/day of red yeast rice extract (3 mg of monacolins) and 10 mg/day of policosanols or placebo	n.3 children on dietary supplement: headache, diarrhea and dyspepsia			
				Duration: 8 weeks	n.2 mild CPK increase		No significant differences in HDL-C and ApoA1 levels	
				Washout period: 4 weeks				
PROBIOTICS	DB-PLACEBO-CO-RCT	n. 38 HyperCT children n. 2 drop-out	Effects of a probiotic formulation containing three Bifidobacterium strains on lipid profiles in children affected by primary dyslipidaemia	Dietary advice: 4 weeks	No relevant adverse effects	Compliance 91% vs 89% probiotics	↓CT: −3.4% ↓LDL-C: −3.8% ↓TG: −1.9% ↑HDL–C: 1.7%	O. Guardamagna et al. Nutrition. 2014
				n.19: Intervention group: Probiotics 1cps/day before dinner (dosage: 1 × 109cfu-oral capsules containing maltodextrin/ silicon dioxide excipient) Duration: 12 weeks	n.3 patients: abdominal discomfort and cramps			
		TOT n° 36 Hyperlipidemic children		n.19: Control group: Placebo-Duration: 12 weeks				
		n. 2 FH children n. 23 FCH children n. 13 HyperCT children		Washout period: 4 weeks				
				Duration: 32 weeks				
		Age: 6.3–15.1 years		Probiotic formulation: B. animalis subspecies lactis MB 2409 (DSM 23733), B. bifidum MB 109 (DSM 23731), and B. longum subspecies longum BL04 (DSM 23233) in lyophilized form. Duration 32 weeks				
		Inclusion criteria: children 6–18 years + TC > 90th percentile age sex specific						

SOY PROTEIN	RCT	n. 23 children n. 7 drop-out TOT n. 16 children n. 13 FH n. 3 Poligenic HyperCT Age: 4–18 years	To assess the effect of 3 month treatment of FH and Poligenic HyperCT children with a soy-substituted diet on serum lipids and lipoproteins	Phase 1: dietary advice Duration: 3 months Phase 2: Includes soy protein of at least 0.25 g/kg body weight into diet substituting soy protein for animal protein. This was achieved by the introduction of soy foods (soy dairy-free milk alternatives) and/or a mixture of other animal proteins	No relevant adverse effects	Drop-out: n.7 Soy protein allergy: n. 2 Not adherence to either phase 1 or phase 2: n. 5	Phase 1: ↓CT: −12.3% ↓LDL-C: −11.8% ↓ApoB: -10.6% No significant reduction in HDL-C and ApoA1 Phase 2: ↓CT: −7.7% ↓LDL-C: −6.4% ↓ApoB: −12.6% No significant reduction in HDL-C. ApoA1 and Lp(a)	D.Weghuber. British Journal of Nutrition. 2008
	CO-RCT	Inclusion criteria: diagnosis of FH and at least one FH family member n. 23 FH/Poligenic HyperCT children (n.12 M; n.11F) Mean age: 9.3 ± ±4.5 years Inclusion criteria: familial or polygenic hypercholesterolemia	To assess the effect on serum lipid and lipoprotein levels of a standard low fat, low cholesterol diet compared with a soy protein-substituted low fat, low cholesterol diet in FH or Poligenic HyperCT children	Duration: 3 months Group 1: received the soy protein diet Group 2 received the low fat, low cholesterol diet Duration: 8 weeks Washout period: 8 weeks	No relevant adverse effects	Not indicated	Soy protein intervention Group 1: ↓CT: −16% ↓LDL-c: − 22% Group 2 ↓CT: −18% ↓LDL-c: − 25% Dietary intervention Group 2: ↓CT: −8% ↓LDL-c: − 7% Group 2 ↓CT: −12% ↓LDL-c: − 13%	K.Widhalm et al. Journal of Pediatric. 1993
	CO-RCT	Children with FH Inclusion criteria: not indicated	Effects of soy protein and cow-milk proteins on plasma lipoprotein concentrations in HyperCT children	Dietary advice Group 1: Soy-protein Group 2: Cow-milk-protein Duration: 4 weeks	No relevant adverse effects	Not indicated	↓ TG and ↓ VLDL-C ↑ HDL-C No changes in TC, LDL-C and Apolipoprotein concentrations	D. Laurin et al. Am J Clin Nutr. 1991

(continued)

Table 13.3 (continued)

Nutraceutical	Type of study	Subjects	Aim of the study	Intervention	Intolerance AND/OR side effect	Compliance	Observed effects	Ref.
PUFA	RCT	n.36 children n. 18 children Intervention group n.18 children control group Inclusion criteria: primary hyperlipidaemia + compliance with dietary guideline	The impact of HSO supplementation on the serum lipid profile and FA composition of RBCs in children with primary hyperlipidaemia	Dietary guidelines Intervention HSO: 3 g/day of HSO (1.4 g of LA and 0.7 g/day of ALA) Duration: 8 weeks	No relevant adverse effects	Not indicated	↓RBC SFAs: −5.02% ↓RBC MUFAs: −2.12% ↑ PUFAs n-3: + 1.57% ↑ PUFAs n-6: + 5.39% ↑ Omega3-Index: +1.18% No changes in serum lipid profile	C. del Bo', Food Res Int. 2019
Nuts	SB-RCT	TOT n. 66 children with primary hyperlipidaemia (n. 2 drop-out) (n. 4 drop-out) Mean age: 11.6 years Inclusion criteria: diagnosis of primary hyperlipidaemia, TC and/ or TG >90th percentile	Effect of dietary intervention with hazelnuts on serum lipid profile, anthropometric parameters and FAs composition of erythrocyte phospholipids	Intervention groups: HZN+S n. 22, HZN-S n. 20, Controls n. 18 15-30 g/day of HZNs Duration: 8 weeks	No relevant adverse effects	Not indicated	HZN + S ↓LDL-C:-6.5% ↑HDL/LDL:+8% HZN-S ↓LDL-C: −6.2% ↑HDL/LDL: + 10% ↓non-HDL-C: −6.6% No changes in serum lipid profile in the control group	V. Deon et al. Clinical Nutrition. 2018
Nuts	SB-RCT	TOT n.60 with primary hyperlipidaemia Inclusion criteria: normal weight + diagnosis of primary hyperlipemia + TC and/or TG > 90th percentile.	Impact of a dietary intervention with hazelnuts on selected oxidative stress markers in children with primary hyperlipidaemia	Intervention groups: HZN+S n. 22, HZN-S n. 20, Controls n. 18 15-30 g/day of HZNs Duration: 8 weeks	No relevant adverse effects	Not indicated	↓Endogenous DNA damage: HZN + S: −18.9% HZN-S: −23.1% No changes in Ox-LDL levels after HZN + S intervention	F. Guaraldi et al. Journal of Nutritional Biochemistry. 2018

NUTS	RCT	TOT n.32 children primary hyperlipidemia	Effects of hazelnut intake on microbiota composition and SCFA levels	Intervention: HZN + S (0.43 g/kg body weight up to a maximum of 30 g)	No relevant adverse effects	Not indicated	Limited changes in fecal microbiota composition but modulation of fecal levels of predominant intestinal SCFAs	Gargari et al. FEMS Microbiology Ecology. 2018
		n. 15 children HZN + S n. 15 normolipidemic controls		Duration: 8 weeks				
		n.32 children SCFAs evaluation						
		Age: 7–17 years						
		Inclusion criteria: normal weight + diagnosis of primary hyperlipemia + TC and/or TG levels highter than age and sex-specific 90th percentile						

SB: Single Blind, *PH*: polygenic hyperlipidaemia, *HyperCT*: hypercholesterolemia, *HZN+S*: Hazelnuts with skin, *HZN-S*: Hazelnuts without skin, *FAs*: Fatty acids, *HSO*: hempseed oil, *LA*: linoleic acid, *ALA*: α-linolenic acid, *RBC*: red blood cells, *SFAs*: saturated fatty acids, *MUFAS*: monounsaturated fatty acids, *PUFAs*: polyunsaturated fatty acids, *IME*: intestinal microbial ecosystem

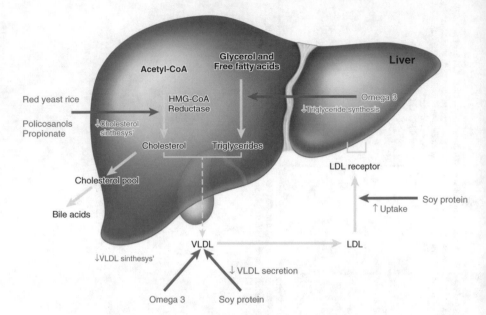

Fig. 13.2 Effects of nutraceuticals on cholesterol and triglyceride synthesis, very low density lipoprotein (VLDL) liver secretion and Low Density Lipoprotein (LDL) uptake
HMG-CoA Reductase- 3-hydroxy-3-methylglutaryl-coenzyme A reductase; *LDL* low density lipoprotein, *LDL-R* low-density lipoprotein receptor, *VLDL* very-low-density lipoprotein

Red Yeast Rice (Monacolin K)

RYR has been largely employed for many centuries in China as an additive to flavour food; it was obtained by fermentation of rice cooked with red wine mash giving the typical red colour. Actually the nutraceutical preparation is obtained by fermentation with the mycete *Monascus purpureus* Went. This compound is then processed 9 days later and gel capsules are available as supplement [87]. RYR contains a series of monacolins. Monacolin K, the bioactive one, shows effects similar to lovastatin [88] as inhibitor of 3-hydroxy-3methylglutaryl-coenzymeA reductase then shows lipid lowering benefits (Fig. 13.2). The efficacy of hypolipidemic effects of Monacolin K has been largely demonstrated in adults. A number of recent metanalysis confirm its safety [89] and addresses the administration of RYR also to intolerant statin subjects [90].

At present just one study has been conducted in children at increased cardiovascular risk including children suffering FH and FCH, already on Step II diet [91]. The study design was a double blind, randomized cross-over trial that lasted 6 months. All patient completed the study without relevant adverse effects. At the end of treatment, 8 weeks later, TC, LDL-C and ApoB decrease were −18.5%, −25.1% and −25.3% respectively. HDL-C was unchanged. These results were interesting for compliance, tolerability and effectivness. In particular, considering the Monacolin K, 3 mg/day dosage, the result was impressive as similar to that reached by pravastatin 10 mg/day suggesting a synergic effect of other bioactive components.

With respect to safety the concern should be related to Monacolin, the statin-like molecule, showing real pharmacological benefits as well as potential adverse effects. Children undergoing this supplement need a strict follow-up, in particular in the first weeks of administration, to avoid intolerance, transaminase or creatinphosfokinase changes as miopathy and rabdomyolisis have been described [92, 93]. Another point concerns the quality of capsule content as citrinin, a micotoxin produced by monascus, resulted strongly nephrotoxic and possibly genotoxic and carcinogenic [94] then it should be removed by manifacturers.

In conclusion RYR represents a good choice for high cardiovascular risk children showing hypercholesterolemia but in the practice the administration needs to comply with Guidelines on statin treatment concerning children selection, follow-up to ascetain tolerability and target levels to be observed.

Probiotics

Probiotics or "live microbes which, when administered in adequate amounts, confer a health benefit to the host" as defined by FAO/WHO [95], have been demonstrated useful in reducing lipids in hyperlipidemic adults [93]. This effect is the result of cholesterol assimilation and bile salts hydrolysis (BSH) [97, 96]; the first, triggered by lactic acid bacteria, inhibits the intestinal cholesterol reabsorption and the second impacts on bile salt homeostasis leading to LDL-C and ApoB reduction [96]. Furthermore some Bifidobacteria strains ameliorate blood lipids as transform linoleic acid (LA) into conjugated linoleic acids (CLA) [98].

The combination of different probiotic strains seems to improve results as healthy hypercholesterolemic adults showed TC, LDL-C and ApoB reduction when administered yoghurt, enriched with BSH producing probiotic strains as *Lactobacillus acidofilus*, *L. casei*, *L. reuteri*, *Bifidobacterium longum* [99, 100]. The effects of Lactobacillus acidofilus on TC, LDL-C and on inflammatory markers of hypercholesterolemic adults were further confirmed in two metanalysis, in particular when the medium was yoghurt [101], but also when administered in capsules [102]. A double-blind, randomized, placebo-controlled, cross-over trial, 32 weeks long, was performed in children showing TC exceeding the 90 percentile (age/sex related). The administration of a mixture of three Bifidobacterium strains, active on BSH activity, cholesterol assimilation, and CLA production enhanced a very mild, but significant, decrease of TC (3.4%), LDL-C (3.8%), TG (1.9%) and increased HDL-C (1.7%) levels [103]. Compliance and tolerance were optimal. Concerning the safety it should be remembered that species B. animalis, B. bifidum, and B. breve are currently included in the QPS (qualified presumption of safety) list of European Food Safety Authority (EFSA), based on their history of safety [104].

Poliunsatured Fatty Acids (PUFAs)

The quality of dietary fat affects serum concentrations of lipoprotein profile [105] but the dietary intake of PUFAs is often inadequate in children [106]. PUFAs, and in particular Omega-3 PUFAs and Omega-6 PUFAs, impact on cardiovascular risk markers such as TG (Fig. 13.2), LDL-C, adhesion molecules and show anti-inflammatory properties [107, 108]. The effects of a 5-month daily intake of milk enriched with long-chain PUFAs, and low in saturated fatty acids, were evaluated in a randomized double-blind placebo-controlled trial on 107 healthy children. The functional food reduced markers of endothelial cell activation as adhesion molecules, E-selectin, ICAM-1 and lymphocyte levels decreased while plasma DHA increased [109]. Hempseed oil (HSO) is rich in essential fatty acids Omega-3 PUFAs α-linolenic acid (ALA) and Omega-6 PUFAs linoleic acid (LA). The LA/ALA ratio ranges between 2:1 and 3:1, a favorable proportion then is suitable as dietary supplement [110]. While HSO has been already checked in animals and human adults just a recent RCT 8 week long study was performed in hyperlipidemic children. It increased red blood cell content of total n-3 and n-6 PUFAs and ameliorate the Omega3-index. A significant mean reduction (14%) in LDL-C levels was detected in the HSO group [111].

In conclusion results on PUFAs supplemented diet is of great value to provide and complement the food intake but further studies are necessary to confirm preliminary data.

Soy

The effects of Soy and its derivatives, extensively studied in adults, are referred to the isoflavone content that promotes the expression of LDL receptors [112] (Fig. 13.2). On this basis Soy Proteins have been considered beneficial for subjects suffering hypercholesterolemia. Adults with borderline-high TC levels ameliorate serum TC and LDL-C around 4–6% after the consumption of 25 g/day of Soy protein [113]. Studies in children are scanty but a preliminary one addressed FH children to soy protein versus milk protein. TC and LDL-C did not change significantly while TG decreased and HDL-C increased in the former group [114]. Results similar to those above described in adults were obtained in a prospective study conducted on 16 hypercholesterolemic children, mainly FH affected. TC, LDL-C and ApoB decreased significantly (7.7, 6.4, 12.6% respectively) when Soy Proteins (administerd as soya dairy-free milk, 0·25–0·5 g/kg body weight) were added to STEP I diet for 3 months [115]. This was the more extended study on soy protein in pediatrics, children were compliant to this program but not all subjects (4/16) were responders, although showing the same basal characteristics. In general most studies agree with the efficacy of Soy protein, although safety data are conflicting. Issues concern allergic disorders or the effects of phytoestrogen content which are still questionable mainly in very young subjects [116].

Nuts

Nuts are dry fruits that include almonds, walnuts, hazelnuts, macadamia nuts, pistachios and peanuts. The cardioprotective effects and health benefits of nuts have been largely demonstrated in epidemiologial studies, particularly on walnuts, and attributed to bioactive components like MUFAs and PUFAs, phytosterols, antioxidants, vitamins (e.g. tocopherols), fibers, and polyphenols well represented in hazelnuts [117]. Poliphenols are regarded to improve lipid profile as impact on cholesterol absorption, TG synthesis and secretion, showing antioxidant effects [118]. Furthermore hazelnuts show the highest content of MUFAs when compared to all other nuts [119].

Once more very poor data concern trials in hyperlipidemic children and as far as we know just 3 available randomized studies were addressed to explore the effects of hazelnuts on lipid profile, antioxidative properties and microbiome. Results from these studies confirm the beneficial power and efficacy of a daily intake (0.43 g/ kg of body weight, 15–30 g portions). Hazelnuts with or without skin reduced significantly LDL-C and increased the ratio HDL-C/LDL-C when the hazelnut supplemented group was compared to the control group receiving STEP I diet. Furthermore an increase of MUFA/SFA on red blood cells [119] was demonstrated. On the same cohort hazelnuts lowered the endogenous and oxidatively induced DNA damage, as already known in adults after the intake of almonds or walnuts [120]. The effects on microbiome has been as well demontrated to modulate the abundance of gut microbiota and to modulate the intestinal concentration of SCFAs [121].

Final Considerations

Although randomized and controlled studies considering strong end-point in children are poor, and often occasional, benefits observed at least in the short – mean time, mainly concerning phyto-sterol/stanol and fibre, should be underlined.

Sterol/Stanol and fibre supplementary foods demonstrate usually the efficacy in reducing TC and LDL-C in FH children, but also in poligenic hypercholesterolemia or in children showing metabolic disturbances and mild changes of lipid profile. ApoB as well ameliorate after phytosterols intake while contrasting results concern fibre. On the contrary no favourable variations have been observed on the endothelial function on phyto-sterol/stanol addiction but since only 2 studies concern this topic results are unconclusive. Phyto-sterol/stanol and fibre were well tolerated and the compliance was elevated at least in the short time. The compliance decrease occurring at phytosterol follow-up did not worsen the biochemical parameters. No significant serious adverse effects were detected but abdominal discomfort or diarrhea were the most frequently referred symptoms on fibre supplementation. Functional foods containing phyto-sterol/stanol are related to a significant decrease of carotenoids requiring an uphold intake of vegetables and fruits to avoid nutritional deficiency.

Available data sustain the lipid-lowering effect of phytosterols in subjects suffering lipid disorders, as declared by Pediatric Guidelines, and the EAS Consensus Panel established on 2014 that functional foods with plant sterols/stanols should be considered also in children with FH [122].

In conclusions phytosterol and fiber are safe, as other above mentioned nutraceuticals could be, acceptable and effective complement to dietary therapy. It should be underlined that nutraceuticals should not be considered an alternative to diet or statins when required, as Guidelines suggest. Diet STEP I or STEP II (CHILD I or CHILD II) represent the therapeutic cornerstone in the prevention of dyslipidemia in children and the first basic approach that need to be respected to promote healthy life and outcome.

Acknowledgments Authors thanks Elisabetta Bartoletti for kindly providing drawings. Authours declare no conflict of interest.

References

1. Guardamagna O, Baracco V, Abello F, et al. Identification and management of dyslipidemic children. Minerva Pediatr. 2009;61:391–8.
2. American Academy of Pediatrics Committee on Nutrition. Cholesterol in childhood. Pediatrics. 1998;101:141–7.
3. Expert Panel on Integrated Guidelines for Cardiovascular Health and Risk Reduction in Children and Adolescents, National Heart, Lung, and Blood Institute. Expert panel on integrated guidelines for cardiovascular health and risk reduction in children and ado- lescents: summary report. Pediatrics 2011;128(Suppl 5):S213e56.
4. Kwiterovich PO. Recognition and management of dyslipidemia in children and adolescents. J Clin Endocrinol Metab. 2008;93:4200–9.
5. Slavin JL. Carbohydrates, dietary fiber, and resistant starch in white vegetables: links to health outcomes. Adv Nutr. 2013;4:351S–5S.
6. Giacco R, Clemente G, Cipriano D, Luongo D, Viscovo D, Patti L, et al. Effects of the regular consumption of wholemeal wheat foods on cardiovascular risk factors in healthy people. Nutr Metab Cardiovasc Dis. 2010;20:186–94.
7. Anderson JW, Story L, Sieling B, et al. Hypercholesterolemic effects of oat-bran or bean intake for hypercholesterolemic men. Am J Clin Nutr. 1984;40:1146–55.
8. Bell LP, Hectorne K, Reynolds H, et al. Cholesterol lowering effects of psyllium hydrophilic mucilloid: adjunct therapy to a prudent diet for patient with mild to moderate hypercholesterolemia. JAMA. 1989;261:3419–23.
9. European Food Safety Authority: scientific opinion on dietary reference values for carbohydrates and dietary fiber. EFSA J. 2010;8:1462.
10. Food and Drug Administration. Food Labeling: health claims; oats and coronary heart disease. Maryland: Health and Human Services; 1997.
11. EFSA Panel on Dietetic Products, Nutrition and Allergies (NDA) (2011) Scientific opinion on the substantiation of health claims related to beta-glucans from oats and barley and maintenance of normal blood LDL-cholesterol concentrations (ID 1236, 1299), increase in satiety leading to a reduction in energy intake (ID 851, 852), reduction of post-prandial glycaemic responses (ID 821, 824), and 'digestive function' (ID 850) pursuant to Article 13(1) of Regulation (EC) No 1924/ 2006. EFSA J 9, 2207.
12. Dwyer JT. Dietary fiber for children: how much? Pediatrics. 1995;96:1019–22.

13. Kranz S, Brauchla M, Slavin JL, Miller KB. What do we know about dietary fiber intake in children and health? The effects of fiber intake on constipation, obesity, and diabetes in children. Adv Nutr. 2012;3:47–53.
14. Edwards CA, Xie C, Garcia AL. Dietary fibre and health in children and adolescents. Proc Nutr Soc. 2015;74:292–302.
15. Daniels SR, Greer FR, the Committee on Nutrition. Lipid screening and cardiovascular health in childhood. Pediatrics. 2008;122:198–208.
16. Institute of Medicine 2000. Dietary reference intakes: applications in dietary assessment. Washington, DC: National Academy Press pp 306.
17. Bollella M, Williams CL, Strobino B, Brotanek J. Dietary predictors of cardiovascular risk factors among children in a 5-year health tracking study: healthy start. Presented at the American Dietetic Association, Food & Nutrition Conference & Expo, San Antonio, TX, October 25–28, 2003
18. Singh B. Psyllium as therapeutic and drug delivery agent. Int J Pharm. 2007;334:1–14.
19. Gonzalez Canga A, Fernandez Martınez N, Sahagun AM, Garcıa Vieitez JJ, Dıez Liebana MJ, Calle Pardo AP, et al. Glucomannan: properties and therapeutic applications. Nutr Hosp. 2004;19:45–50.
20. Butt MS, Tahir-Nadeem M, Khan MKI, Shabir R, Butt MS. Oat: unique among the cereals. Eurn J Nutr. 2008;47:68–97.
21. Zavoral JH, Hannan P, Fields DJ, Hanson MN, Frantz ID, Kuba K, Elmer P, Jacobs D. R. the hypolipidemic effect of locust bean gum food products in familial hypercholesterolemic adults and children. Am J Clin Nutr. 1983;38:285–94.
22. Vuksan V, Jenkıns AL, Rogovık AL, Fairgrieve CD, Jovanovski E, Leiter LA. Viscosity rather than quantity of dietary fibre predicts cholesterol-lowering effect in healthy individuals. Br J Nutr. 2011;106:1349–52.
23. Jane M, McKay J, Pal S. Effects of daily consumption of psyllium, oat bran and polyGlycopleX on obesity-related disease risk factors: a critical review. Nutrition. 2019;57:84–91.
24. Gunness P, Gidley MJ. Mechanisms underlying the cholesterol lowering properties of soluble dietary fibre polysaccharides. Food Function. 2010;1:149–55.
25. Shinozaki K, Okuda M, Sasaki S, Kunitsugu I, Shigeta M. Dietary fiber consumption decreases the risks of overweight and hypercholesterolemia in Japanese children. Ann Nutr Metab. 2015;67:58–64.
26. Davidson MH, Dugan LD, Burns JH, Sugimoto D, Story K, Drennan K. A psyllium-enriched cereal for the treatment of hypercholesterolemia in children: a controlled, double-blind, crossover study. Am J Clin Nutr. 1996;63:96–102.
27. Sanchez-Bayle M, Gonzalez-Requejo A, Asensio-Anton J, Ruiz-Jarabo C, Fernandez-Ruiz ML, Baeza J. The effect of fiber supplementation on lipid profile in children with hypercholesterolemia. Clin Pediatr (Phila). 2001;40:291–4.
28. Martino F, Martino E, Morrone F, Carnevali E, Forcone R, Niglio T. Effect of dietary supplementation with glucomannan on plasma total cholesterol and low density lipoprotein cholesterol in hypercholesterolemic children. Nutr Metab Cardiovasc Dis. 2005;15:174–80.
29. Gold K, Wong N, Tong A, Bassin S, Iftner C, Nguyen T, et al. Serum apolipoprotein and lipid profile effects of an oat-bran-supplemented, low-fat diet in children with elevated serum cholesterol. Ann N Y Acad Sci. 1991;623:429–31.
30. Williams CL, Bollella MC, Strobino BA, Boccia L, Campanaro L. Plant stanol ester and bran fiber in childhood: effects on lipids, stool weight and stool frequency in preschool children. J Am Coll Nutr. 1999;18:572–81.
31. Glassman M, Spark A, Berezin S, Schwartz S, Medow M, Newman LJ. Treatment of type IIa hyperlipidemia in childhood by a simplified American Heart Association diet and fiber supplementation. Am J Dis Child. 1990;144:193–7.
32. Taneja A, Bhat CM, Arora A, Kaur AP. Effect of incorporation of isabgol husk in a low fibre diet on faecal excretion and serum levels of lipids in adolescent girls. Eur J Clin Nutr. 1989;43:197–202.

33. Dennison BA, Levine DM. Randomized, double-blind, placebo-controlled, two-period crossover clinical trial of psyllium fiber in children with hypercholesterolemia. J Pediatr. 1993;123:24–9.
34. Williams CL, Spark A, Haley N, Axelrad C, Strobino B. Effectiveness of a psyllium-enriched step I diet in hypercholesterolemic children. Circulation. 1991;84:II–6.
35. Clauss SB, Kwiterovich PO. Long-term safety and efficacy of low-fat diets in children and adolescents. Minerva Pediatr. 2002;54:305–13.
36. The DISC Collaborative Research Group. The efficacy and safety of lowering dietary intake of total fat, saturated fat, and cholesterol in children with elevated LDL-C: the Dietary Intervention Study in Children (DISC). JAMA. 1995;273:1429–35.
37. Williams CL, Bollella M, Spark A, Puder D. Soluble FIber enhances the hypercholesterolemic effect of the step I diet in childhood. J Am Coll Nutr. 1995;3(14):251–7.
38. Ribas SA, Cunha DB, Sichieri R, Santana da Silva LC. Effects of psyllium on LDL-cholesterol concentrations in Brazilian children and adolescents: a randomised, placebo-controlled, parallel clinical trial. Br J Nutr. 2015;113:134–41.
39. EFSA Panel on Dietetic Products, Nutrition and Allergies. Scientific opinion on the substantiation of health claims related to konjac mannan (glucomannan) and reduction of body weight (ID 854, 1556, 3725), reduction of post-prandial glycaemic responses (ID 1559), maintenance of normal blood glucose concentrations (ID 835, 3724), maintenance of normal (fasting) blood concentrations of triglycerides (ID 3217), maintenance of normal blood cholesterol concentrations (ID 3100, 3217), maintenance of normal bowel function (ID 834, 1557, 3901) and decreasing potentially pathogenic gastro-intestinal microorganisms (ID 1558) pursuant to Article 13(1) of Regulation (EC) No 1924/2006. EFSA J 2010; 8(10):1798
40. Guardamagna O, Abello F, Cagliero P, Visioli F. Could dyslipidemic children benefit from glucomannan intake? Nutrition. 2013;29:1060–5.
41. Sood N, Baker WL, Coleman CI. Effect of glucomannan on plasma lipid and glucose concentrations, body weight, and blood pressure: systematic review and meta-analysis. Am J Clin Nutr. 2008;88:1167–75.
42. Livieri C, Novazi F, Lorini R. The use of highly purified glucomannan- based fibers in childhood obesity. Ped Med Chir. 1992;14:195–8.
43. Ho HVT, Jovanovski E, Zurbau A, Blanco Mejia S, Sievenpiper JL, Au-Yeung F, Jenkins AL, Duvnjak L, Leiter L, Vuksan V. A systematic review and meta-analysis of randomized controlled trials of the effect of konjac glucomannan, a viscous soluble fiber, on LDL cholesterol and the new lipid targets non-HDL cholesterol and apolipoprotein B. Am J Clin Nutr. 2017;105:1239–47.
44. Blumenschein S, Torres E, Kushmaul E, Crawford J, Fixler D. Effect of oat bran/ soy protein in hypercholesterolemic children. Ann N Y Acad Sci. 1991;623:413–5.
45. Catapano AL, Graham I, De Backer G, Wiklund O, Chapman MJ, Drexel H, Hoes AW, Jennings CS, Landmesser U, Pedersen TR, Reiner Z, Riccardi G, Taskinen MR, Tokgozoglu VWMM, Vlachopoulos C, Wood DA, Zamorano JL. 2016 ESC/EAS guidelines for the Management of Dyslipidaemias. Eur Heart J. 2016;37:2999–3058.
46. Vido L, Facchin P, Antonello I, Gobber D, Rigon F. Childhood obesity treatment: double blinded trial on dietary fibres (glucomannan) versus placebo. Padiatr Patol. 1993;28:133–6.
47. Maki CK, Davidson HM, Ingram AK, et al. Lipid responses to consumption of a beta-glucan containing ready- to-eat cereal in children and adolescents with mild- to-moderate primary hypercholesterolemia. Nutr Res. 2003;23:1527–35.
48. Theuwissen E, Mensink RP. Water-soluble dietary fibers and cardiovascular disease. Physiol Behav. 2008;94:285–92.
49. Food and Drug Administration, F.D.A. Issues a Safety Warning On Imported Jelly Cup Candies., August 17, 2001.
50. Ho HVT, Sievenpiper JL, Zurbau A, Mejia SB, Jovanovski E, Au-Yeung F, Jenkins AL, Vuksan V. A systematic review and meta-analysis of ran- domized controlled trials of the effect of barley b-glucan on LDL-C, non-HDL-C and apoB for cardiovascular disease risk reduction (i-iv). Eur J Clin Nutr. 2016;70:1239–45.

51. Kwiterovich PO, Chen SC, Virgil DG, et al. Biochemical and clinical characterization of obligate heterozygotes for phytosterolemia and their response to a low-fat diet and to a plant sterol ester dietary challenge. J Lipid Res. 2003;44:1143–55.
52. Third report of the national cholesterol education program (NCEP) expert panel on detection, evaluation, and treat- ment of high blood cholesterol in adults (Adult Treatment Panel III) final report. Circulation. 2002;106:3143–421.
53. Thompson G, Grundy MS. History and development of plant sterols and stanol esters for cholesterol lowering purposes. Am J Cardiol. 2005;96(1):3D–9D.
54. Clifton P, Noakes M, Sullivan D, Erichsen N, Ross D, Annison G, et al. Cholesterol-lowering effects of plant sterol esters differ in milk, yoghurt, bread and cereal. Eur J Clin Nutr. 2004;58(3):503e9.
55. Gylling H, Miettinen TA. New biologically active lipids in food, health food and pharmaceuticals. Lipidforum; Scandinavian forum for lipid research and technology, 19th Nordic Lipid Symposium, Ronneby, Sweden, June 1997; 81–86.
56. Jones PJ, Raeini-Sarjaz M, Ntanios FY, Vanstone CA, Feng JY, Parsons WE. Modulation of plasma lipid levels and cholesterol kinetics by phytosterol versus phytostanol esters. J Lipid Res. 2000;41:697–705.
57. Tammi A, Rönnemaa T, Gylling H, Rask-Nissilä L, Viikari J, Tuominen J, et al. Plant stanol ester margarine lowers serum total and low-density lipoprotein cholesterol concentrations of healthy children: the STRIP project. J Pediatr. 2000;136:503–10.
58. Gylling H, Miettinen TA. Inheritance of cholesterol metabolism of probands with high or low cholesterol absorption. J Lipid Res. 2002;43:1472–6.
59. Miettinen TA, Tilvis RS, Kesäniemi YA. Serum plant sterols and cholesterol precursors reflect cholesterol synthesis and absorption in volunteers of a randomly selected male population. Am J Epidemiol. 1990;131:20–31.
60. Gylling H, Siimes MA, Miettinen TA. Sitostanol ester margarine in dietary treatment of children with familial hypercholesterolemia. J Lipid Res. 1995;36:1807–12.
61. Ribas SA, Sichieri R, Moreira ASB, Souza DO, Cabral CTF, Gianinni DT, Cunha DB. Phytosterol-enriched milk lowers LDL-cholesterol levels in Brazilian children and adolescents: double-blind, cross-over trial. Nutr Metabol Cardiovasc Dis. 2017;27:971–7.
62. Tammi A, Rönnemaa T, Miettinen TA, Gylling H, Rask-Nissilä L, Viikari J, Tuominen J, Marniemi J, Simell O. Effects of gender, apolipoprotein E phenotype and cholesterol lowering by plant stanol esters in children: the STRIP study. Special Turku coronary risk factor intervention project. Acta Paediatr. 2002;91(11):1155–62.
63. Amundsen AL, Ose L, Nenseter MS, Ntanios FY. Plant sterol ester-enriched spread lowers plasma total and LDL cholesterol in children with familial hypercholesterolemia. Am J Clin Nutr. 2002;76:338–44.
64. Amundsen ÅL, Ntanios F, van der Put N, Ose L. Long-term compliance and changes in plasma lipids, plant sterols and carotenoids in children and parents with FH consuming plant sterol ester-enriched spread. Eur J Clin Nutr. 2004;58:1612–20. https://doi.org/10.1038/sj.ejcn.1602015.
65. Garoufi A, Vorre S, Soldatou A, Tsentidis C, Kossiva L, Drakatos AS, Marmarinos, Gourgiotis AD. Plant sterols–enriched diet decreases small, dense LDL-cholesterol levels in children with hypercholesterolemia: a prospective study. Ital J Pediatr. 2014;40:42.
66. Ketomäki AM, Gylling H, Antikainen M, Siimes MA, Miettinen TA. Red cell and plasma plant sterols are related during consumption of plant stanol and sterol ester spreads in children with hypercholesterolemia. J Pediatr. 2003;142:524–31.
67. Guardamagna O, Abello F, Baracco V, Federici G, Bertucci P, Mozzi A, Mannucci L, Gnasso A, Cortese C. Primary hyperlipidemias in children: effect of plant sterol supplementation on plasma lipids and markers of cholesterol synthesis and absorption. Acta Diabetol. 2011;48:127–33.
68. Jakulj L, Vissers MN, Rodenburg J, Wiegman A, Trip MD, Kastelein John JP. Plant stanols do not restore endothelial function in prepubertal children with familial hypercholesterolemia despite reduction of low-density lipoprotein cholesterol levels. J Pediatr. 2006;148:495–500.

69. de Jongh S, Vissers MN, Rol P, Bakker HD, Kastelein JJP, Stroes ESG. Plant sterols lower LDL cholesterol without improving endothelial function in prepubertal children with familial hypercholesterolaemia. J Inherit Metab Dis. 2003;26:343–51.
70. Malhotra A, Shafiq N, Arora A, Singh M, Kumar R, Malhotra S. Dietary interventions (plant sterols, stanols, omega-3 fatty acids, soy protein and dietary fibers) for familial hypercholesterolaemia (Review). Cochrane Database Syst Rev. 2014;(6):Art. No.: CD001918.
71. Demonty I, Ras RT, Van der Knaap HCM, Meijer L, Zock PL, Geleijnse JM, et al. The effect of plant sterols on serum triglyceride concentrations is dependent on baseline concentrations: a pooled analysis of 12 randomised controlled trials. Eur J Nutr. 2013;52:153e60.
72. Miettinen TA, Gylling H. Effect of statins on noncholesterol sterol levels: implications for use of plant stanols and sterols. Am J Cardiol. 2005;96:40–6.
73. Vuorio A, Kovane PT. Decreasing the cholesterol burden in heterozygous familial hypercholesterolemia children by dietary plant stanol esters. Nutrients. 2018;10:1842.
74. Davidson MH, Maki KC, Umporowicz DM, Ingram KA, Dicklin MR, Schaefer E, et al. Safety and tolerability of esterified phytosterols administered in reduced-fat spread and salad dressing to healthy adult men and women. J Am Coll Nutr. 2001;20:307–19.
75. Brink EJ, Hendricks HFJ. Long-term follow-up study on the use of a spread enriched with plant sterols, TNO report, vol. 99. Zeist: TNO Nutrition and Food Research Institute Report; 2000. p. 869.
76. AbuMweis SS, Barake R, Jones PJH. Plant sterols/stanols as cholesterol lowering agents: a meta-analysis of randomized controlled trials. Food Nutr Res. 2008;52:1–17.
77. Miettinen TA, Puska P, Gylling H, Vanhanen H, Vartiainen E. Reduction of serum cholesterol with sitostanol-ester margarine in a mildly hypercholesterolemic population. N Engl J Med. 1995;333:1308–12.
78. Hallikainen MA, Sarkkinen ES, Uusitupa MI. Plant stanol esters affect serum cholesterol concentrations of hypercholesterolemic men and women in a dose-dependent manner. J Nutr. 2000;130:767–76.
79. Katan MB, Grundy SM, Jones P, Law M, Miettinen T, Paoletti R. Efficacy and safety of plant stanols and sterols in the management of blood cholesterol levels. Mayo Clin Proc. 2003;78:965–78.
80. Glueck CJ, Speirs J, Tracy T, Streicher P, Illig E, Vandergrift J. Relationships of serum plant sterols (phytosterols) and cholesterol in 595 hypercholesterolemic subjects, and familial aggregation of phytosterols, cholesterol, and premature coronary heart disease in hyperphytosterolemic probands and their first-degree relatives. Metabolism. 1991;40:842–8.
81. Assmann G, Cullen P, Erbey J, Ramey DR, Kannenberg F, Schulte H. Plasma sitosterol elevations are associated with an increased incidence of coronary events in men: results of a nested case- control analysis of the prospective cardiovascular Munster (PRO- CAM) study. Nutr Metab Cardiovasc Dis. 2006;16:13e21.
82. Thiery J, Ceglarek U, Fiedler GM, Leichtle A, Baumann S, Teupser D, Lang O, Baumert J, Meisinger M, Loewell H, Doering A. Elevated campesterol serum levels—a significant predictor of incident myocardial infarction: results of the population-based MONICA/KORA follow-up study 1994–2005. Circulation. 2006;114:II–884.
83. Mannucci L, Guardamagna O, Bertucci P, Pisciotta L, Liberatoscioli L, Bertolini S, Irace C, Gnasso A, Federici G, Cortese C. Beta-sitosterolaemia: a new nonsense mutation in the ABCG5 gene. Eur J Clin Investig. 2007;37(12):997–1000.
84. Wilund KR, Yu L, Xu F, Vega GL, Grundy SM, Cohen JC, Hobbs HH. No association between plasma levels of plant sterols and atherosclerosis in mice and men. Arterioscler Thromb Vasc Biol. 2004;24(12):2326–32.
85. Fassbender K, Lutjohann D, Dik MG, Bremmer M, Konig J, Walter S, Liu Y, Letie'mbre M, von Bergmann K, Jonker C. Moderately elevated plant sterol levels are associated with reduced cardiovascular risk–the LASA study. Atherosclerosis. 2008;96(1):283–8.
86. Lutjohann D, Bjorkhem I, Ose L. Phytosterolaemia in a Norwegian family: diagnosis and characterization of the first Scandinavian case. Scand J Clin Lab Invest. 1996;56:229–40.
87. Ma J, Li Y, Ye Q, Li J, Hua Y, Ju D, Zhang D, Cooper R, Chang M. Constituents of red yeast rice, a traditional Chinese food and medicine. J Agric Food Chem. 2000;48:5220–5.

88. Journoud M, Jones PJ. Red yeast rice: a new hypolipidemic drug. Life Sci. 200474:2675–83.
89. Cicero A, Colletti A, Bajraktari G, Descamps O, Djuric DM, Ezhov M, Fras Z, Katsiki N, Langlois M, Latkovskis G, Panagiotakos DB, Paragh G, Mikhailidis DP, Mitchenko O, Paulweber B, Pella D, Pitsavos C, Reiner Z, Ray KK, Rizzo M, Sahebkar A, Serban MC, Sperling LS, Toth PP, Vinereanu D, Vrablík M, Wong ND, Banach M. Lipid lowering nutraceuticals in clinical practice: position paper from an International Lipid Expert Panel. Arch Med Sci. 2017;13(5):965–1005.
90. Pirro M, Vetrani C, Bianchi C, Mannarino MR, Bernini F, Rivellese AA. Joint position statement on "Nutraceuticals for the treatment of hypercholesterolemia" of the Italian Society of Diabetology (SID) and of the Italian Society for the Study of Arteriosclerosis (SISA). Nutr Metab Cardiovasc Dis. 2017;27:2–17.
91. Guardamagna O, Abello F, Baracco V, Stasiowska B, Martino F. The treatment of hypercholesterolemic children: efficacy and safety of a combination of red yeast rice extract and policosanols. Nutr Metab Cardiovasc Dis. 2011;21:424–9.
92. Lapi F, Gallo E, Bernasconi S, Vietri M, Menniti-Ippolito F, Raschetti R, et al. Myopathies associated with red yeast rice and liquorice: spontaneous reports from the Italian surveillance system of natural health products. Br J Clin Pharmacol. 2008;66:572–4.
93. Prasad GVR, Wong T, Meliton G, Bhaloo S. Rhabdomyolysis due to red yeast rice (Monascus purpureus) in a renal transplant recipient. Transplantation. 2002;74:1200e1.
94. European Food Safety Authority. EFSA J. 2012;10:2605–87.
95. Joint FAO/WHO Working Group. Guidelines for the evaluation of probiotics in food. London; 2002.
96. Jones ML, Tomaro Duchesneau C, Martoni CJ, Prakash S. Cholesterol lowering with bile salt hydrolase-active probiotic bacteria, mechanism of action, clinical evidence, and future direction for heart health applications. Exp Opin Biol Ther. 2013;13:631–42.
97. Bordoni A, Amaretti A, Leonardi A, Boschetti E, Danesi F, Matteuzzi D, et al. Cholesterol-lowering probiotics: in vitro selection and in vivo testing of bifidobacteria. Appl Microbiol Biotechnol. 2013;97:8273–81.
98. Dilzer A, Park Y. Implication of conjugated linoleic acid (CLA) in human health. Crit Rev Food Sci Nutr. 2012;52:488–513.
99. Jones ML, Martoni CJ, Parent M, Prakash S. Cholesterol-lowering efficacy of a microencapsu- lated bile salt hydrolase-active Lactobacillus reuteri NCIMB 30242 yoghurt formulation in hypercholesterol- aemic adults. Br J Nutr. 2011;107:1505–13.
100. Jones ML, Martoni CJ, Prakash S. Cholesterol lowering and inhibition of sterol absorption by Lactobacillus reuteri NCIMB 30242: a randomized controlled trial. Eur J Clin Nutr. 2012;66:1234–41.
101. Sun J, Buys N. Effects of probiotics consumption on lowering lipids and CVD risk factors: a systematic review and meta-analysis of randomized controlled trials. Ann Med. 2015;47:430–40.
102. Shimizu M, Hashiguchi M, Shiga T, Tamura HO, Mochizuki M. Meta-analysis: effects of probiotic supplementation on lipid profiles in normal to mildly hy- percholesterolemic individuals. PLoS One. 2015;10:e0139795.
103. Guardamagna O, Amaretti A, Puddu PE, Raimondi S, Abello F, Cagliero P, Rossi M. Bifidobacteria supplementation: effects on plasma lipid profiles in dyslipidemic children. Nutrition. 2014;30:831–6.
104. European Food Safety Authority (EFSA). Scientific opinion on the maintenance of the list of QPS biological agents intentionally added to food and feed (2012 update). EFSJ. 2012;10:3020.
105. Schwab US, Callaway JC, Erkkilä AT, Gynther J, Uusitupa MI, Järvinen T. Effects of hempseed and flaxseed oils on the profile of serum lipids, serum total and lipoprotein lipid concentrations and haemostatic factors. Eur J Nutr. 2006;45:470–7.
106. Patch CS, Tapsell LC, Mori TA, et al. The use of novel foods enriched with longchain n-3 fatty acids to increase dietary intake: a comparison of methodologies assessing nutrient intake. J Am Diet Assoc. 2005;105:1918–26.

107. Jacobson TA, Glickstein SB, Rowe JD, Soni PN. Effects of eicosa- pentaenoic acid and doco-sahexaenoic acid on low-density lipoprotein cholesterol and other lipids: a review. J Clin Lipidol. 2012;6:5–18.
108. Calder PC. n-3 polyunsaturated fatty acids, inflammation, and inflammatory diseases. Am J Clin Nutr. 2006;83:1505–19.
109. Romeo J, Wärnberg J, García-Mármol E, et al. Daily consumption of milk enriched with fish oil, oleic acid, minerals and vitamins reduces cell adhesion molecules in healthy children. Nutr Metab Cardiovasc Dis. 2009; https://doi.org/10.1016/j.numecd.2009.08.007.
110. Rodriguez-Leyva D, Pierce GN. The cardiac and haemostatic effects of dietary hempseed. Nutr Metab (Lond). 2010;7:32.
111. Del Bo' C, Deon V, Abello F, Massini G, Porrini M, Riso P, Guardamagna O. Eight-week hempseed oil intervention improves the fatty acid composition of erythrocyte phospholipids and the omega-3 index, but does not affect the lipid profile in children and adolescents with primary hyperlipidemia. Food Res Int. 2019;119:469–76.
112. Tokede OA, Onabanjo TA, Yansane A, Gaziano JM, Djousse L. Soya products and serum lipids: a meta-analysis of randomised controlled trials. Br J Nutr. 2015;114(6):831–43.
113. Anderson JW, Johnstone BM, Cook-Newell ME. Meta-analysis of the effects of soy protein intake on serum lipids. N Engl J Med. 1995;333(5):276–82.
114. Laurin D, Jacques H, Moorjani S, Steinke FH, Gagne C, Brun D, Lupien PJ. Effects of a soy-protein beverage on plasma lipoproteins in children with familial hypercholesterolemia. Am J Clin Nutr. 1991;54:98–103.
115. Weghuber D, Widhalm K. Effect of 3-month treatment of children and adolescents with familial and polygenic hypercholesterolaemia with a soya-substituted diet. Br J Nutr. 2008;99:281–6.
116. Rizzo G, Baroni L. Soy. Soy foods and their role in vegetarian diets. Nutrients. 2018;10:43.
117. Ros E. Health benefits of nut consumption. Nutrients. 2010;2:652–82.
118. Sanchez-Gonzalez C, Ciudad C, Noe V, Izquierdo-Pulido M. Health benefits of walnut poly-phenols: an exploration beyond their lipid profile. Crit Rev Food Sci Nutr. 2017;57:3373–83.
119. Deon V, Del Bo' C, Guaraldi F, Abello F, Belviso S, Porrini M, Riso P, Guardamagna O. Effect of hazelnut on serum lipid profile and fatty acid composition of erythrocyte phos-pholipids in children and adolescents with primary hyperlipidemia: a randomized controlled trial. Clin Nutr. 2018;37:1193–1201.
120. Guaraldi F, Deon V, Del Bo' C, Vendrame S, Porrini M, Riso P, Guardamagna O. Effect of short-term hazelnut consumption on DNA damage and oxidized LDL in children and adolescents with primary hyperlipidemia: a randomized controlled trial. J Nutr Biochem. 2018;57:206–11.
121. Gargari G, Deon V, Taverniti V, Gardana C, Denina M, Riso P, Guardamagna O, Guglielmetti S. Evidence of dysbiosis in the intestinal microbial ecosystem of children and adoles-cents with primary hyperlipidemia and the potential role of regular hazelnut intake. FEMS Microbiol Ecol. 2018;94:fiy045.
122. Gylling H, Plat J, Turley S, Ginsberg HN, Ellegård L, Jessup W, Jones PJ, Lütjohann D, Maerz W, Masana L, Silbernagel G, Staels B, Borén J, Catapano AL, De Backer G, Deanfield J, Descamps OS, Kovanen PT, Riccardi G, Tokgözoglu L, Chapman MJ; European Atherosclerosis Society Consensus Panel on Phytosterols. Plant sterols and plant stanols in the management of dyslipidaemia and prevention of cardiovascular disease Atherosclerosis 2014;232:346–60.

Chapter 14
Future Perspectives in Nutraceutical Research

Arrigo F.G. Cicero and Manfredi Rizzo

Introduction

In the previous chapters, we have seen that many nutraceuticals have been identified, exerting possible positive effects on cardiovascular disease risk factors in humans [1]. Some of them, namely the one active on heart failure metabolism, have also an impact on functional parameters and clinical outcomes in severe patients [2]. Moreover, for a few compounds we have cumulated strong clinical evidence of efficacy and safety, so that they have been considered as advisable by international guidelines [3]. In this context, what could be the future perspectives in nutraceutical research? There are many issues that should be considered (Table 14.1). In fact, currently, the research process on nutraceuticals is relatively chaotic, with different research groups working on similar (not always the same) compounds, with different methodologies, without interaction and often furnishing interesting results but non included in a congruous research plan, as usually done with chemical drugs.

A. F.G. Cicero (✉)
Medicine and Surgery Sciences Department, Alma Mater Studiorum University of Bologna, Bologna, Italy

Italian Nutraceutical Society (SINut), Bologna, Italy
e-mail: arrigo.cicero@unibo.it

M. Rizzo
PROMISE Department, School of Medicine, University of Palermo, Palermo, Italy

Italian Nutraceutical Society (SINut), Bologna, Italy

© Springer Nature Switzerland AG 2021
A. F.G. Cicero, M. Rizzo (eds.), *Nutraceuticals and Cardiovascular Disease*,
Contemporary Cardiology, https://doi.org/10.1007/978-3-030-62632-7_14

Table 14.1 Issues that should be considered by the future nutraceutical research

Identification of new bioactive compounds
Clear definition of pharmacodynamics
Definition of the potential usefulness of the nutraceutical
Clear definition of pharmacokinetics (in humans)
Well-designed and repeated randomized clinical trials
Meta-analysis of randomized clinical trials

Table 14.2 Parameters to be considered at the end of the preclinical phase before to continue clinical research on nutraceuticals

Availability and cost of the active compound source
Possibility to standardize extraction and/or concentration of the product
Cost of extraction and/or concentration of the product
Innovativeness of the mechanism of action (comparison with available nutraceuticals and drugs)

Identification and Characterization of New Bioactive Compounds

First, new bioactive compounds could be discovered from epidemiological observation or from in vitro testing. Once the bioactive compound identified and chemically characterized, the procedure to extract and/or concentrate it should be strictly standardized. Then, the mechanism of action by which it should exert a positive effect on human health has to be defined in vitro and (always less frequently) in animal models [4]. This is also relevant in order to understand eventual safety risk related to the mechanism of action and of potential pharmacodynamics interactions with other drugs [5]. At this stage, it should be needed to consider the available evidence and evaluate a relatively large number of parameters. (Table 14.2).

Anyway, all these issues have to be considered also for already known bioactive compounds, often available on the market, for which the previous steps have not be so fully considered.

Bioavailability in Humans

A relatively large number of bioactive compounds with interesting mechanism of action and strong effect in vitro or ex-vivo models do not show clinically proportional effects in humans. This is the known case of powerful molecules such as curcumine, resveratrol and berberine that, anyway, exert some effects in humans [6]. Therefore, now, the research have to clarify if the identified compound is orally available in humans, and if there could be a pharmaceutical technique able to improve its bioavailability if naturally insufficient. The most effective and safe way to improve the absorption of large molecule is the use of emulsion, in particular nanoemulsion [7]. Then, the nutraceutical industry also often associated to bioactive compounds some so called "bioavailability enhancers" reducing the density of mucus on intestinal wall, accelerating the opening velocity of the intestinal intercellular tight junctions and/or inhibiting the activity of intestinal P-glycoprotein and/or cytochromes [8, 9]. Recently it has been also shown that the modulation of bowel microbioma could improve the bioavailability of some bioactive compounds (for instance, phytoestrogens). Anyway, the bioavailability of the bioactive compounds (alone or associated to pharmaceutical techniques to theoretically improve their absorption) has to be demonstrated in humans. The main limitation to do it is that the researcher needs to have a method to measure the bioavailability of the tested active compound or of its known metabolite. Alternative methods could be to comparatively measure the known effect of the natural compound and the pharmaceutically transformed version with an adequate study design (see below).

Study Methodology

Frequently, promising nutraceuticals do not clearly confirm their efficacy in clinical trials. However, it should be recognized that a relatively large part of trials carried out on nutraceuticals is not adequately powered and correctly designed. Usually, the gold standard for clinical research is a double-blind, placebo-controlled, randomized clinical trial. The only reason not to calculate the sample size of a trial is that the tested product has never been clinically tested before standard deviation of the expected change of a studied parameter is unavailable. The outcome/outcomes of the study could be largely different and the methods used to reach them have a very variable cost (Table 14.3) [10].

Statistical planning should follow the ICH E9 Guidance. Given the multifactorial effects of nutraceuticals on different organ and tissues, one should consider the possibility of carrying out multivariate analysis procedures such as multivariate analysis of variance, principal component analysis, nonmetric multidimensional scaling or the Wei-Lachin test[11] to assess whether the treatment has a beneficial effect simultaneously on multiple outcomes.

The results obtained by a research group should be then verified by other research groups in similar or different kind of subjects. Then, when more clinical trials have been carried out on a same nutraceutical, preferably with similar dosage and pharmaceutical forms, meta-analyses of clinical trials should be carried out in order to strength the obtained information [12, 13].

Table 14.3 Possible study outcomes in nutraceuticals clinical research

Outcomes	Instrument	Advantages	Difficulties
Soft	Anthropometric measures	Non-invasive, non expensive	None
	First level haemodynamic evaluation	Non-invasive, non expensive	High pre-test variability
	Vascular aging evaluation	Non-invasive, not excessively expensive	Usually middle-term, Need for expertise
	Validated questionnaires	Non-invasive, non-expensive	Often time-consuming
	Standardized laboratory parameters	Mildly invasive	Very variable costs
Hard	Disease prevention	Health claim support	Long/Very long term, Very high costs (mainly related to the high sample size required)

Adequately designed randomized clinical trials and their meta-analysis constitutes the basis for the suggestion of nutraceutical use in clinical practice by the main international expert consensus [14, 15].

Consequently, the future of nutraceutical research is to follow always more strictly the rules of the research applied to conventional drugs and in particular the rules of the Good Clinical Practice. The research should also extend from the study of short term effects on anthropometric/laboratory parameters to middle-term effects on functional/instrumental parameters and, if and when possible, to long-term effect on disease prevention. Moreover, the tested products should reflect the products available on the market and the subjects enrolled in the trials should represent the final consumers of the nutraceutical themselves.

References

1. Cicero AFG, Fogacci F, Colletti A. Food and plant bioactives for reducing cardiometabolic disease risk: an evidence based approach. Food Funct. 2017;8(6):2076–88. https://doi.org/10.1039/c7fo00178a.
2. Cicero AFG, Colletti A. Nutraceuticals and dietary supplements to improve quality of life and outcomes in heart failure patients. Curr Pharm Des. 2017;23(8):1265–72. https://doi.org/10.2174/1381612823666170124120518.
3. Catapano AL, Graham I, De Backer G, Wiklund O, Chapman MJ, Drexel H, Hoes AW, Jennings CS, Landmesser U, Pedersen TR, Reiner Ž, Riccardi G, Taskinen MR, Tokgozoglu L, Verschuren WM, Vlachopoulos C, Wood DA, Zamorano JL. ESC/EAS guidelines for the management of dyslipidaemias: The task force for the management of dyslipidaemias of the European Society of Cardiology (ESC) and European Atherosclerosis Society (EAS) Developed with the special contribution of the European Assocciation for Cardiovascular Prevention & Rehabilitation (EACPR). Atherosclerosis. 2016;253:281–344. https://doi.org/10.1016/j.atherosclerosis.2016.08.018.

4. Sut S, Baldan V, Faggian M, Peron G, Dall Acqua S. Nutraceuticals, a new challenge for medicinal chemistry. Curr Med Chem. 2016;23(28):3198–223.
5. Cicero AFG, Colletti A. An update on the safety of nutraceuticals and effects on lipid parameters. Expert Opin Drug Saf. 2018;17(3):303–13. https://doi.org/10.1080/14740338.201 8.1429404.
6. McClements DJ, Li F, Xiao H. The nutraceutical bioavailability classification scheme: classifying Nutraceuticals according to factors limiting their Oral bioavailability. Annu Rev Food Sci Technol. 2015;6:299–327. https://doi.org/10.1146/annurev-food-032814-014043.
7. Fratter A, Semenzato A. New association of surfactants for the production of food and cosmetic nanoemulsions: preliminary development and characterization. Int J Cosmet Sci. 2011;33(5):443–9. https://doi.org/10.1111/j.1468-2494.2011.00652.x.
8. Fratter A, Frare C, Uras G, Bonini M, Casari Bariani E, Ragazzo B, Gaballo P, Longobardi P, Codemo C, Paoli A. New chitosan salt in gastro-resistant oral formulation could interfere with enteric bile salts emulsification of diet fats: preliminary laboratory observations and physiologic rationale. J Med Food. 2014;17(6):723–9. https://doi.org/10.1089/jmf.2013.0131.
9. Fratter A, Mason V, Pellizzato M, Valier S, Cicero AFG, Tedesco E, Meneghetti E, Benetti F. Lipomatrix: a novel ascorbyl palmitate-based lipid matrix to enhancing enteric absorption of Serenoa Repens oil. Int J Mol Sci. 2019;20(3):E669. https://doi.org/10.3390/ijms20030669.
10. Cicero AF, Petrini O, Prasad C. Clinical studies with nutraceuticals and how to carry them out. Curr Topics Nutr Res. 2017;15(2):63–6.
11. Lachin JM. Applications of the Wei-Lachin multivariate one-sided test for multiple outcomes on possibly different scales. PLoS One. 2014;9:e108784.
12. Fogacci F, Grassi D, Rizzo M, Cicero AFG. Metabolic effect of berberine-silymarin association: a meta-analysis of randomized, double-blind, placebo-controlled clinical trials. Phytother Res. 2019;33(4):862–70. https://doi.org/10.1002/ptr.6282.
13. Fogacci F, Banach M, Mikhailidis DP, Bruckert E, Toth PP, Watts GF, Reiner Ž, Mancini J, Rizzo M, Mitchenko O, Pella D, Fras Z, Sahebkar A, Vrablik M, Cicero AFG. Lipid and Blood Pressure Meta-analysis Collaboration (LBPMC) Group; International Lipid Expert Panel (ILEP). Safety of red yeast rice supplementation: a systematic review and meta-analysis of randomized controlled trials. Pharmacol Res. 2019;143:1–16. https://doi.org/10.1016/j.phrs.2019.02.028.
14. Banach M, Patti AM, Giglio RV, Cicero AFG, Atanasov AG, Bajraktari G, Bruckert E, Descamps O, Djuric DM, Ezhov M, Fras Z, von Haehling S, Katsiki N, Langlois M, Latkovskis G, Mancini GBJ, Mikhailidis DP, Mitchenko O, Moriarty PM, Muntner P, Nikolic D, Panagiotakos DB, Paragh G, Paulweber B, Pella D, Pitsavos C, Reiner Ž, Rosano GMC, Rosenson RS, Rysz J, Sahebkar A, Serban MC, Vinereanu D, Vrablík M, Watts GF, Wong ND, Rizzo M. International Lipid Expert Panel (ILEP). The role of nutraceuticals in statin intolerant patients. J Am Coll Cardiol. 2018;72(1):96–118. https://doi.org/10.1016/j.jacc.2018.04.040.
15. Cicero AFG, Colletti A, Bajraktari G, Descamps O, Djuric DM, Ezhov M, Fras Z, Katsiki N, Langlois M, Latkovskis G, Panagiotakos DB, Paragh G, Mikhailidis DP, Mitchenko O, Paulweber B, Pella D, Pitsavos C, Reiner Ž, Ray KK, Rizzo M, Sahebkar A, Serban MC, Sperling LS, Toth PP, Vinereanu D, Vrablík M, Wong ND, Banach M. Lipid-lowering nutraceuticals in clinical practice: position paper from an International Lipid Expert Panel. Nutr Rev. 2017;75(9):731–67. https://doi.org/10.1093/nutrit/nux047.

Index

© Springer Nature Switzerland AG 2021
A. F.G. Cicero, M. Rizzo (eds.), *Nutraceuticals and Cardiovascular Disease*,
Contemporary Cardiology, https://doi.org/10.1007/978-3-030-62632-7

Printed in the United States
by Baker & Taylor Publisher Services